THE MOST COMPREHENSIVE, COMFORTING, AND FACT-FILLED GUIDE EVER PUBLISHED— NEWLY REVISED AND UPDATED FOR TODAY'S EXPECTANT PARENTS

Here is what The New York Times *said about this celebrated guide:*

"Dr. Alan F. Guttmacher is the Dr. Spock of unborn children. His wisdom, refreshing honesty and practical advice have helped lead countless mothers through worry-free pregnancies and happy childbirth experiences. He is the kind of physician who never talks down to his patients, who tells what he thinks and also what others who may disagree with him think. His book should help assuage the fears and answer the questions of expectant mothers and sustain them between monthly visits to the obstetrician."

ALAN F. GUTTMACHER, M.D., was one of the most distinguished figures in the world of medicine. He was associate professor of obstetrics at Johns Hopkins, chief of obstetrics and gynecology at Mt. Sinai Hospital, emeritus professor of obstetrics and gynecology at Mt. Sinai Medical School, visiting professor at Albert Einstein College of Medicine, President of Planned Parenthood Federation of America, and on the board of directors of the Margaret Sanger Research Bureau.

IRWIN H. KAISER, M.D., was Dr. Guttmacher's student and his friend. Currently professor of obstetrics and gynecology at Albert Einstein College of Medicine, he has been professor and head of department of obstetrics and gynecology at the University of Utah as well as director of the department of gynecology and obstetrics at The Hospital of the Albert Einstein College of Medicine.

Pregnancy, Birth & Family Planning

The Definitive Work
by Alan F. Guttmacher, M.D.

Revised and Brought Up-To-Date
by Irwin H. Kaiser, M.D.

with drawings by
Glenna Deutsch

A PLUME BOOK

NEW AMERICAN LIBRARY

NEW YORK AND SCARBOROUGH, ONTARIO

PUBLISHER'S NOTE

The ideas, procedures, and suggestions contained in this book are not intended as a substitute for consulting with your physician. All matters regarding your health require medical supervision.

NAL BOOKS ARE AVAILABLE AT QUANTITY DISCOUNTS WHEN USED TO PROMOTE PRODUCTS OR SERVICES. FOR INFORMATION PLEASE WRITE TO PREMIUM MARKETING DIVISION, NEW AMERICAN LIBRARY, 1633 BROADWAY, NEW YORK, NEW YORK 10019.

A hardcover edition of *Pregnancy, Birth and Family Planning* has been published simultaneously by E. P. Dutton, a division of New American Library, 2 Park Avenue, New York, New York 10016, and, in Canada, by Fitzhenry & Whiteside Limited, Toronto.

 PLUME TRADEMARK REG. U.S. PAT. OFF. AND FOREIGN COUNTRIES REGISTERED TRADEMARK—MARCA REGISTRADA HECHO EN FORGE VILLAGE, MASS., U.S.A.

Library of Congress Cataloging-in-Publication Data

Guttmacher, Alan Frank, 1898–1974
  Pregnancy, birth, and family planning.

  Includes index.
  1. Pregnancy. 2. Childbirth. 3. Birth control.
I. Kaiser, Irwin H. II. Title. [DNLM: 1. Family
Planning—popular works. 2. Obstetrics—popular
works. 3. Pregnancy—popular works. WQ 150 G985p]
RG525.G82 1986   618.2'4   86-706
ISBN 0-525-24420-4
ISBN 0-452-25827-8 (pbk.)

Designed by Leonard Telesca

First Plume Printing, June, 1986

1 2 3 4 5 6 7 8 9

PRINTED IN THE UNITED STATES OF AMERICA

To Leonore G. Guttmacher and Barbara L. Kaiser

—I.H.K.

ACKNOWLEDGMENTS

I have had gracious assistance in preparation of the text from Teri Darwish, Rachline Habousha, Florence Haseltine, Anna G. Loeb, Barbara Machado, Karen Schlam, Johanna Shulman, Shelley Schwartzbaum, Esther Steinhauer, and Sylvia Wassertheil.

Secretarial support was efficiently provided by Donna Gerardi and Evelyn Tolliver.

It was gratifying to work with Glenna Deutsch in preparing the illustrations, which are all new in this edition.

Particular sections of the text were reviewed by Nancy Devore, Ruth Merkatz, Lucy Perotta, and Sidney Shulman. The entire responsibility for the text is of course mine.

I am particularly indebted for the hours of editorial review of the manuscript by Barbara L. Kaiser.

Hugh Rawson, my editor, was of assistance and support in all stages of the writing of this volume. His enthusiasm for the text and his ability to identify jargon and ambiguity combined to make my task much easier than it might have been.

—I.H.K.

It is with deep pleasure that I thank Dr. Irwin Kaiser for his excellent revision—both in style and substance—of my husband's now classic book, *Pregnancy, Birth and Family Planning*. I take special pride in the selection of Dr. Kaiser for this particular job, which he accepted with such grace and performed so well.

He was trained, in part, by my husband, and I must add that, to me, Irwin Kaiser represents the very best of his medical specialty—Obstetrics—as did his mentor, Alan Guttmacher.

LEONORE GUTTMACHER
(*Mrs. Alan F. Guttmacher*)

Contents

Illustrations

FOREWORD

Why a new edition of an established classic?

A book intended as a guide to pregnancy, birth, and family planning must deal primarily with medical and scientific facts. But these do not exist abstractly; they deal with major events in our lives that have heavy emotional weight and long-enduring consequences. The social circumstances under which the previous edition was written no longer exist; new attitudes have replaced many of the old assumptions, and some of what we formerly thought were facts have proved not to be so.

In the years since the 1973 edition of this book, the number of women working outside the home has increased. The role of these women in the family has necessarily been redefined. Many have postponed childbearing in order to pursue careers.

To do so, they have made use of the continuing technical improvement in the efficiency and safety of methods of contraception, of surgical sterilization, and of the availability of safe abortion by choice. Today, when women report for prenatal care expecting to carry their pregnancies to term, we can be fairly sure that they do want the child.

The women's health movement has also had a significant impact. Traditionally, up to the recent past, all medical care was authoritarian and paternalistic. Nowhere was this more so than in the care of women, and nowhere has it changed more than in the recognition of patients' rights. One feature of this change has been the steadily increasing number of women practitioners of obstetrics and gynecology. Women are still a minority in the specialty but it is no longer appropriate to refer to an obstetrician casually as "he."

It was clear a generation ago that the future of obstetrics lay primarily in the study of the fetus. The full appreciation of the basic science foundation of fetal medicine has had to await several technical developments. One is the continuing improvement of sonography, which allows us to see the fetus inside the uterus. Another is the steady increase in the scope of prenatal genetic diagnosis. Many medical and surgical fetal diagnoses, unthinkable fifteen years ago, are made routinely now. Monitoring of acute and chronic changes in fetal condition also is firmly established as an integral part of pregnancy care. The mother of a healthy fetus need no longer wait apprehensively until the birth of her baby to learn of its condition, since these and related techniques can provide her with reassurance well in advance of delivery.

Simultaneous with these changes, major advances have been made in the last decade in neonatology—the care of the newborn. For instance, we are now able to prevent serious bowel and respiratory problems in premature infants and to treat elevated bilirubin levels with noninvasive techniques.

Along with these events has come the growing practical acknowledgment of an increasingly active role for the pregnant woman in her own care. This has been manifested by increased attention to preparation for pregnancy and labor, for breastfeeding, and for newborn hygiene with its emphasis on maternal-infant bonding and rooming-in. It has also involved drawing the woman's partner and her other children into the drama. In many hospitals, what used to be the postpartum ward now often looks like a cross between a nursery school and a classroom.

In many ways, then, obstetrics has changed. New categories of providers of care have been added. For example, certified nurse midwives are increasingly entering an area previously reserved exclusively for physicians. What is being called family-centered care is gaining acceptance, implying an active participation of other members of the family in childbearing experiences. However, I must add that I do not share the current interest in home birth as a way of achieving this ideal, since

I see it as gambling with the survival of the fetus in the event of unpredictable catastrophes. My preference is to tackle the problem by making birthing areas more comfortable and home-like while maintaining the immediate accessibility of emergency medical support and equipment.

With all the advances I have noted, parents are encouraged to expect that pregnancy must have a perfect outcome. But such perfection cannot be guaranteed. When it is not achieved, even when this could not have been prevented, the disappointment of the parents, their anger and frustration and sense of failure, calls for special understanding and support.

The parents may be moved to cast blame on the care given, often through the mechanism of a malpractice or negligence action. Ironically, it seems that recent increases in the number of these legal actions have come hand in hand with, and possibly because of, the rapid pace of improvements in techniques and in overall results. Some physicians have tended to subscribe to Dick the Butcher's advice in Shakespeare's Henry VI, part 2: "First thing we do, let's kill all the lawyers." But the "litigation explosion" is not caused by the lawyers; it results rather from the fact that our society does not make any provision for meeting the extraordinary cost of lifelong care for a dependent defective child other than the insurance of a physician who is found responsible for the condition. Litigation also results in part from a failure of practitioners to build understanding, in pregnant women and their families, of the processes of pregnancy and birth, and of the fact that there are still areas in which our control of the outcome is not perfect. I do not suppose we can eliminate the malpractice action without some sort of radical restructuring of the ways in which we deliver medical care; nor, probably, in the present system, would it be advisable to do so. But I do think we practitioners can do our part to ameliorate the situation by improving our own performance and by working to improve our personal relationships with our patients—whose welfare, after all, is and should be our first concern.

I have never ceased to be amazed by the birth of a baby. This tiny person develops from an egg so small that it cannot be seen by the naked eye and from an even smaller sperm.

The two unite in the nourishing fluid in a woman's fallopian tube to form an embryo. At that moment, inside this minute sphere, there is the information required to form a living, independent, thinking, human being. Where the liver will form, on which side the left leg is to go, how fast the heart will beat, what the blood type will be, the color of the eyes, and a myriad of myriads of other decisions on growth and development— all these are already established. The most complex devices yet created by human beings are simple in comparison with a human embryo. Nine months from its beginning in the fertilized egg a baby emerges: it looks around, reacts to its mother, breathes, cries, urinates, sucks, and on a few glorious occasions, smiles at the world. There is nothing else like it.

The process of pregnancy is unique. A human being, the fetus, grows inside another, the mother. In the first three months, its organs and its limbs and muscles form, and its heart beats and it moves about in an ingeniously protected liquid world. It spends the succeeding six months becoming larger and perfecting the systems that will work after birth to make possible independent existence.

At the proper time, the mother's uterus undertakes the task of propelling the baby, so carefully guarded up to this moment, through the cervix and vagina and out into the world. It can be a perilous journey, but in most cases the mother, even when she does this for the first time, with no opportunity to practice, accomplishes it rapidly and safely for her baby as well as herself.

The obstetrician and midwife differ from all other health care providers because we are responsible for two patients simultaneously—the mother and the fetus—whose interests late in pregnancy are almost always identical. When a labor ends with a healthy mother and baby, there is a sense of triumph—curiously so because the odds are heavily in favor of a happy outcome. I nevertheless never fail to get this sense of accomplishment at such a moment.

For so long in our urban twentieth-century society, birth was accepted as the doctor's accomplishment. The mother and certainly her partner were regarded somehow as passive participants. Our first child was born with her mother sound asleep for hours before and for hours afterward. I had been banished from the labor room and actually did not know of the outcome until our daughter was an hour old.

Present concepts of care are radically different. We encourage mothers to learn everything they can about childbearing, ideally starting even before they initiate sexual activity. Their partners are brought into the educational process as early as possible, so they can join in prenatal visits, classes for pain relief, education in child care, and, in fact, in the entire range of preparation.

And so the parents now have the center of the stage. This is exactly as it should be.

This book is dedicated to their education. I have tried to avoid making the text provincial—specifically, I have described medical concepts with particular care to present controversial issues clearly while stating my own conclusions. The facts of conception, pregnancy, labor and birth, family planning, infertility treatment, and abortion are laid out. There is some repetition, so that important concepts can be presented in several contexts. It is intended to gratify the needs of curiosity—a first pregnancy particularly must raise many questions. Most of these can be answered by common sense, but it can still be of value to have a trusted book of reference to validate what your instincts teach. It is not surprising that in such emotional matters as sex and pregnancy there is a whole catalog of myths. I have tried to discuss the common "old wives'" tales—to confirm a few and explain the fallacies of the others.

The progenitor of this volume, *Into This Universe*, was published by Alan Guttmacher in 1937. Revised paperback editions appeared in 1947 and 1950 under the title *Having a Baby*. A complete revision entitled *Pregnancy and Birth* appeared in 1956 and was revised again in 1962. Alan played a prominent role in calling the attention of the public to the need for effective contraception and for revision of the nation's antiquated abortion laws. So, in 1973, a lengthy and authoritative section on family planning was added to the text, which itself was also extensively revised at that time.

Alan Guttmacher died of leukemia in 1974. In 1983 I completed an update of the text intended to eliminate out-of-date recommendations without altering the text. In the present revision I have gone further. There have continued to be technical advances in obstetrics, endocrinology, the investigation of infertility, and new diagnostic procedures which need presentation and explanation. Some concepts have become outmoded. A large proportion of the text has therefore been rewritten.

Alan Guttmacher recruited me into obstetrics and was my first teacher and role model in this field. His knowledge was encyclopedic, and he was skilled at conveying that wisdom to others. I have striven to maintain the standards that he embodied in his life and work.

1

You Were a Long Shot

When babies grow up to be winners of marathons or authors of great books or presidents, they are considered to have done so in part as a result of chance. Yet in none of these happenings does chance play so large a part as in the miracle of birth. The selection of parents is most fortuitous; if your father and mother had not been who they were, you would not be you. Then, too, at the moment of conception any one of four hundred million male cells—spermatozoa—had an equal chance of becoming your particular biological father; only one did. And no two of these four hundred million spermatozoa were exactly alike. Each had a slightly different chromosomal makeup. The chromosomes containing helixes of deoxyribonucleic acid, DNA, are those constituents of the body cells which carry the blueprint of the offspring. When the two sets of blueprints— one from the father and one from the mother—are followed, a unique product results. In your case, by one chance in four hundred million, that unique product was you. If any other of those four hundred million spermatozoa had fertilized the ovum from which you were created, you certainly would have been a strikingly different person, perhaps of the opposite sex.

The complex, seemingly magical process of fashioning a baby is by now quite well understood—a process that is a far cry from the primordial beginnings of life on this planet. The earliest life was probably a single-celled organism that reproduced by division into two similar organisms. And when those

1

two organisms had grown to adult size, each of them divided into two. There were no special sex cells and no separate sexes. Some simple animals still adhere to this primitive reproductive pattern.

The Biological Advantage of Two Sexes

Later in the process of evolution sexual differentiation arose, and the fusion and mixing of elements from two separate adult cells were required for the fabrication of a new young cell. The existence of separate sexes is of great advantage to both the survival and development of a species. That advantage lies in variability. If a single parent cell simply divides into two new cells, and they split into two and all the new individuals also reproduce by division, each of the progeny in this species is an exact or almost exact duplicate of the original parent. Then if some adverse environmental influence comes along, such as drought or extreme cold, and the organism is especially susceptible to it, the whole species will be wiped out. This is far less likely if elements from two separate parent cells fuse and this combination of genetic materials then divides; for the progeny is never an exact duplicate of either parent, but has some characteristics of both. When this progeny mates with a similar organism from a set of different parents, still greater variation results.

The process of the union of the sex cells, as it occurs in humans and other mammals, did not just happen; it evolved through many steps, some of which we can trace. More primitive forms of life, simple marine animals like the starfish, have a very wasteful form of sexual reproduction. There are two sexes, but the sperm and eggs are discharged haphazardly without any physical awareness or even propinquity between the two parents. A more advanced stage in the evolution of the union of the sex cells is illustrated by fish. In them there is strong physical awareness between male and female during mating, but absence of physical contact. The male swims above the female, and as she discharges her eggs he discharges his sperm. In the frog, which has a still more advanced pattern of mating behavior, there is not only sex awareness but actual physical contact. The male clasps the back of the female with a specialized clasp organ, and as she discharges her eggs he discharges his sperm upon them. All varieties of external insemination, however, are relatively wasteful and inefficient.

Internal insemination as practiced by humans, by the other mammals, and by many submammalian forms, is far more efficient. In this pattern of reproduction a special organ of the male, the penis, is inserted into a special organ of the female, the vagina. In addition to depositing the semen well on the way to the precise area where it is to function, this method of introducing the male ejaculatory organ deep within the body of the female protects the spermatozoa by releasing them in a highly favorable environment. Such conditions as temperature and moisture within the cervical canal, the uterus, and the fallopian tubes of the female reproductive tract are optimal for the conservation of spermatozoa.

Libido

The ageless, unhurried process of evolution has granted animals immense protection by making vital functions pleasurable. It is pleasant to eat, drink, void, defecate, sleep—and impregnate or be impregnated. This pleasure in sex is termed libido, and the libido is created by body chemicals, the sex hormones. So closely interwoven are reproduction and sexual pleasure that the sex cells that unite to form the embryo and the sex hormones that create the appetite for mating in each of the sexual partners are produced in one and the same organ—in the ovary of the female and in the testis of the male.

Mating among mammals may be restricted to a single annual season, as in deer, bears, and seals; or it may take place in isolated recurrent estrus periods (mating periods), as in cats, dogs, and the domesticated rodent: rats, mice, and rabbits. Still a third type of sexual rhythm is demonstrated by the primates—humans, apes, and monkeys: a willingness to mate at all times without restriction of season or estrus period, though, to be sure, with fluctuations of desire, particularly on the part of the female. In many women libido seems to bear a close time relationship to the stage of the menstrual cycle, being most intense just before the menses, during its waning days, and immediately following it. This is difficult to understand from the viewpoint of survival of the species, since these three periods occur during the least fertile days of the month. Another oddity in the sexual behavior of primates is the female's acceptance of the male during pregnancy. Since mating at this time serves no apparent physiological function one must postulate that primates have discovered its emotional value to both participants. Nonprimate animals do not copulate after pregnancy has begun. However, some species mate almost immediately after birth has occurred.

No doubt through the timeless process of evolution primates have gradually emancipated mating from many of the modifying influences that still affect subprimate species, and in making love we are the most emancipated of the primates. In some baboons the skin of the vaginal area goes through a cycle of color changes dependent upon the ovarian hormones, estrogen and progesterone, and when the color is a scarlet red the female is most receptive to the male. Estrogen and progesterone are hormones produced by the ovary in all mammals, but each at different times and in differing amounts depending upon the stage in the reproductive cycle. In monkeys it has been shown that the male develops sexual interest in a spayed female (one in which the ovaries have been removed) only if she is given estrogen, but remains uninterested if progesterone is injected.

Some subprimate mammals breed only in the spring, the time of breeding regulated by the proportion of light to darkness. If such an animal is captured and artificially subjected to ten hours of light and fourteen of darkness the female's heat period does not occur, but when the proportion of light is increased to fourteen hours, mating occurs. Other animals breed in the fall, the act of breeding triggered by a daily excess of darkness over light. It has been found that the brain measures the light-darkness ratio, and when a proper seasonal mix is reached a message from the brain activates the ovary.

In some animals there are social factors that affect mating. Among several strains of mice, if a large group of sexually active females are put into a cage without males, a gradual disappearance of mating cycles occurs. The inhibiting factor was found to be the odor of the other females' urine. Disappearance of mating cycles does not occur if a female is caged alone unless urine from another female is frequently smeared

on her nose. The presence of males, due to the sexually stimulating influence of the odor of male urine, will neutralize such
inhibiting influences from the smell of female urine. Realization that the mating instinct is so sensitively influenced in
many other animals makes it easier to comprehend human
sexual difficulties.

Doctor William H. Masters and Mrs. Virginia E. Johnson,
in their excellent studies of human sexual inadequacy, under-
scored the fact that sexual difficulties among human beings
are almost never caused by an organic lesion but are ordinarily
psychological in origin. That is why it is so important that
adolescents be introduced to the miracle of sexual reproduction
in a sensitive, intelligent fashion by the home and the school.
The Masters-Johnson study proves that it is dangerous to create
an aura of sin, dirt, and taboo about human sexual activity.
Sexuality should be viewed as a beautiful gift which when used
intelligently with freedom, joy, and consideration greatly en-
riches all facets of life.

The Sex Cells—Eggs and Spermatozoa

The eggs of all the higher mammals are similar in both size
and appearance—round, with a clear, thin, shell-like capsule,
as rigid as stiff jelly. The capsule encloses liquid in which are
suspended hundreds of fat droplets, protein substances, and
other materials, including the nucleus. The egg, the largest
cell of the whole body, is approximately $\frac{1}{200}$ of an inch in
diameter—about one-fourth as large as the period punctuating
the end of this sentence. The eggs of mice, rabbits, gorillas,
dogs, pigs, whales, and humans are all about the same size.
It is incredible but true that the whale's tons and the mouse's
ounces spring from a round speck of matter with relatively the
same diameter and weight.

The spermatozoa of different species show greater differences in form than do ova. The human spermatozoon consists
of an oval head $\frac{1}{6000}$ of an inch in diameter, mostly occupied
by the nucleus. With the aid of additional magnification provided by the electron microscope, it has become evident that
the head is covered by a saclike structure called the acrosome
and this provides an outer membrane, the acrosomal mem-

brane. This is attached by a short neck to a cylindrical middle piece that terminates in a thin tail about ten times as long as the head. The tail, which consists of several hairlike fibrils resembling a horse's tail, is capable of rapid side-to-side lashing movements, by means of which the spermatozoon is propelled.

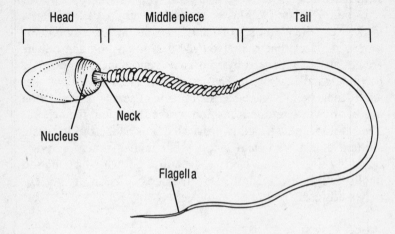

A human spermatozoon enlarged 5,000 times.

The motor that moves the tail is located in the middle piece. A spermatozoon is 1/600 of an inch long from the top of its head to the end of its flagellum, a short, hairlike structure protruding from the end of the tail. A spermatozoon can swim an inch in four to sixteen minutes depending on whether it is traversing watery uterine or tubal fluid or relatively viscid cervical mucus. Easily blocked by the slightest obstruction because of its small size, its path is seldom in a straight line, and frequently it takes more than the minimum time to progress an inch.

When ejaculated, spermatozoa are suspended in seminal plasma, a thick mucoid fluid produced by the male during sexual orgasm. Semen, which arises from the prostate, the seminal vesicles, and the other accessory reproductive glands, is a homogeneous fluid immediately upon ejaculation. Within a few minutes it sets to a gel, the coagulum. After about fifteen to twenty minutes this is fully redissolved into a viscous fluid. In some cases this is not complete and then the semen is very viscous and it may have tapiocalike lumps.

The amount of semen ejaculated depends in part upon the interval between successive ejaculations; in humans the normal quantity varies from one-half to one and one-half teaspoons. In the stallion the quantity is ordinarily two ounces, ten to thirty times as much as in the human. A fresh drop of semen seen under a microscope suggests the rush of traffic in a crowded city street. Myriads of spermatozoa dash here and there, now steering straight ahead, now halted by a speck of dust, now free again to scurry out of the microscopic field. It is a spectacle surcharged with dramatic interest. The average human ejaculate contains almost a half billion spermatozoa—a seemingly extravagant superfluity of numbers, since only one spermatozoon fertilizes the egg.

Fertilization

The essential step in the initiation of a new life is fertilization, the penetration of the ovum by a spermatozoon and the fusion of a portion of the two cells into a new single cell. From this united parent cell originate all the billions of cells that form the infant. The part of each cell that fuses is the nucleus, that glob of material in a cell which stains dark with aniline dyes in properly prepared microscopic slides. The nucleus is not a solid mass of tissue, as it may appear under low magnification, but is made up of a network of little dark-staining rods called chromosomes, which were referred to at the beginning of this chapter. There is a specific number of chromosomes characteristic for each species, and every cell of the body of each animal belonging to the particular animal family contains this number of chromosomes. Chromosomes are paired. One species of primate has its genetic material divided in forty pairs of chromosomes, while in one species of rodent it is divided into seventeen pairs. The famous fruit fly, which has contributed so selflessly to our knowledge of genetics, possesses only four pairs of chromosomes. In humans there are forty-six single chromosomes, but each has a counterpart; thus there are twenty-three different pairs. Before fertilization is accomplished the chromosome number of each parent cell, sperm and ovum, has been halved, in the human from forty-six to twenty-three, one member of each of the twenty-three pairs remaining in the fully mature sex cell. Thus, when the two mature human sex cells fuse, each brings twenty-three chromosomes to the process of fertilization, and their union restores the human species number of forty-six. Research has shown that these minute microscopic rods are the all-powerful agents in the transmission of hereditary characteristics. To them each of us owes not only his sex but his body build, coloring, and, in large measure, his mentality, emotional makeup, and longevity.

Chromosomes in reality are chains of smaller genetic units termed genes. The total number of genes in our twenty-three pairs of chromosomes is estimated at between fifty and one hundred thousand. Since the individual genes are the ultimate determinants of genetic inheritance, the almost infinite variety of combinations explains why all humans differ so markedly, unless they are identical, one-egg twins. One-egg twins have exactly the same chromosome-gene makeup, since the egg after fertilization divides and from each half an independent embryo develops. Thus since a pair of one-egg twin children contain the same chromosomes and genes they are genetic duplicates of each other.

2

Impregnation

For conception to occur it is necessary that a sperm cell make contact with and penetrate an egg cell. Where are the two sex cells produced, and how is contact between them established?

The Testes and Sperm Production

Throughout a man's reproductive life, which in rare cases continues after the age of eighty or ninety, spermatozoa are constantly being formed by the two testicles suspended in the scrotum, a thin-walled sac of skin. The scrotum is a highly specialized structure which, because of its external location and its large area of skin surface, constantly maintains the testicles at a temperature about six degrees Fahrenheit below that of the interior of the body. In warm weather the scrotum is large and flaccid, exposing a large skin area for heat loss through evaporation, while in a cold temperature the scrotum is small and contracted to conserve heat. In truth, the scrotal pouch is a highly effective air conditioner. The sperm-making cells of the testicle are extremely sensitive to heat, and within twenty-four hours after being exposed to a temperature as high as that of the body's interior, cease producing spermatozoa.

In early fetal life the testicles are situated high up within the abdomen, and they gradually migrate downward, reaching the scrotum about eight weeks before birth. Occasionally boys delivered at full term are born with undescended testicles; in some, the condition corrects itself within the first few months or years of life. If lack of descent persists, at four to five years of age the child is given injections of the gonadotrophic hormone recovered from the urine of pregnant women. This hormone stimulates the testicles to grow, and because of the resulting increase in weight they may then gravitate spontaneously into the scrotum. Cases in which this does not occur require a surgical operation to guide the testicle into the scrotum and sew it in place. The operation is successful in preserving potential fertility in most but not all cases. The ideal time to perform such an operation is between the ages of five and six years. Otherwise, by the time of full adolescence, the sperm-producing tissue of the testicle is already so irreparably damaged by chronic exposure to the relatively high intra-abdominal temperature that reposition has uncertain value. A few mammals possess no scrotum, notably the bull elephant, whose testicles remain intra-abdominal. As far as I know, the relationship of sperm production to temperature has not been studied in these species.

Endocrine Glands and Hormones

The structures that produce hormones are known as endocrine glands (Greek: *endo*, "internal"; *crine*, "secretion") because their chemical products circulate within the body and have specific influences on particular target organs.

Hormones are these chemical messengers, produced in several locations in the body. One set of hormones, manufactured in the brain, regulates the formation of secondary messengers. An example of this is gonadotropin- (Greek: *gonad*, "sex organ"; *tropin*, "acting upon") releasing hormone GnRH, which is formed in the hypothalamus at the base of the brain and from there transported to the pituitary gland. The pituitary is about the size of a seedless grape. It is located in a socket in the skull and is attached to the base of the brain by a short stalk. The function of GnRH is to stimulate the pituitary to release two of the several hormones it produces. One of these, follicle-stimulating hormone FSH, causes the ripening of an ovarian follicle and the egg it contains and the secretion of estrogen. The other, luteinizing hormone LH, causes the ripe follicle to rupture, thereby releasing the egg into the fallopian tube. LH further stimulates the ovary to convert the empty follicle into a corpus luteum (Latin: *corpus*, "body"; *luteum*, "yellow"), which secretes the estrogen and progesterone responsible for the ripening of the lining of the uterus and the initial maintenance of pregnancy. In males, FSH stimulates the formation of sperm and LH the production of testosterone.

There is still another hormone of importance: chorionic gonadotropin (hCG). The chorion is the layer of the embryo from which the placenta and the outer of the two membranes develop. hCG is produced first by the fertilized egg and later by the placenta. It maintains the corpus luteum and prevents menstruation from occurring.

The hormonal effects are thus in sequence. The brain influences the formation of GnRH. It in turn releases FSH and LH and these then affect the production of sperm or eggs and the formation of the steroid sex hormones. In later life the amount and relative proportions of estrogen, progesterone, and testosterone bring about puberty, secondary sexual development, and the possibility of reproduction.

When designating hormones by their initials, a lower case "h" often is used to distinguish naturally occurring human hormones from synthetic ones. Thus, human chorionic gonadotropin always is designated hCG in medical literature. As time goes on, this system seems likely to become standard in all medical writing.

The Testicles

In the human adult the two testicles have the shape and size of plums. Their functions, the production of sperm cells and the manufacture of the masculinizing hormone, testosterone, are accomplished by separate types of cells.

Spermatogenesis, the creation of sperm cells, is a continuous process commencing in early adolescence and usually not ceasing until death. Each testicle contains hundreds of thousands of little round chambers, lined with cells called spermatogonia from which spermatids, the forerunners of spermatozoa, are derived. When the formation of a spermatozoon has been completed, it is delivered into a collecting duct that interconnects with larger ducts, through which it finally passes into the epididymis, a long, narrow, much-coiled tube lying above each testicle. The canal of the epididymis is continuous with the canal of the *vas deferens*, a tube which runs from the upper scrotum through the body to the urethra of the penis, from which the sperm cells are ejaculated. Millions of sperm cells enter the *vas* daily to be stored there until ejaculation.

At ejaculation the muscle cells in the wall of the seminal vesicle go through a series of contractions, expelling its fluid swarming with spermatozoa into the urethra. Other glands, most notably the prostate, also contract during orgasm, expelling their fluids as well. All these secretions form the semen. Because of their tiny size, the hundreds of million sperm cells make up a negligible amount of the semen. Therefore, male sterilization, tying and severing each *vas* near the testicle to obstruct the upward journey of the sperm cells from the testicle, does not appreciably diminish the volume of ejaculated semen. The seminal vesicles, prostate, and other glands still discharge their fluids during orgasm, precisely as they did before the operation. The volume and quality of the semen is the same if ejaculated during coitus or masturbation.

The second type of testicular cell, the interstitial, or Leydig, cell, produces testosterone, which is absorbed directly into the bloodstream from its place of origin in the testicle. Carried in the blood, it affects such masculine characteristics as body form, libido, sexual potency, voice register, and body and facial hair. Leydig cells are not sensitive to heat and, unlike spermatogonia, continue to function normally in an intra-abdominal testicle. Therefore, males with undescended testicles are wholly masculine except for the absence of spermatozoa in ejaculated semen. In the castrated or eunuchoid male, however, the removal of the testicles causes profound modification of masculine characteristics because of the lack of testosterone in the bloodstream.

The Journey of Spermatozoa Up the Male Ducts

From each testicle the spermatozoa slowly pass upward through the epididymis. The trip through the ducts requires two to four weeks, the spermatozoa maturing as the journey progresses. If the male is continent for some time, the spermatozoa that complete the journey are stored in the ducts and epididymis and may suffer effects of senility. Therefore, the first ejaculation after a long interval may produce cells of impaired motility. For this reason, doctors prescribe moderately frequent intercourse for most couples desirous of pregnancy who are having difficulty in conceiving.

Spermatozoa do not make their own way up the male ducts, since they are motionless at this stage, but are propelled upward by imperceptible contractions of the muscular tissue forming the walls of the epididymis and *vas*. It is only after the mass of sperm cells is diluted during orgasm by addition of fluid from the prostate and other glands of the male that they are thrown into vigorous movement. Spermatozoa remain actively motile in the seminal fluid at room temperature for twenty-four hours or longer after ejaculation and as long as seventy-two hours in the upper reaches of the female reproductive tract.

Function and Structure of the Penis

The penis, the male depository organ, has a conical end, the glans, which in the uncircumcised male is partially protected by a thin, elastic, retractile skin cover, the foreskin. The urethra, the tube from which the urine ordinarily flows and from which semen is ejaculated during orgasm, runs through the center of the shaft of the penis and terminates in a small elliptical opening at the tip of the glans. When relaxed and flaccid, the penis of the average man measures about four inches in total length and has a diameter of about an inch. When completely erect under the stimulus of sexual excitement, it measures slightly more than six inches and is an inch and one-half in diameter. Erection is accomplished by the rapid and greatly increased inflow of blood into the special spongy tissue that forms the organ, and by the temporary imprisonment within it of this increased blood under pressure—which comes about through the closure of exit valves in the veins that return the blood from the penis back into the general circulation.

Orgasm consists of a series of muscular contractions involving the whole male tract, which drives out the semen in spurts, after which the valves of the veins open, releasing the imprisoned blood and allowing the penis to soften and wilt.

During the process of erection, a temporary valvelike structure forms at the junction of the bladder with the urethra, which prevents urine from being discharged with the semen during ejaculation.

Function and Structure of Female Sex Organs

The reproductive organs of the female serve a fivefold purpose. First, they provide a receptacle for the male semen; second, they produce the ovum; third, they serve as a trysting site for sperm and egg; fourth, they furnish a place where the fertilized ovum can develop into a fetus; and fifth, they manufacture two chemicals, estrogen and progesterone, essential for carrying out the female's role.

The vagina is the body cavity adapted to the reception of the semen. In actuality, the vagina is a potential cavity. Unless distended by the penis or by passage of an infant during birth, the front and rear walls are virtually in apposition to each other. In the virgin, its entrance is, in most cases, partly closed by the hymen, a skinlike membrane that stretches across the vaginal entrance, containing one or more small openings. Normally the membrane is destroyed at the initial sexual intercourse. However, the hymen is a highly variable structure, being absent at birth in some cases and complete without any opening in others; therefore, caution is necessary in attaching medico-legal importance to its condition as evidence of virginity.

The entrance to the vagina is guarded on either side by a small and a large fold of skin, called the labia, or lips of the vagina. Since one pair is relatively small and the other large, they are termed labia minora and majora. At the outer end of the vagina, just above the urethra from which the urine exits, is the clitoris, the homologue of (i.e., roughly, but not exactly, corresponding to) the male's penis. When unerected, it is usually about a half-inch in length, and when erected, almost twice as long. In its unerected state the clitoris is virtually completely covered by a hood of skin, equivalent to the male foreskin, or prepuce. The sole function of the clitoris is to react to sexual stimulation, enhancing the female's pleasure and response.

The two ovaries, almond-sized and -shaped organs that lie in the lower part of the abdominal cavity, produce the ova. Ordinarily, one ovum matures each month, beginning with the onset of the menses and continuing until the menopause, except during the nine months of pregnancy and a few months thereafter. Since usually there is but one ovum a month, only one of the ovaries matures an egg every four weeks, the two ovaries dividing the task with no discernible plan. Sometimes they alternate; at other times the same ovary produces the ovum several months in succession. If one ovary is surgically removed, the remaining one takes over the complete burden of egg production, maturing an ovum each month, usually with no reduction in fertility.

Perhaps in 5 to 10 percent of cycles, two eggs are ovulated, one from each ovary or both from the same one. If both eggs are fertilized and then implant and develop, which occurs in less than 1 percent of cycles, two-egg, or nonidentical, fraternal twins result. Since two eggs and two sperms are involved, the twins are no more alike than single-born siblings would be at the same age. One could say that fraternal twinning is not true twinning, since the term comes from "getwin," dividing into two. Quite properly fraternal twinning could be termed "littering," a litter of two babies at once.

The ovary, like the testicle, is an endocrine gland. It manufactures the two steroid female hormones, estrogen and progesterone, in quantities that depend upon the phase of the monthly cycle. The ovary in addition produces folliculostatin, also called inhibin, a nonsteroid hormone that opposes the hormone FSH, produced by the pituitary gland, which initially stimulates the growth of primordial follicles in the ovary.

The two fallopian tubes, or oviducts, one on either side of the uterus, lead from the abdominal cavity near each ovary to the interior of the uterus. Their length is approximately five inches each. They form the pathway for the upward trek of the spermatozoa and the downward journey of the ovum. The tubal canal, or channel, is constantly moist with secreted fluid, the amount of which increases significantly at the time of ovulation. Finally, there is the pear-sized, pear-shaped, two-to-three-ounce, muscular uterus, enclosing a slitlike, highly distensible cavity. It is here that the fertilized ovum embeds and the fetus develops.

Fertilized ova are able to implant elsewhere in the reproductive tract. These are ectopic (Greek: *ektopos*, "out of place") pregnancies, which at present are increasing in occurrence. They almost all abort early but may cause severe internal bleeding.

Ovulation

During fetal life the ovaries contain hundreds of thousands of eggs, which are scattered around in the connective tissue of the ovary. The largest proportion of these eggs disappear prior to birth. As the girl grows older some of them are surrounded by specialized cells that eventually form a capsule called the follicle, much like the shell of a hen's egg. As sexual maturity approaches, the pituitary gland, located at the base of the skull, under the stimulation of hormones coming from the brain itself, begins to secrete human follicle-stimulating hormone FSH. Under the influence of this hormone some of the follicles now develop a fluid, and those that are near the surface may bulge through it. They are now called graafian follicles. In an entirely random manner, one or at most a few grow far larger than the rest, which, in their turn, simply shrivel and disappear. When a certain level of growth is reached, the graafian follicle falls under the influence of another hormone from the pituitary gland. This one, luteinizing hormone LH, then stimulates the development of the follicle further until it bursts through the surface of the ovary and pops the egg with its surrounding mantle of follicle cells into the awaiting folds of the fallopian tube.

The exquisite interplay and miraculous coordination of multiple mechanisms to make reproduction work successfully never cease to amaze me. A good example is the coordination of activities of the fallopian tubes with follicular rupture. The fallopian tube resembles a cornucopia. The wide bowllike ovarian end is fringed with many fingerlike processes, termed fimbria. During most of the monthly cycle, the fimbria are flaccid and inert. Just preceding ovulation they become erect and constantly lick the surface of the adjacent ovary like hungry tongues seeking to sweep the surface of the freshly ruptured follicle and lick the egg into the open end of the tube. If by mischance the tiny egg is spilled into the abdominal cavity near the vicinity of the tube, the tube acts like a siphon and attempts to suck the spilled egg into it.

In humans ovulation is totally independent of sexual intercourse, occurring with equal frequency in the sexually developed virgin and the sexually active woman. If fertilization does not occur—obviously its occurrence is relatively infrequent—the tiny unfertilized egg quickly dies and fragments into many pieces, which white blood cells scavenge.

To be fruitful, sexual intercourse must take place within seventy-two hours before ovulation or within twenty-four hours after its occurrence, since a sperm cell is capable of causing fertilization for no more than seventy-two hours after being deposited in the female and an egg if unfertilized survives less than twenty-four hours after ovulation. If we can place ovulation in a definite relationship to some easily observed recurrent phenomenon of the reproductive cycle, such as menstruation, we are well on the track of knowing when sexual intercourse is most likely to result in pregnancy. Significant data on ovulation have been collected by several methods—by the examination of ovaries at the operating table and in surgically removed specimens; by the actual washing of an egg from the fallopian tube; by observation of pregnancies following a single, accurately dated copulation; and by observation of results from artificial insemination.

Even more precise timing information has come from sonography and laparoscopy observations of the ripening of ovarian follicles. Sonography is a visualizing method that uses the fact that various body tissues echo sound waves differently from one another. These echoes can be converted into an image. Laparoscopy is a technique in which an optical instrument is introduced into the abdominal cavity after it has been distended with gas; the internal organs are then directly inspected.

From such observations it appears that ovulation most often occurs between eight and nineteen days after the onset of the menses, the exact day being influenced by the length of the menstrual interval. Women with short menstrual intervals—for example, twenty-five days—are likely to ovulate early, and

those with long intervals—such as thirty-one to thirty-five
days—late. Actually, a woman ovulates about fourteen days
before the onset of her next menses. However, when an egg
is fertilized there is no next menstrual period, ovulation occurring about fourteen days before she would have menstruated
had she not become pregnant.

Since most women menstruate approximately every twenty-
eight days, if one counts the first menstrual day as day one,
the usual time of ovulation is day thirteen or day fourteen,
which explains the fact that impregnation is most likely to
occur in mid-cycle, midway between the menses. In very rare
instances, however, impregnation may result from intercourse
at virtually any time during the menstrual month—which implies that ovulation in exceptional cycles occurs at exceptional
times. There is evidence that female orgasm infrequently may
trigger an aberrant ovulation in some women. Three mammals,
the cat, ferret, and rabbit, regularly ovulate only after copulation. They lack the spontaneous ovulation of the human and
other mammals, which ovulate cyclically, irrespective of copulation. All clinicians of experience can cite examples of patients becoming pregnant at odd periods in the cycle. There is
in fact no truly safe period. Anecdotal reports of pregnancies
being established during the menses and very early and very
late in the nonbleeding part of the cycle abound. In truth, such
pregnancies are quite rare.

The two periods in the month when impregnation is least
likely, the relatively "safe periods" for sex relations without
causing conception, are the first week of the cycle including
the menses, and the last week, that is, the week prior to menstruation. The smallest number of conceptions takes place at
these times.

The Egg's Journey Down the Tube

After ovulation, the egg, having passed from an ovary into the
fallopian tube, travels down the five-inch tube. The passage
takes from three to five days. The muscular walls of the tube
encircle a canal which is wide at the ovarian end and at the
uterine end narrows to a bore as small as a broomstraw. The
mechanism that propels the egg downward through the tube

toward the uterus seems to be a combination of fluid currents and rhythmic muscular contractions like those which carry food and excreta through the intestinal tract. Many of the cells lining each fallopian tube are ciliated: they possess hairlike projections from the surface that beat vigorously. Under the microscope they remind me of a field of wheat being blown by the wind. The beating of the cilia causes a fluid current which mostly flows down the tube from the ovarian toward the uterine end. When the ovum is ovulated from a ripe ovarian follicle, it is surrounded by a thick, loosely adherent covering of some three thousand small cells, the cumulus cells that envelop it completely during its residence in the follicle. Some of the cells are brushed loose by the egg's contact with the sides of the tube, especially with the ciliated cells of the tubal wall.

The Upward Journey of the Spermatozoa

The mid-portion of the tube is the rendezvous for egg and sperm. Explanations of how spermatozoa ascend from the vagina into the uterus, and from the uterus to the meeting place in the tube, have shifted as knowledge of the subject has increased and clarified. A hundred years ago a spermatozoon was believed to be endowed with instinctive, bloodhoundlike qualities which directed it along the proper path to insure fertilization.

Today it is known that the fate of the several hundred million spermatozoa depends in part on the phase of the recipient's menstrual cycle.

During the three or four days before ovulation and the day of ovulation itself, the canal of the cervix, the entrance passage into the uterus from the vagina, is filled with a profuse, transparent, watery mucus which furnishes a highly favorable environment for sperm cells and through which they swim with ease. The appearance of this profuse mucus explains why some women notice a colorless vaginal discharge each month during three to five days in mid-cycle. Some women occasionally stain or even bleed lightly for forty-eight hours in mid-month, this being synchronous with the time of ovulation. Many report pain in occasional cycles for four or five hours on one side or the other of the lower abdomen, depending on whether the egg that particular month was ovulated from the right or left ovary. At all other times of the month except for these several days in mid-cycle, the cervical canal contains a scant, sticky, opaque mucus, much less easily penetrated by spermatozoa, and many are entrapped and halted in it like flies on flypaper.

During intercourse the spermatozoa are catapulted into the upper vagina, into the region of the cervix. When ejaculated, the semen contains discrete gelatinous material, but rapidly becomes uniformly liquefied. The sperm cells swim haphazardly in all directions, some into the upper recesses of the vagina, some toward the outside, others away from the middle of the vagina far to one side or the other. The bulk of the spermatozoa never reach the protective confines of the cervical canal, but remain in the vagina, exposed to the hostile environment of vaginal secretions, which are quite acid in reaction. Sperm cells are sensitive to an acid medium, and those remaining in the vagina become motionless and dead within a few hours. A relatively few by sheer spatial accident immediately gain the sanctuary of the cervical mucus. This was demonstrated by studies in which cooperating couples notified the physician as soon as male orgasm had been accomplished. The physician then took samples of mucus from high up in the cervical canal. Much to the surprise of the scientific community, the cervical mucus tested was already swarming with sperm cells.

The cervical mucus is weakly alkaline and sperm cells thrive in it. On occasion it is acidic, and this may be a factor in infertility. Unfortunately, despite everybody's hopes this is not corrected by alkaline douches.

Some of the sperm swim straight up the one-inch, mucus-filled canal with almost purposeful success, while others bog down on the way, getting hopelessly stranded in tissue bays and coves. A small proportion of the total number ejaculated eventually reach the cavity of the uterus and begin their upward two-inch excursion through its length. Whether this progress results solely from the swimming efforts of the spermatozoa or whether they are aided by fluid currents and muscular contractions of the uterus is still unknown. The undaunted ones, those not stranded in this veritable everglade, reach the openings of the two fallopian tubes—one on each side of the triangular-shaped, slitlike uterine cavity, the base of the triangle being up—and continue their journey upward from the uterus into one of the tubes.

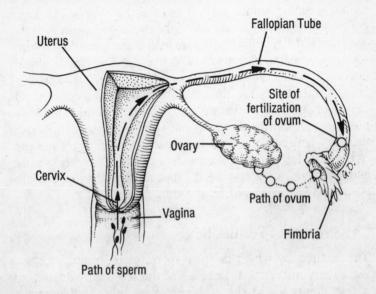

The female internal reproductive organs. A window cut into the wall of the uterus shows the path taken by sperm through the uterus enroute to the site of fertilization. The drawing also shows the path of the ovum from the ovary to where it meets the sperm in the tube.

If the egg is discharged from the right ovary and has reached the mid-portion of the right tube, two or three inches above the utero-tubal junction, a spermatozoon swimming up the left tube has, of course, no chance of impregnating it. It is calculated that only a few thousand of the four hundred million cells ejaculated ever reach the trysting site, the mid-segment of the fallopian tube containing the egg. The one sperm that achieves its destiny has won against gigantic odds, several hundred million to one. The baby it engenders has a far greater mathematical chance of becoming president than the sperm had of fathering a baby. No one knows just what selective forces are responsible for the victory. Perhaps the winner had the strongest constitution; perhaps it was the swiftest swimmer of all the contestants entered in the race. Perhaps it was merely the luckiest in finding a fluid current leading straight to the ovum. According to experimental evidence, this total five-inch journey requires approximately thirty or forty minutes. If ovulation occurred within several minutes to twenty-four hours before the sperm's journey ends, the ovum will be in the tube, awaiting fertilization; if ovulation took place more than twenty-four hours before insemination, the egg cell will have already begun to deteriorate and fragment, rendering it incapable of being fertilized by the time the spermatozoon reaches it. On the other hand, if ovulation has not yet occurred, but takes place within two or three days after intercourse, living spermatozoa will be cruising at the tubal site waiting for the egg.

We have followed the sperm and egg to their meeting place, and we can now observe what happens when they meet—that is, the actual process of fertilization.

The Process of Fertilization

The method by which the tiny sperm cells locate the egg is not clearly understood. Because of the few spermatozoa, just a few thousand, in the relatively long tube at the time of fertilization, many investigators feel some process other than random encounter is involved. It has been suggested that the egg exerts a chemical trapping effect, increasing sperm concentration by making them swim more rapidly when they are headed toward it and less rapidly when going away from it. When sperm-egg collision occurs the sperm becomes immediately bound to the egg's surface.

There is species specificity in the process of fertilization. All animal groups within the same species interbreed and are normally fertile with each other, as is illustrated by the bizarre results in the crossing, most usually by accident, of diverse canine strains. Related species are occasionally fertile with each other: horse and jackass (mule); zebra and donkey (dobra); cattle and buffalo (cattalo); and lion and tiger (liger). However, offspring from related species are almost invariably infertile.

Before fertilization can be accomplished the sperm must undergo the process of capacitation, that is, gaining the capacity to fertilize. Freshly ejaculated spermatozoa are in fact incapable of causing fertilization, which has nothing to do with their motility, as uncapacitated spermatozoa swim quite handsomely. Capacitation is accomplished by exposure of the sperm to secretions of the uterus, the fallopian tube, or the ovary's graafian follicle. Capacitation requires as little as two hours in the hamster and as long as eleven hours in the rabbit. There is suggestive evidence that it requires eight hours in human beings. Through electron microscopy, which permits magnification from ten thousand to more than one hundred thousand times, it has been determined that each sperm head is surrounded by two membranes, a plasma membrane closely applied to it and the loose, veillike acrosomal membrane mentioned earlier. Capacitation permits two very essential activities by the sperm cell, first penetration of the multilayered halo of cumulus cells, which surround and adhere to the surface of the egg, the zona pellucida. As far as can be observed, a capacitated sperm appears the same as a sperm before capacitation. However, several hours' exposure to fluids of the female reproductive tract enables it to undergo the acrosomal reaction, which ruptures the outer membrane surrounding the sperm head and releases an enzyme beneath the membrane that can dissolve cumulus cells, cutting a path through the surrounding halo to the egg's surface, where it softens the capsule so that a sperm can penetrate it. In the process of fertilization it is believed that hundreds of sperm cells jointly contribute this essential enzyme material.

The egg capsule, the zona pellucida, is relatively firm and rigid; its thickness is approximately one-tenth the diameter of the egg. Precisely how a spermatozoon penetrates the capsule is not completely known. The sperm does not swim its way through the capsule with the point of its head foremost, but appears to attack the egg with the side of its head. The path it makes through the zona is not straight but oblique. It is possible that the egg cooperates in the process by thrusting out a streamerlike process that engulfs the sperm head and draws it inward.

In the human it is not known whether the head alone or the whole spermatozoon, including the tail, enters the egg. However, supernumerary sperm are often lodged or trapped in the gelatinous zona pellucida. Some enter the perivitelline space, the narrow zone between the covering of the egg and its true contents, the cytoplasm with its nucleus. However, only a single sperm penetrates the perivitelline membrane to pair the twenty-three chromosomes of its nucleus with the twenty-three chromosomes of the nucleus of the egg.

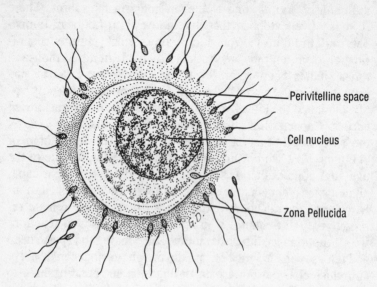

Perivitelline space

Cell nucleus

Zona Pellucida

Whether rat or human, the infant animal is formed by a marvelously intricate and orderly arrangement of billions of cells.

Fusion of the Two Nuclei

In the rat during the first nineteen hours after fertilization, both the male and female nuclei enlarge and migrate toward the center of the cell. The next step is the fusion of the two nuclei into one parent nucleus. When this has been accomplished, fertilization is completed, and the fertilized ovum then begins to divide into two cells; the two cells divide into four, the four into eight, and so on, creating after twenty-one days a newborn rat weighing less than an ounce. In the human the same process, after an average of 266 days from the moment of fertilization or 280 days from the beginning of the last menstrual period, creates a seven-and-a-half-pound baby.

The Enigma of When the Fetus First Becomes a Living Being

The revision of the laws restricting elective abortion has had the consequence of reviving discussions as to when life begins. In many cultures and in a number of religions life is not considered to begin until either the mother becomes aware of independent fetal movement or at some other time when ensoulment is assumed to have taken place. Others who have thought about this consider that human life begins with the union of the sperm and the egg and the reestablishment of the normal number of chromosomes and therefore the potential of a unique human being. For still others this is not the beginning of life, since a free-floating structure such as a fertilized egg must accomplish implantation in the wall of the mother's uterus before developing the true potential of independent existence. Another large group of people believes that life commences only at the point when the fetus is able to maintain an independent existence. At present, with the improvement in perinatal care this is somewhere in the vicinity of the twenty-sixth week of pregnancy; in extraordinarily rare instances, fetuses of this developmental age have in fact survived to adulthood. Many others believe that the fetus achieves life only when it is actually born and has left its mother's body.

My own conviction is that the only scientific resolution to all this is that life is a continuum; that the sperm and the unfertilized egg are living structures and that, although their union creates a unique individual, it does not create life. Unfortunately this conviction does very little to resolve the practical, social, and political problems that are related to this discussion. I doubt that these problems can indeed be resolved on a scientific basis.

The Early Hours of the Fertilized Egg

In the mouse the two-cell egg appears twenty-four hours after fertilization, and the four-cell stage after thirty-eight to fifty hours. In the human a two-cell stage has been observed within twelve hours after fertilization and sixty-four-cell development in seventy-two hours. By the fifth day the human embryo is made up of about five hundred cells, the cells having doubled their number about every twelve hours since the time of fertilization.

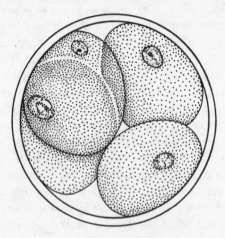

A 4-cell human embryo, ready for transfer to the uterus in the course of in vitro fertilization

In all mammals the developing egg in its earliest phase, while still a traveler down the fallopian tube, is a solid mass of cells, aptly termed a morula (Latin: *morum*, "mulberry," which it resembles). It is still round and has increased little if at all in diameter, its contents merely having divided into smaller units. In this respect it is like a real estate development. At first a road bisects the whole area; then a crossroad divides it into quarters, and later other roads into eighths and twelfths. This happens without the addition of any land, simply by subdivision of the original tract.

The egg passes from the tube into the uterus on day four or five, when it is no longer a solid mass of cells, the cells having arranged themselves about the outer surface of the sphere, the center now being occupied by fluid. It is then termed a blastocyst (Greek: "sprouting bladder"). By the fifth day the multicellular conceptus begins to increase in size. It floats about the slitlike uterine cavity for three or four more days and then adheres to its inner cell lining, which has been exquisitely prepared by the special hormone progesterone, fed by the ovary into the bloodstream from whence it reaches the uterus. Progesterone has made the lining succulent and swollen with a network of new and enlarged blood channels coursing through it. The developing egg, possessing an enzyme that digests away the surface cells to which it has adhered, then sinks down into the depths of the uterine lining. The process is something like hoeing the firm, dry earth above to plant the corn in the soft, moist, rich earth beneath. Implantation occurs on the eighth day in man and on the fifth day in the mouse, despite the fact that pregnancy in the mouse is only $\frac{1}{18}$ as long as in man. By the twelfth day the human egg is already firmly implanted, but the damaged, superficial uterine lining cells through which it passed have only partially healed to roof over the tissue nest in which the egg now rests. About six out of ten pregnancies implant on the posterior, or rear, wall of the uterine cavity, and four in ten on the anterior, or front, wall.

On microscopic study the twelve-day egg already shows a

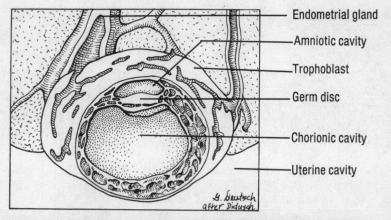

Endometrial gland

Amniotic cavity

Trophoblast

Germ disc

Chorionic cavity

Uterine cavity

G. Dautsch
after Didusch

A cross section of a 12-day-old human embryo and the site in the uterine lining in which it has implanted. The tubular structures are maternal blood vessels, two of which have opened into that portion of the embryo destined to become the placenta, inside which the fluid-containing membranes are taking shape. In the very midst of all this is the germ disc, the part of the embryo which will become the fetus. The actual measurement of the structures shown in this illustration is about $\frac{1}{64}$ of an inch across.

specialized accumulation of cells which later will form the embryo. The remaining cells become the afterbirth and membranes.

Impregnation is now completed, as yet unbeknown to the woman. She has not even had time to miss her first menstrual period, and other symptoms suggestive of pregnancy are still several days distant.

It is important to point out that many more eggs are fertilized than babies born. Fertilization, implantation, and early development of the ovum are each so complex that something frequently goes wrong and then further growth ceases. If this occurs within the first ten to twelve days, the menstrual period is not even late. If development of the ovum is arrested, say around the fifteenth day, the menses are delayed a week or so but no recognizable tissue is passed. However, if pregnancy progresses several weeks before it comes to a halt a discernible miscarriage occurs. It is estimated that at least 50 percent of fertilizations never end up as a baby.

3

Are You Pregnant?

Ordinarily diagnosis of pregnancy presents no problem to patient or physician. In contrast to most conditions for which people seek a doctor, pregnancy is usually prediagnosed by the patient. Yet on rare occasions its diagnosis may be puzzling. The correct answer to such a puzzle is then determined from three types of data: the patient's symptoms, certain bodily changes determined by the physician, and specific laboratory tests.

For practical purposes we consider the number of weeks of pregnancy as the weeks that have elapsed since the first day of the last normal menstrual period. Since most months are longer than four weeks, the estimations by weeks and months do not correspond in a simple way. The commonest length of pregnancy is 280 days after the start of the last period. This is forty weeks or nine months and one week. Counting from the day of conception, the duration of pregnancy is 266 days, or thirty-eight weeks, or one week less than nine months.

Symptoms

Absence of Menses

Failure to menstruate (amenorrhea) is usually the earliest evidence of pregnancy. A missed menstrual period in a woman between fifteen and forty-five with previously regular cycles who has been having sexual intercourse suggests pregnancy as the most likely possibility, though not the only one, since there are many other causes for a delayed or even a skipped period.

Age must be taken into account, since the periods may be quite irregular toward the onset and the termination of a woman's menstrual career. Recent childbirth, especially when a woman is nursing, may eliminate the menses temporarily or lengthen the interval between them. Illnesses, including severe anemia, untreated diabetes, disturbances of the thyroid gland, high fever from infection, and a host of other disease states may create menstrual disturbances. Malnutrition may lead to an absence of menstruation; the failure of many female war prisoners in World War II to menstruate during incarceration was probably mainly for this reason. Amenorrhea may occur in women who have lost weight rapidly on a very strict anti-obesity regimen.

It is now well known that among ballet dancers and women athletes, particularly among those who train intensely for long-distance running, absence of menses is a frequent phenomenon. Psychological stress may also be responsible for the temporary disappearance of menses. Among the stresses, one might list adjustment to living in a new country or to a change of occupation. Amenorrhea is not uncommonly observed among young women who go away from home to start a college education. Emotional upsets such as the death of a loved one can precipitate this phenomenon. Another common cause is the sudden fear that an unwanted pregnancy has occurred, and, at the other end of the spectrum, the conviction by a woman with a long history of infertility that she has now finally achieved pregnancy although it has not in fact occurred. This is referred to as pseudocyesis, which in extreme cases can mimic pregnancy sufficiently to mislead not only family but medical attendants.

Menses in Early Pregnancy

You may be pregnant and still appear to menstruate during the early months. On close observation, such menstrual periods are different. Ordinarily they are shorter and scantier. In the typical instance the woman menstruates three days instead of five at the normal time her period is due. A month later she menstruates half a day, the following month for an hour, and then the menses cease entirely during the remainder of pregnancy. Not infrequently women may develop menstrual cramps at the first missed period without any bleeding or staining. They fully expect to menstruate each hour, but do not. The discomfort lasts for three or four days, then ceases.

Breast Changes

Many women suffer a pronounced fullness of the breasts premenstrually, which subsides rapidly just before or with the onset of menstruation. When pregnancy occurs, this fullness continues instead of disappearing, and becomes even more marked. At the same time the pregnant woman may feel a tingling in the breasts, and they may become tender, the nipples being hypersensitive. These sensations usually are of short duration; the breasts remain large, but the feelings of tenseness and tenderness disappear. In preparation for lactation the mammary glands actually continue to increase in size during the remainder of pregnancy, the enlargement in part being due to growth of the milk-secreting glandular tissue and in part to a greatly enriched blood supply. This latter is often manifested in the second half of pregnancy by the appearance of a delicate tracery of blue veins beneath the skin on the chest, especially noticeable in women with very fair skin. The nipple and the colored circle of skin surrounding it—the areola—enlarge, and their pigmentation darkens. Arranged in a circular fashion around the periphery of the areola, near the skin edge, are a number of small, roundish elevations, oil glands—in the inimitable words of Montgomery, their discoverer, "a constellation of miniature nipples scattered over a milky way." In some women breast enlargement is accompanied by the formation of stretch marks in the skin—striae; since they appear more extensively over the abdomen they will be discussed later in this chapter under "Abdominal Changes."

Nipple Secretion

After the first few months a sticky, yellowish, watery fluid—colostrum—may be expressed from the nipples by gently stripping the breast. This finding is not absolute evidence of pregnancy, for women who have borne and suckled children may retain colostrum in the breasts for years. In the later months of pregnancy drops of colostrum may flow from the nipples spontaneously. As term is approached, the colostrum takes on an opaque, whitish appearance, more resembling milk.

Nausea and Vomiting

Nausea and vomiting in pregnancy—"morning sickness," as they are so cheerfully termed in popular speech—are going out of fashion. Thirty years ago most pregnant women appeared to suffer from morning sickness. This is no longer true; if one eliminates slight cases of occasional, unimportant queasiness, today's pregnant women are infrequently plagued by it. It is difficult to explain this. Perhaps the improvement is associated with better all-year-round diet, improved health, a higher incidence of planned conceptions, and a changed attitude toward pregnancy and labor. The last few decades have witnessed a marvelous revolution in the way the average woman regards childbirth. She was tense, fearful, apprehensive; but now she is relaxed, reassured, and confident. Multiple causes are responsible for the change in attitude. The pregnant woman realizes that obstetrics has improved vastly, so that pain, illness, and death for those bringing life are virtually relics of the past. Then, too, she is no longer kept in ignorance about the process of birth. Books like this one, government pamphlets, magazine articles, school lectures, maternity classes, and personal teaching by physicians, all have contributed to make the laity more knowledgeable regarding obstetrics.

Morning sickness usually begins when the pregnant woman's menstrual period is several days overdue, and then gradually disappears six to eight weeks later. In the beginning the patient awakens with a feeling of gastric instability, a little uncertain as to whether she is going to vomit or not. The uncertainty is replaced in a few days by the actuality, which usually occurs as soon as she lifts her head from the pillow. As the morning lengthens, the nausea and vomiting diminish, and by lunchtime she eats an ordinary meal. There are exceptions to this pattern; some women vomit only in the evening, and others at irregular times or all day long. Some are actively nauseated during early pregnancy by odors from the kitchen, and others by tobacco smoke.

It is not uncommon for the woman who vomits during pregnancy to observe that her vomitus is flecked or streaked with blood. This should not cause concern, as repeated vomiting from any source may rupture a tiny blood vessel in the throat or esophagus. Such a small vessel soon clots and heals spontaneously.

Many instances are recorded of particularly suggestible husbands who vomit with their pregnant wives; there are even cases in which the husband vomited though his wife did not.

Excessive salivation (ptyalism) to the amount of three or four quarts a day is sometimes a concomitant of pregnancy. It is likely to begin two or three weeks after the first missed period, persist throughout pregnancy, and disappear promptly after delivery. Treatment in the main is unsatisfactory. Mild sedatives, strong mouthwashes, and sucking peppermint candies may bring relief.

Changes in Appetite

It is not uncommon for the newly pregnant woman to note a temporary diminution in appetite, and ordinary amounts of food make her feel overfull and bloated; without the advice of a physician, she is likely to substitute frequent small feedings for scheduled meals.

Some pregnant women develop a craving for one particular food almost to the exclusion of anything else. When one reads the obstetrical texts of a few centuries ago and observes the space and emphasis they gave to what they termed "pica," or aberrations of appetite, one gains the impression that the condition is probably only one-fiftieth as common today as it was then. Unquestionably diets are more diversified and better balanced today, and the opportunity to obtain milk, fruits, and vegetables at all seasons of the year is greater. Food cravings during pregnancy probably have their genesis in dietary omissions.

In my own experience I have seen different women crave soup, pretzels, and dill pickles. We have all encountered patients who have minor versions of this kind of specialized craving. (Many years ago the wife of a young Johns Hopkins Hospital staff member, who was on a very stringent budget, developed a particular taste for, of all possible foods, lobster. Two or three evenings a week the couple would go downtown and the young doctor enviously watched his wife devour a lobster. Prior to that they had occasionally gone to the theater or a concert, but those funds were completely consumed in the form of lobsters!) At the present time the rarity of this particular kind of food craving and the increase in the remuneration of young hospital staff members is such that the couples can probably dine out, and go to a show too, without putting an undue burden on their budgets.

One remarkable present-day form of pica is geophagia. It consists of eating mud or related thick materials like moistened laundry starch. The best evidence is that the taste for these is at least in part the result of dietary shortages, especially a deficiency of iron and trace elements. The women are invariably markedly anemic. Geophagia is most frequently observed among blacks in the southern United States and their relatives who have migrated north. It occurs less among those pregnant women who can get nutritional supplements.

Excessive Need of Sleep

In some women one of the early symptoms of pregnancy is an unusual degree of sleepiness. This is not too much of a problem for women who do not already have children and who spend most of their time at home. It can be a great nuisance for women who are professionally active. This generally disappears after the end of the first three months, or trimester, of pregnancy.

Frequent Urination

Sometimes frequency of urination begins as early as the first missed period. This condition disappears about the tenth or twelfth week, often to recur a few weeks before delivery.

Abdominal Changes

As pregnancy progresses, the woman herself is likely to become more conscious of the gradual filling of her lower abdomen, manifest at first by an inability to hold her abdominal wall in as well as she could before she was pregnant. The next thing she is likely to notice is that she can feel a small, soft mass just above the pelvic bone, particularly when her bladder is full. Of course, the bladder is simply pushing the pregnant uterus up to a point where it can be felt through the relaxed abdominal wall. The uterus then gradually grows upward during the remainder of the pregnancy, reaching the level of the navel at about the twentieth week. To external observation the patient begins to "show" at some time between the fourteenth and twentieth weeks. This varies greatly from woman to woman. I have had patients who were obviously pregnant at the fourteenth week while wearing ordinary street clothes, and others who wore skintight blue jeans through the sixth month and who barely looked pregnant at all to the casual observer. What may disclose the presence of the pregnancy to the patient's friends is that her wardrobe begins to change as she enters the fourth and fifth months, to accommodate the changes in her shape that her friends may not yet have noticed.

As the size of the uterus increases, stretch marks may appear. This common term is actually something of a misnomer. The marks are only partly due to the mechanical stress of the growing uterus on the skin and connective tissue of the abdominal wall. They result also from the hormonal influences of pregnancy, and in fact appear in areas where there is no actual physical stretching. Above the navel they tend to look something like the upper half of a circle; around the navel they form a circular pattern; and in the lower abdomen they characteristically form lines slanting downward and inward. The marks are very slightly depressed below the level of the normal skin, making the skin look frayed.

Stretch marks may appear no matter how little weight a woman gains. They tend to increase up to term, and have a red color from the proliferation of tiny blood vessels. After delivery they gradually fade as the blood vessels become less prominent. Then they become shiny and pearl-white, and narrower than they were during pregnancy, but they do not entirely vanish.

Despite the great enlargement of the size of the uterus, at rest the intra-abdominal pressure in a pregnant woman is completely normal. During the bearing-down movements of the second stage of labor, however, it is markedly increased and the navel may protrude remarkably. The weakness of the abdominal wall at the navel results from the laxity at that point during intrauterine life. The umbilical artery and vein which make up the cord and run from fetus to placenta pass through the abdominal wall there, and it is essential that there be ample space for the blood's unobstructed passage.

The end of the breastbone, the xiphoid, is attached to the lower end of the sternum by a hinged joint. Under ordinary circumstances, this bone cannot be felt, but in late pregnancy it may loosen up and rotate outward so that a bump can be felt in the V-shaped space between the lower margins of the ribs. The presence of this is quite normal.

The long muscles of the abdominal wall, which run from the rib cage down to the pubic bone, located behind the sexual hair, are stretched and separated by the growing uterus. As a result, in the midline of the pregnant abdomen, the abdominal wall consists of skin, some thinned-out connective tissue, and a little bit of fat covering the lining of the peritoneal cavity, which in turn contains the abdominal organs. When the abdomen is filled with the pregnant uterus, this is not particularly noticeable, but as soon as the baby is delivered, then separation of the muscles and the weakness of the abdominal wall—the diastasis recti—is quite obvious.

Quickening

Somewhere between the sixteenth and the twenty-second week, the mother is first able to feel the movements of the fetus. Fetal movements are felt more readily when the placenta is attached to the rear wall of the uterus. A woman having her first baby will probably notice the movements about two weeks farther along than she will in later pregnancies, when she may recognize them as early as the sixteenth week. The subjective sensation of these first movements has been likened poetically to the faint flutter of a caged bird's wings and, more prosaically, to the bursting of a bubble of thick syrup.

At the onset the movement is so gentle, particularly since the baby is floating in an amount of water greater than its size, that the patient may not be certain as to what she has felt. Only after these light taps against her uterine wall have been repeated several times can she be certain that this is fetal movement. Of course, later in pregnancy, the movements of the arms and legs, the stretching of the trunk, and the movement of the baby's head become very much more powerful, to the point where anyone is able to feel the fetal movements by placing a hand on the mother's abdominal wall. Sometimes the movements are so active that patients become convinced that they are carrying twins or triplets. It is worthwhile to report to your doctor when you first definitely feel the fetus move because this can help to time the pregnancy.

Once women perceive fetal movements they come to expect to feel them every day, but at the beginning, several days may pass when they are not felt at all. In later pregnancy, certainly by the twenty-fourth week, fetal movements are felt daily. The fetuses in general tend to be more active late in the day, after supper and stretching into bedtime, to the point where they may sometimes make it difficult for the patient to fall asleep. Ultrasound examinations have confirmed that at quiet times the fetus is in fact asleep. In general, cycles of sleeping and awakening tend to run on about a ninety-minute schedule, but the fetus's physical activity is much more appreciated when the mother herself is inactive. Late in pregnancy if a fetus goes more than twenty-four hours without manifesting activity, it is wise to report this, since it may be an early warning signal of fetal distress.

False Pregnancy (Pseudocyesis)

The woman with a false pregnancy may present any and all of the symptoms of a true pregnancy. A positive diagnosis of pregnancy, therefore, cannot be made solely on the basis of the patient's reports but depends on the evidence of a living fetus by ultrasound. A positive pregnancy test in urine or blood, which detects the presence of hCG, the hormone produced by the placenta, may be present due to certain rare tumors. I distinctly recall a shy adolescent who developed abdominal enlargement and a positive pregnancy test and was pronounced pregnant despite her firm insistence that she had not had any sexual exposure. It was only after some five months, during which this child was made extremely miserable by the doctors and her parents with constant badgering to admit what they assumed to be the case, that an X-ray demonstrated that she had a tumor of the ovary that was the source of all the findings. Fortunately for her, it was possible to cure her, and I subsequently had the pleasure of receiving the announcement of her first child.

The diagnosis of false pregnancy depends on physical and pelvic examination and repeated negative hCG tests and sonographic examinations.

Physician's Findings on Physical Examination

Virtually every organ and tissue of the body is affected in some measure by the physiologic changes induced by pregnancy. These changes result, directly or indirectly, from the action of the chemicals produced by the afterbirth, the placenta (from the Latin, meaning a flat cake). Considering the fact that the placenta's primary function is to strain out food essentials from the mother's bloodstream for the baby and to excrete the baby's waste products, it is amazing that it is also such an efficient chemical factory.

The most striking pregnancy changes occur in the generative organs. Therefore, for a diagnosis of pregnancy, the reproductive organs are examined to determine whether any of the anticipated changes have occurred.

Examination of the Breasts

The initial physical examination in pregnancy ordinarily begins with the breasts. They are inspected first to see whether they have enlarged and if there is any change in the pigmentation of the nipple and the areola. The patient is usually able to confirm the fact that her breasts are distinctly fuller. The doctor or midwife may ask how they fit into the brassiere she usually wears. The breasts are then palpated to be certain that the increase in size is due to glandular tissue and not fat. Since the breasts do change in pregnancy, early signs of cancer of the breast may be inadvertently disregarded. When present, they are no different from those which the patient could find for herself were she not pregnant. It is important on this first examination therefore to search for lumps and plugged milk ducts, which should be found and noted.

The patient may have noticed, particularly in later pregnancies, a leakage of some colostrum from the nipple; and the examiner can confirm this by massaging the gland toward the nipple to see whether colostrum is in fact present. Patients who have previously nursed, particularly if they have done so recently, may have milk in the breast in small amounts even in the absence of pregnancy.

Abdominal Examination

Palpation in your upper abdomen directs attention to the liver and spleen, which are up under the ribs on the right and left sides respectively. When you take a deep breath and your diaphragm drops, the liver is pushed down to the examiner's hand, but the spleen cannot be felt unless it is enlarged. The lowermost part of a normal kidney can sometimes be felt deep in the abdomen of a slender woman during a deep breath. The other organs, such as the stomach and the small and the large intestine, cannot be felt unless they contain masses.

The examiner next checks for ruptures at the navel and in the groins. If you have had a previous pregnancy, the muscles of your abdominal wall may still be spread apart and this should be called to your attention.

In each area of the abdomen the examiner is alert for the presence of unusual lumps.

Next to be examined is the lower abdomen which, beyond the thirteenth or fourteenth week, will contain the rising uterus. The uterus at first is a small, vaguely definable midline swelling, globular and quite soft. It can usually be distinguished from tumors such as uterine fibroids and ovarian cysts, both of which feel quite different to the experienced examiner's hand.

At about the twentieth week the uterus generally has risen to the level of the navel. One month later it may become possible to feel the fetus as a separate structure within the uterus. The first portion of the fetus that can be felt with any certainty is its head. This has been compared to feeling a doll through several thicknesses of blanket. Clearly the larger the doll the easier it will be to be certain of its outline; the thinner the blanket the more certain the identification of its various parts. By the twenty-eighth week it may be possible to make out the extremities and to locate the buttocks, which feel substantially softer than the head. Past the thirty-second week it is ordinarily possible to outline the fetus with considerable certainty in slender patients, and even more easily in women having later pregnancies, since their uteri are more relaxed than they were the first time around.

Pelvic Examination

This is the examination of the external and internal genitalia. You should empty your bladder before it is carried out, as a full bladder can be mistaken for a pregnant uterus.

You will be asked to lie on your back, with your buttocks at the edge of the examining table, your heels close to the buttocks, probably in a footrest, and your knees relaxed and wide apart. You may find yourself more comfortable with your head and back propped up. Many patients feel very exposed and vulnerable in this position and have trouble relaxing. For this reason, I have found it helpful to get the patient to participate in the examination and directly observe what I am doing, with the help of a hand-held mirror. This is sometimes the first opportunity the patient has had to see her own external genitalia; I like to take this chance to acquaint her with her own anatomy and give her a clear notion of the location of the urethra, the anus, and the opening of the vagina. For this reason, and also because drapes tend to be a barrier preventing eye contact between patient and examiner, I prefer to use minimal drapes for pelvic examination. Thus, when I insert a speculum to visualize the cervix, I can show it to the patient in the mirror and let her see the color associated with the pregnant state.

If you find this style of pelvic examination appealing, and those providing your care to do not customarily employ it, there is no reason why you cannot request it. You can consider taking your own mirror with you to the examination.

The principal changes in the vagina during pregnancy are threefold: increased blood supply, softening of the tissues, and augmented secretions. Pelvic circulatory changes appear early in pregnancy, usually before the second missed period, and often serve as a valuable aid for the establishment of the diagnosis. The tissues about the entrance of the vagina and within it take on a purplish, dusky color instead of the normal pink (Chadwick's sign). The color deepens as pregnancy advances, and is likely to be more striking in those who have already borne children.

As pregnancy advances, the vagina becomes increasingly elastic and distensible because of the softening of the tissues which form its walls. This change facilitates the performance of a vaginal examination.

The increase in vaginal discharge that is usually concomitant with pregnancy is in large part due to the normal excess in activity of the mucus-secreting glands of the cervix.

To perform a pelvic examination, one finger is first inserted into the vagina to establish some estimate of the size of the entrance. Over the years I have actually seen three patients who arrived at the end of pregnancy with intact hymens, so that I know that one cannot assume that pregnancy alone is a guarantee of adequate space to insert a speculum. The initial finger examination also feels the muscles surrounding the introitus (the entrance to the vagina) and the bones of the lower portion of the pelvis.

Following this initial one-finger exploration, I insert a second finger and press against the muscles surrounding the vagina—but not before telling the patient that this is what I am about to do. The purpose of this maneuver is to prepare to introduce the speculum, which, because it is made of steel and likely to be cold, I warm under running water. I then visualize the cervix, and take material for a Pap smear. I put a cotton-tipped applicator stick into the opening in the cervix, to harvest some cells from this area. Some examiners prefer to press a small wooden scraper, much like a butter spreader, against the cervix to gather the cells. Next, a second applicator is wiped in the rear corner of the vagina to gather cells which have been shed from the cervix and have collected there. The sampling is completely painless and takes less than a minute.

The harvested cells are spread on a glass slide and sprayed to fix them to the glass. In the laboratory they are stained and studied under the microscope by a cytologist who looks for cancer cells and other abnormalities. The cytologist's report may not be ready until several days after the smear is obtained.

After the cell sampling is completed I remove the speculum and reinsert the two fingers into the vagina to feel the internal organs. The cervix can be felt as a firm structure protruding into the upper vagina and attached to the uterus, which is more or less enlarged and softened depending on the duration of the pregnancy. I then feel the tissues on either side of the cervix for thickening or any evidence of scarring that might fix the cervix in position. Finally, the tissues to either side of the uterus are palpated to identify the ovaries, if possible, and any abnormal structures, such as ovarian cysts or fibroids.

The next step is to feel the uterus itself, not only to confirm the pregnancy but also to find out whether the size of the uterus is consistent with the supposed duration of the pregnancy. In very early pregnancy the body of the uterus may remain firm and the mid-portion between the body and the cervix soften. This is called Hegar's sign and is suggestive of the diagnosis of pregnancy. Still later on, the body of the uterus softens and becomes increasingly spherical and, in the presence of a single fetus, enlarges in an entirely predictable manner. By the eighth week of pregnancy the bulk of the uterus is approximately doubled and by the twelfth week it is tripled.

If the uterus is smaller than expected, the pregnancy may be abnormal or the dates may be off. On the other hand, an unexpectedly large uterus may indicate fibroids or a multiple pregnancy, or just that the dates are off in the opposite direction. The correct diagnosis is established by watchful waiting or by sonography.

At the time of pelvic examination, the examiner makes an estimation of the adequacy of the bony pelvis for the passage of a normal-sized infant. Nowadays contraction of the bony pelvis sufficient to obstruct birth is an exceedingly rare event, unless the fetus is extraordinarily large. When I was an intern we spent much time measuring the bony pelvis to try to decide about pelvic capacity. This, along with most of the X-ray studies for the same purpose, has nearly vanished from obstetrics. Congenital abnormalities of bony pelvic shape are rare, and the marked deformities seen three generations ago, due to rickets and malnutrition, simply no longer exist.

Indisputable Evidence of Pregnancy

The changes in the vagina, cervix, and uterus found on pelvic examination are only presumptive evidence of pregnancy, since other conditions also can cause them. The earliest conclusive proof of pregnancy is the demonstration by sonography of a live embryo. It can ordinarily be visualized at the seventh week of pregnancy, surrounded by the gestational sac and the uterus.

By the ninth or tenth week of pregnancy the fetal heart can be heard by the use of an ultrasound detector. Sound waves encounter tissues and bounce back in an echo phenomenon, and moving tissues will change the pitch of the sound. This is the Doppler effect. Ultrasound waves at 2 million cycles per second, the frequency that is used, are not heard by the unaided human ear. Changes in the pitch of their echoes from a moving object can be converted by electronic means and made audible. By this means the beating heart of the fetus can be "heard."

Still later in pregnancy, the movement of the fetus can be felt by the mother and by an outside observer using a hand on the mother's abdomen; its heartbeat can be heard with an ordinary stethoscope by the twentieth week.

Pregnancy Tests

When early diagnosis of pregnancy is important, even before a physical examination or detection of a fetal heartbeat by ultrasonography provides proof, a laboratory test for pregnancy can be done. The blastocyst begins to produce human chorionic gonadotropin when it is four days old. The hCG spreads in body water to all tissues and hence is found in the blood, the urine, spinal fluid and all other body fluids. It can be detected in minute amounts and with great accuracy, at first in the blood and shortly thereafter in the urine.

The very high level of accuracy of blood tests for hCG has resulted in their increasing use, although the urine tests continue to be valuable for screening purposes. They certainly are less expensive than the blood tests. In normal patients, determination of hCG in the blood is not worth the expense. There are, however, several circumstances in which availability of the test has markedly improved care of uncommon but serious illnesses. In ectopic pregnancy the implantation, being outside the uterus, is commonly defective, and so the normal very rapid rise in hCG titer is not observed; low values are reported instead. This usually corroborates the mother's impression that she may be pregnant but that it doesn't feel right. Since it also proves the presence of placental tissue somewhere in the mother, it becomes incumbent on the physician to find out where the tissue is located. As was mentioned above, by ultrasonography it is now possible to find very early pregnancies. The combination of these two diagnostic methods has greatly accelerated our detection of ectopic pregnancies—a significant advance at a time when the incidence of ectopic pregnancy is steadily rising. The hCG hormone is also formed in the presence of a few rare tumors of the ovary, and can then be used as a marker in following the treatment of these patients. And, as mentioned below, the hCG is also positive in the presence of tumors of the placenta such as hydatidiform moles (Greek: *hydatid*, "watery vesicle"; *form*, "shape").

Urine Tests for Pregnancy

A number of simple, easily done tests exist for determining if hCG is present in the urine. They all depend on a reaction between the hCG and an anti-hCG antibody. A second reaction is then invoked as a marker to detect whether the first reaction has taken place. This may produce a color.

Slide tests using the clumping of red blood cells or of coated latex beads as the marker can be read in two minutes after the solutions have been mixed on the slide. Test-tube tests on the same principle are more sensitive and can be read in two hours.

In patients who are four to seven days overdue for an expected period and pregnant, 77 percent have a positive test. If the woman is fourteen days overdue, these tests are close to 100 percent correct and are therefore reliable either as positive or negative. The color-producing test is even more sensitive, developing earlier in pregnancy and being more reliable. If a pelvic examination and a urine test do not agree, the wise move is to wait a week and repeat the test.

The sensitivity of the test can be increased by running it on the first urine voided in the morning, because this urine is ordinarily more concentrated than the urine voided during the day and therefore has a higher proportion of hCG in it.

Over-the-Counter Tests

At present, pregnancy testing kits are available in neighborhood drug stores. If these are applied to study of the mother's urine ten days or more after she has missed an anticipated period, something like 95 percent accuracy is available almost regardless of the brand of the test. Other tests based on the same principle may be available at clinics or doctors' offices at less cost, barring an additional fee for the office visit.

Progesterone Test

This test is mentioned in the interest of completeness. If a patient is not pregnant but simply a bit off in her cycle, she may be delayed in menstruating and very much puzzled. Given doses of either natural progesterone by injection or one of the synthetic progestins by mouth for a few days, she will probably respond by bleeding if not pregnant. If pregnant, the patient will not bleed, and therefore this was formerly used as a "provocative" test for pregnancy. It is outmoded now. For one thing, the hCG immunologic tests are faster and more accurate. For another, administration of the synthetic progestins in pregnancy may be associated with anomalies in the embryo.

4

Duration of Pregnancy

Patients almost always ask when the baby is due to be born. I generally reply by saying that it is very difficult to select a precise date but that I can give the patient an estimate of the approximate one. I then follow this up with a question: "When did your last menstrual period begin?"

Let us say that you then reply, "Well, let's see, it was the day of the last concert we went to. Let me see, wasn't that Wednesday, March 18?" Without any further ado I can then tell you that your baby is most likely due to be born on Christmas Day. This is a very impressive performance, particularly when it is carried out early in May and predicts an event at what seems to be an almost indecent distance in the future. How is this done?

The calculation of the expected date of confinement is very simple, absurdly simple. I hesitate to divulge the formula for fear of revealing a guild secret. The rule is: Add seven days to the first day of the last normal menstrual period. Count back three months. In this case, I added seven to March 18, and then counted back—February, January, December. That made the expected date of confinement December 25. The mystic formula is now exposed. In reality, this formula affords a short-cut for counting 280 days from any fixed date. In other words, a woman delivers approximately nine months and seven days from the beginning date of her last menstrual period.

It must be stressed that the 280 days is an average figure,

47

which means that a vast number of pregnancies terminate before the 280th day, a vast number after it, and only relatively few on the exact day. At best the calculated or expected date of confinement is an approximate date. This is an important fact for the pregnant couple as well as relatives and other interested persons to remember. It is all too common for panic to become general when "B" day arrives, then passes, and yet there is no sign of labor. Telephones soon begin ringing, and on each occasion the patient is unhappily greeted by the salutation, "Haven't you gone to the hospital yet?"

Calculating the Delivery Date from the Day of Insemination

In calculating the expected date of confinement from 425 cases in which a purported single, fruitful coitus led to impregnation, it was found that the average patient delivered 269.9 days after insemination. However, there was wide variation, extending from 231 to 329 days. A second study, involving fifteen cases of artificial insemination, yielded an average duration of pregnancy of 272 days from the day of treatment, with a span of 261 to 288 days. It is obvious that calculating the anticipated delivery date from coital data has little or no advantage over the more standard technique of utilizing the first day of the last menstruation.

Calculating the Delivery Date from the Onset of Fetal Movements

Another method of computing the "due date" is to count eighteen or twenty weeks from the time the patient first feels fetal movements; however, this is even less exact than the calculations from menstrual and coital data.

After sifting all available modern scientific data, we come to the conclusion that the generalization first made decades ago about the duration of pregnancy is relatively correct. If the date is calculated from the onset of the last menses, almost 50 percent will deliver within the week before or after the 280th day, and 75 percent within two weeks of it.

What Are the Chances of Delivering on Time?

In over 17,000 cases of pregnancy carried beyond the twenty-seventh week, 54 percent delivered before 280 days, 4 percent on the 280th day, and 42 percent later. Forty-six percent had their babies either the week before or the week after the calculated date, and 74 percent within a two-week period before or after the anticipated day of birth.

On the basis of these data one can calculate the likelihood which the average woman faces when carrying a single infant, not twins, of having her baby, during each week after the twenty-seventh week from the first day of her last menstrual period.

Weeks	Days	Approximate Chance
28	189-196	1:625
29	196-203	1:625
30	203-210	1:525
31	210-217	1:240
32	217-224	1:240
33	224-231	1:135
34	231-238	1:115
35	238-245	1:58
36	245-252	1:39
37	252-259	1:22
38	259-266	1:11
39	266-273	1:5
40	273-280	1:3½
41	280-287	1:5⅔
42	287-294	1:12
43	294-301	1:34
44	301-308	1:74

Another reliable study has shown that 40 percent of women go into labor within a ten-day period—five days before and five days after the calculated date, and nearly two-thirds within plus or minus ten days of the expected time.

Factors Affecting the Delivery Date

Ordinarily the woman with a consistent, regular menstrual cycle is more likely to have a baby at the 280th day than the woman who menstruates irregularly. Furthermore, a short menstrual interval, such as twenty-five days, is frequently associated with delivery a few days early, and a lengthy menstrual cycle with birth beyond the due date. The calculated date increases or decreases by about one day for each day the patient's average menstrual cycle exceeds or falls short of twenty-eight days. Neither age, race, size, nor the previous number of children seems to influence the length of pregnancy.

In a study of almost fifteen thousand first births of a single infant in Aberdeen, Scotland, 24 percent of patients with a male infant delivered during the thirty-ninth week and 28 percent in the fortieth week (total 52 percent). Twenty-three percent of mothers in a first labor who gave birth to daughters bore them during the thirty-ninth week and 30 percent in the fortieth week (total 53 percent). This slight difference in delivery dates between boys and girls is not statistically significant.

A study of over twenty thousand total births at the University of Chicago showed that babies weighing over ten pounds averaged pregnancies of 288 days instead of 280 days.

A twin conception shortens pregnancy by about three weeks; actually, the average woman who carries twins delivers them on the 258th day instead of the 280th day. Triplet and quadruplet pregnancies are usually briefer than this, triplets commonly arriving five weeks early and quadruplets six weeks before time. Mrs. Dionne delivered her famous quintuplets on the 219th day (thirty-one weeks).

A Prolonged Pregnancy

A pregnancy carried more than two weeks beyond the calculated date is considered prolonged, and the resulting infant designated as postmature. Such a delivery occurred in 8 to 12 percent of the pregnancies in the two studies previously cited.

There are apparently medically authentic cases in which pregnancy extended to 336 and 337 days, and one in which the duration was 343 days (forty-nine weeks). When pregnancy is excessively protracted there are three possibilities: an error in menstrual dates; ovulation several weeks later than the usual fourteenth day of the cycle, impregnation therefore not taking place until forty or fifty days after the onset of the last menses; or actually several extra weeks of pregnancy beyond the usual forty weeks before labor commences. In most cases the true answer is never known, but it is generally believed that in most instances error is at fault. It is believed that at the most 4 percent of pregnancies are truly carried two weeks or more beyond the average time.

Evidence is accumulating that a baby in the uterus gains little weight after the term date of 280 days is reached, so that the birth of a baby of excessive size adds little proof of true postmaturity. As a matter of fact, babies may actually lose weight in the uterus after the due date is reached, and it is thought by some authorities that the typical postmature baby is thin, scrawny, and odd-looking, with loose, baggy skin, long nails, abundance of scalp hair, and a singularly alert look. They may also show desquamation, or peeling, of the superficial skin of the palms and soles. After birth such infants gain back the weight they lost and soon appear normally chubby and well padded. In addition, in such cases the surface of the placenta often displays thick deposits of calcium, perhaps evidence of its relative senility.

Legal Problems Associated with Duration of Pregnancy

Beyond the medical importance of knowing the duration of pregnancy there is its legal aspect, involving such matters as inheritance and child support. The laws and the court decisions are in an almost constant state of flux and are not the same from one country to another. Some recognize legitimacy for any baby born after the marriage of the parents. In some countries as many as half the women are pregnant at the time of marriage and this is so widely accepted that it no longer provides grist for the gossip mills. Elsewhere legitimacy is accepted only if the baby is born eight months or more after the date of the marriage.

Babies born as long as 355 days after the supposed fertile contact have been declared legitimate, and in one celebrated case, according to the testimony the date of the last coitus between the couple preceded birth by 360 days. This particular decision was overthrown, on appeal by the husband, as being medically unreasonable.

Extremely brief pregnancies sometimes involve not only the reputation of the mother, but the father as well. In Scotland in 1835 the Reverend and Mrs. Jardine had a living baby born five months and three weeks after marriage (twenty-four and a half weeks). Charges of immorality against the reverend couple were brought by the Presbytery of Kirkcaldy, and after four years of investigation a doubtful verdict was rendered. Both sides appealed to the General Assembly of the Church of Scotland, which found the charge of immorality unproved, absolving the couple.

Laboratory Tests for Paternity

When a dispute as to paternity arises, recourse may be had to genetic testing. By either blood or tissue typing it is possible to prove that either or both the presumed father and mother cannot be the actual biologic parents.

Blood typing is a test for proteins on the surface of red blood cells. More than thirty different such proteins have been identified. Tests for tissue types detect proteins common to all the cells of the body. These are called human leukocyte antigens (HLA) and are present in many different combinations from one person to the next. They are used in matching donor to recipient prior to organ transplanation, because rejection of a graft is more likely in the event of a mismatch. Inheritance of blood and tissue types follows the strict rules of genetics. A child's type must come in part from each parent. If the child has a type, red cell or tissue, not present in a presumed parent, that person is excluded. So many types can be tested for that a high likelihood of parenthood can be demonstrated; however, it takes only one mismatch to exclude it.

The Effect of Prolonged Pregnancy on the Fetus

A consensus exists that prolongation of pregnancy beyond forty-two weeks can jeopardize fetal welfare. Such fetuses may tolerate the stress of labor poorly. They often have diminished amniotic fluid. They are prone to pass meconium (the thick green material that fills the fetal large intestine) into the amniotic fluid, making a dense mixture. In addition, they tend to gasp in response to the stress of uterine contractions and thus to breathe in the meconium. It is very irritating to the lung tissue and results in respiratory difficulty after birth. Fetal and newborn problems are more likely to occur among older women having their first babies and women with other high-risk factors when pregnancy is prolonged.

When postmaturity (prolongation) is a potential problem, the first steps are to review the menstrual history and the patient's weight curve. If she is still gaining weight, it is unlikely that she is much past true term. The adequacy of amniotic fluid amount is estimated by abdominal examination, which can be assisted by sonography. In most instances these measures will give ample evidence as to fetal welfare.

When more information is needed, it is obtained by fetal monitoring, described in detail in Chapter 16. A non-stress test (NST) is carried out. There is no agreement whether to intervene if the NST is normal. If, however, it is equivocal, induction of labor can be considered. Induction is usually done after examination of the patient to determine the presentation of the fetus and the ripeness of the cervix. If the baby's head is well down in the pelvis and the cervix is soft, shortened, and partly dilated, the membranes can be ruptured by means of a fine plastic hook passed through the cervix. Labor ordinarily ensues within a few hours.

If the woman does not go into labor within a reasonable time (the exact length is a matter of judgment) the administration of oxytocics (Greek: *oxy*, "sharp"; *tokos*, "childbirth") such as oxytocin and prostaglandin may be added to bring about effective uterine contractions. Induction of labor by oxytocics has what I am sure is an undeserved bad reputation. It is true that in the past obstetricians who were in a hurry found it possible to force labor by using excessive doses of oxytocin. This was surely as painful as it was unnecessary. When we induce because of a concern for fetal welfare, oxytocics are given in very small amounts and increased very gradually to the least amount to produce effective labor. Such labor is no different in its effect on mother and child than an equally effective natural labor.

Cesarean as a treatment for postmaturity should not be done simply because of the patient's dates unless fetal assessment has given evidence of serious fetal distress and induction will be difficult.

Breast and nipple stimulation for the induction of labor has attracted attention in the past few years. There is no question that there is a prompt reflex for the release of oxytocin from the pituitary and that the uterus responds to it by contracting. It has been claimed that postmaturity is less likely to occur and readiness for induction more likely to be found in women who have used breast and nipple stimulation late in the third trimester. It is therefore important to warn women who are liable to premature labor to avoid any of the methods suggested for preparing their breasts for nursing.

Sometimes when the NST is equivocal, we proceed to stimulate the uterus, while monitoring, to see how the fetus tolerates the stress of uterine contractions. This has been called the contraction stress test (CST), or the oxytocin challenge test (OCT). It is carried out while contractions are produced by administering small amounts of oxytocin. We try to observe the effect on the fetal heart rate of several contractions in a brief period. On occasion, in sensitive patients, the test itself suffices to bring on labor.

5

The Fetus

The origin and growth of the fetus was a simple thing to our medical forefathers. In 1548 all embryology could be put on a single page; today it cannot be crammed into a library of hundreds of volumes. I venture the guess that more pages have been written about the obscure fetus than about the illustrious Shakespeare.

The biological life of an embryo begins with fertilization, as stated in the first chapter. At that moment the precursor of the child is of almost microscopic size, a speck of tissue so very tiny that it is just barely visible to the naked eye of the expert—a mass so light that its weight cannot be expressed in even thousandths of an ounce. Within nine months this minute dot of tissue develops into a twenty-inch, seven-and-a-half-pound screaming infant. The initial ten days in the life of the future citizen are reported in Chapter 2. As described there, the ovum implants itself into the substance of the uterus, excavating the permanent home that it will occupy for more than eight months by digesting its way into the interior lining of the uterus. In the process it taps very, very small maternal blood vessels and soon finds itself surrounded by a veritable lake of its mother's blood, into which it dips vigorous, hungry cells. These cells, which grow like streamers from the surface of what is called the blastocyst at this state of development, absorb minerals, vitamins, carbohydrates, proteins, and fats essential to growth. With absorption of nourishment the fertilized ovum increases rapidly in size. At a certain region on the inside of the covering a thickened mass of cells now appears; this mass is called the inner cell mass or embryonic area, and it is from these cells that the embryo itself develops.

Summary of Fetal Development for Each Period of Pregnancy

Let me now summarize the development of the fetus, always designating the weeks or months since the onset of the last menses. If one assumes that fertilization takes place on the fourteenth day of the cycle, then there is a constant difference of two weeks between the actual age of the conceptus and the duration of pregnancy, since the latter is calculated from the beginning of the last menses. To prevent confusion I shall discuss embryonic and fetal development in terms of duration of pregnancy, not in actual fetal age, for potential parents think in terms of weeks and months of pregnancy.

End of second week: Fertilization occurs. First day in the life of fertilized ovum.

End of third week of pregnancy; *first week after conception*: Fertilized ovum traveling down tube; on 17th day enters uterus as a round, solid, mulberrylike mass of cells; then transforms into blastocyst, an outside cover of hundreds of cells with fluid in the center, like a tiny hollow rubber ball filled with fluid instead of air. Floats in uterus (17th–22nd day). Blastocyst about 1/100 of an inch in diameter.

Beginning of fourth week: Implantation (21st day), i.e., 7 days after fertilization. Egg still barely visible to naked eye. After implantation fertilized ovum begins to grow rapidly, doubling its size every twenty-four hours. Cells forming the embryonic area (from which embryo will grow) appear on inner wall of blastocyst. The placenta begins to form on that part of outer wall of blastocyst deepest within maternal tissues.

Beginning of fifth week: The embryo itself is a minute piece of uniform gray-white flesh. The primitive streak that will become the spine is laid down. The embryonic sac containing

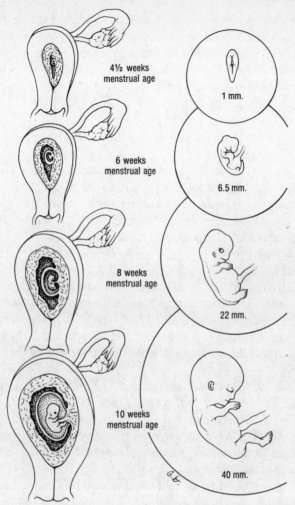

4½ weeks
menstrual age

1 mm.

6 weeks
menstrual age

6.5 mm.

8 weeks
menstrual age

22 mm.

10 weeks
menstrual age

40 mm.

The fetus early in its development and its size relative to the uterus. Only one tube and one ovary are shown.

A. 5 weeks after the start of the last normal period—21 days after fertilization: $^{78}/_{1,000}$ of an inch long.

B. 6 weeks after last menses—4 weeks ovulation age; ¼ of an inch long.

C. 8 weeks after last menses; $^{8}/_{10}$ of an inch.

D. 10 weeks after last menses. The fetus is almost fully formed; 1 $^{6}/_{10}$ inches long.

the embryo is ⅖ inch in diameter, and already contains some fluid in addition to the germ disc.

End of fifth week: Backbone forming, five to eight vertebrae laid down. Nervous system and spinal canal forming. By end of fifth week the foundation for the child's brain, spinal cord, and entire nervous system will have been established, as well as rudiments of its eyes (20 days after conception). Tubular S-shaped primitive heart beginning to beat. Embryo ¼ inch long.

Beginning of sixth week: Head forming. Beating heart visible, located on outside of body, not yet within chest cavity. Intestinal tract forming; growth starts from mouth cavity downward. Mouth closed. Human embryo at this stage cannot be differentiated through its appearance from a pig, a rabbit, a chick, or an elephant embryo. Has a rudimentary tail, extension of its spinal column.

End of sixth week: All of backbone laid down and spinal canal closed over. Brain increasing conspicuously. Tail of embryo visible. Beginnings of arms and legs visible. Depressions beneath skin where eyes and ears are to appear. Length, ½ inch. Germ cells, to become either an ovary or testis, have appeared.

Seventh week: Chest and abdomen completely formed. Heart internal. Eyes clearly perceptible through closed lids. Face flattening, shell-like external ears. Mouth opens. Lung buds appear. Big toes have appeared. Tail has almost disappeared. May begin to move body slightly. The great bulge of its brain predicts that this creature is destined to feel, think, and strive beyond the capacity of all other animals on this earth. Length, ⅝ inch. Weight, 1/100 of an ounce.

Eighth week: Face and features forming. Jaws are now well formed, and the teeth and facial muscles forming. Rudiments of fingers and then toes become evident. Ovaries or testicles taking form. In the male the penis begins to appear. Cartilage and bone may both be seen in the forming skeleton. Length, ¾ inch. Weight, 3/100 ounce (1 gram)—less than an aspirin tablet.

Ninth week (end of second month): Face completely formed. Arms, legs, hands, and feet partially formed. Stubby toes and fingers. Abdominal-wall muscles of fetus, if removed from womb, will contract when touched. By microscopic examination of gonad sex can be determined. Clitoris of female appears. From this time on, looks very much like a miniature infant. Length, 1 + inch. Weight, $\frac{1}{10}$ ounce (3 grams).

Tenth week: The eyes, which were at side of head, moving to front. Face quite human except for jaws, not fully developed. Heart forming four chambers. Scrotum appearing. Palate to form roof of mouth closing. Major blood vessels assuming final form and muscle wall of intestinal tract forming. Fetal heart beating 120 to 160 per minute. Electrocardiogram of live born fetus of this age shows pattern of various waves similar to adult.

Fetus resembles miniature doll, slightly more than one inch in height with a very large head, which is almost half of the fetus, gracefully formed arms and legs, slitlike closed eyes, small ear lobes, protuberant abdomen. Fetus looks top heavy.

End of third month (13½ weeks): Arms, legs, hands, feet, fingers, and toes fully formed. Nails appear. Ears completely formed. External genital organs begin to show clear differences, and by 11th week trained observer can determine sex with naked eye. Now when the brain signals, muscles respond and the fetus kicks, even curling its toes. Arms bend at wrists and elbows, and fingers close to form tiny fist. The face with its tightly shut eyes squints, purses its lips, and opens its mouth. It may swallow amniotic fluid, excreting it back into the amniotic fluid as urine. Movements reflex from spinal cord. Brain not yet sufficiently organized to control them. Length, 3 inches. Weight, 1 ounce (40 grams).

End of fourth month (18 weeks): Casual observer could now distinguish sex in infants delivered at this phase of development. By end of month fetal movements felt by mother and heart can be heard with stethoscope. Fine, downlike hair all over, skin less transparent and pinker. Eyebrows and eyelashes appear. Length, 8½ inches. Weight, 6 ounces (180 grams).

End of fifth month (22½ weeks): Hair appears on head, fat being deposited under skin, although fetus very lean. If born, may live a few minutes, in rarest of instances reported to have survived. Length, 12 inches. Weight, 1 pound (453 grams).

End of sixth month (27 weeks): Fetus covered with cheeselike secretion, vernix caseosa. Skin wrinkled. Hair on head fairly well developed. Eyes open. When given expert premature infant care, approximately two in three born in the 27th week survive. Length, 14 inches. Weight, 2 pounds (906 grams).

End of the seventh month (31½ weeks): In male fetus, testicles usually descend into scrotum. Child born alive during this month has slightly better than 85 percent chance for survival. The age-old superstition that a baby born in the seventh will do better than one born in the eighth is entirely fallacious. Each day nearer term makes the child's chances for survival that much better. Length, 16 inches. Weight, 3 pounds, 12 ounces (1,600 grams).

End of eighth month (35¾ weeks): Child has better than 97 percent likelihood for survival. Length, 18 inches. Weight, 5¼ pounds (2,400 grams).

End of ninth month (40 weeks): Full term. Skin smooth, polished-looking, and still covered by cheeselike secretion. No downlike hair except over shoulders and arms. Head hair 1 inch long. Nails protrude beyond ends of fingers and toes. Eyes usually a slate color; impossible to predict their final tone. Average circumference of head equals circumference of shoulders (13 inches). Length, 20 inches. Weight, 7 pounds, 6 ounces (3,350 grams). When born alive, 99 out of 100 survive.

At birth the various body systems of the newborn human are sufficiently organized to carry on the necessary activities for its survival outside of the uterus, provided it is protected and nourished. But the baby is far from being an independent individual. The complicated muscular coordination necessary for sitting must wait six months and for walking a year or more, until the nerves and brain have developed sufficiently. This is in bold contrast to lower animals. A newly born chick trots off almost at once in search of food. The newborn wildebeest on the plains of Africa is delivered during herd migrations and five minutes after its birth must trudge after its mother if it is to survive. In truth human parents have the privilege and duty to watch with their own eyes the final stages of fetal development in the nursery.

Life in the Uterus

The Amniotic Fluid

The colorless amniotic fluid with which the fetus is surrounded serves many purposes. It prevents the walls of the uterus from cramping the fetus and allows it unhampered growth and movement. It is particularly necessary for the development of the lungs. It encompasses the fetus with a fluid of constant temperature which is a marvelous insulator against cold and heat. Above all it acts as an excellent shock absorber. A blow on the mother's abdomen merely jolts the fetus, and it floats away.

It is easy to appreciate a pregnant woman's special concern if she falls violently, is struck a hard blow on the abdomen, or is badly shaken in an accident. Of course pregnancy does not lessen her chance for injury, but external trauma rarely harms the unborn child. If there is no vaginal bleeding within an hour after the accident, it is almost an infallible rule that no damage has resulted to the pregnancy. Very rarely an accident may initiate premature labor, usually by an associated rupture of the membranes. One may state unequivocally that accidents occurring during pregnancy never cause birthmarks, malformations, or (save in the rare cases in which they cause miscarriage) any other ill effects to the child itself. The exception is an object that penetrates the abdomen and uterus, such as a bullet or a knife.

Amniotic fluid is by no means stagnant, about one-third being replenished every hour. It is constantly being reabsorbed into the mother's blood system and excreted into the sac by the cells of the amniotic membrane, the inner of the two membranes forming the fetal sac. The chorion is the outer membrane. During intrauterine existence the fetus swallows amniotic fluid and voids fetal urine into it. It has been determined that the fetus swallows about one pint a day, and it voids a similar quantity. The fetus does not defecate under normal conditions before birth. At the twelfth week of pregnancy the volume of amniotic fluid in the uterus measures two ounces, in mid-pregnancy a quart, and at term (the end of nine months) a little less than a quart, though amounts up to eight gallons have been observed. When the amount of fluid exceeds two quarts the abnormal condition is called hydramnios. The amniotic fluid contains skin cells shed by the fetus, fetal hairs, specks of vernix (the oily, cheeselike material that covers much of the fetal skin), various minerals and sugar in weak solution, products of fetal urine, such as uric acid and creatinine, and a wide variety of the chemicals, normal and abnormal, which are excreted in the urine.

The Navel Cord

The umbilical cord runs from the navel of the fetus to the inner or fetal surface of the placenta. It is the lifeline of the fetus,

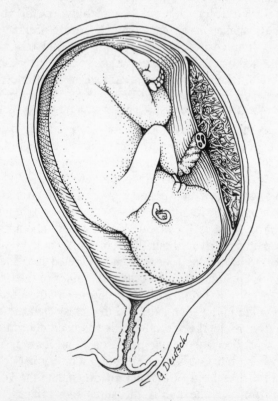

A fetus at about 28 weeks menstrual age. The placenta and umbilical cord have assumed their final shape.

in reality a vital cable circulating fetal blood low in oxygen and high in waste products through its two umbilical arteries to the placenta, where the blood is purified and takes up oxygen and food stuffs. The cleansed, well-oxygenated, placental blood, rich in nutrients, then returns to the fetus through the one umbilical vein. The umbilical cord, a moist, dull white, semi-transparent, jellylike rope, averages twenty-two inches in length at term, although cords from a half-inch to fifty inches have been reported. Some are straight, others twisted, and some, in rare instances, are even knotted by fetal gymnastics *in utero*. The diameter of the cord is about three-quarters of an inch.

The Placenta and Its Function in Fetal Nutrition

The placenta is a complex organ through which the fetus absorbs food and eliminates its waste products. The blood of the mother and the blood of the fetus come in close proximity in the substance of the placenta, and materials pass over from one blood system to the other. If, for example, the mother's blood contains more sugar than that of the fetus, the excess passes over into the fetal blood until relative equality between the two is reached. In this way sugar that the mother eats is fed to her baby. On the other hand, the excess carbon dioxide of the fetal blood goes over to the mother's blood and is exhaled by her lungs. Thus, the mother breathes for her child. Other waste products of the fetus are likewise absorbed by the mother's blood and voided by her kidneys. It is to be noted that not all vitamins, minerals, and hormones are in exact equality in the two circulations. For example, the amount of vitamin C in the fetal blood is several times that in the maternal blood. As another example, calcium to build fetal bones passes to the fetus from the mother at twenty times the rate it passes back from the fetus to the mother. This delicate interchange between mother and fetus is further illustrated by the observation that cigarette smoking by the mother temporarily increases the rate of the fetal heart. The maximum effect occurs from seven to twelve minutes after the cigarette is first lighted.

Intrauterine growth is largely governed by the development and functioning of the placenta. The placenta stops growing completely between thirty-four and thirty-eight weeks, and with cessation of placental growth fetal growth slows but nevertheless continues. It has been observed that women with relatively large placentas are usually delivered later than women with smaller ones. In some abnormal situations the placenta performs poorly, causing a condition termed placental insufficiency, which may adversely affect the growth and well-being of the fetus.

The Bloodstreams of Mother and Fetus Are Separate

The bloodstreams of the mother and fetus are ordinarily quite separate, and the interchange of materials is carried on through a multicelled membranous partition. Some of the smaller molecules pass intact back and forth through the separating membrane; the larger ones, such as fats and antibodies and other proteins are broken down on one side of the barrier, and then pass through to be reconstituted on the other side. This all sounds quite remarkable, and it is. To feed a rapidly growing organism, to keep it supplied with oxygen, and to excrete its waste products is a huge complex task. The placenta, a relatively small organ, weighing one-fifth to one-sixth as much as the fetus, does this with unmatched efficiency.

Before the end of the eighteenth century it was held that the blood cells of the mother intermingled freely with those of the fetus. However, at this time a famous English obstetrician injected a dye into the blood vessels of a woman who had died undelivered, and the dye did not appear in the blood vessels of her fetus. This was thought to prove the independent integrity of the two vascular systems, and the scientific world believed that mother and fetus never interchanged blood.

Blood Cells Can Cross the Placenta

In the 1940's, when the disease erythroblastosis was first described, some doubt was thrown on this concept, for in order to cause erythroblastosis an immune response has to be produced in the mother to some factor present in the fetal red-blood cells—a factor which she would ordinarily lack. Theoretically, this required the passage of fetal red-blood cells into the maternal circulation.

We now know that a transfusion of fetal blood into the mother may occur when the placenta is torn away from the uterine wall after the birth of the baby. In that process the placenta itself can tear, allowing fetal blood to leak into the uterine cavity. The uterine contractions, so necessary to halt maternal bleeding from the placental site, may squeeze some of the fetal blood into the mother's circulation.

But during pregnancy leaks of fetal blood into the mother can also occur. On rare occasions these internal hemorrhages may be large enough to cause severe fetal anemia and even fetal death. If the fetus has Rh-positive red blood cells inherited from its father, and its mother is Rh-negative, the transfer of small amouunts of fetal cells can result in sensitization of the mother to Rh. The maternal antibodies can then leak back across the placenta and damage the Rh-positive fetus.

To prevent the sensitization, a dose of human anti-Rh gamma globulin (a blood protein), Rhogam, the anti-Rh antibody, is administered to the mother at about the twenty-eighth week of pregnancy, whenever an amniocentesis is done, or if an abortion occurs, unless the father is known to be Rh-negative.

Maternal cells are also transferred across the placenta to the fetus. We are not quite sure how this transfer works but it is certain that red and white blood cells of maternal origin have been demonstrated in the newborn, having been transferred during pregnancy. The mother and her fetus cannot be incompatible except for fetal characteristics inherited from the father, so transfer from mother to fetus cannot result in sensitization.

Heat Exchange

The placenta, with rapid flow of blood on both sides of its separating membrane, also acts as a heat exchanger. Normally, the fetal temperature is a fraction of a degree above the maternal. When the maternal temperature goes up, the temperature of the fetus will rise too, because it has no way to lose the extra heat except through the placenta.

Hormone Production by the Placenta

As mentioned earlier, in addition to all the functions already listed the placenta produces a considerable variety of hormones. The unique one is human chorionic gonadotropin (hCG), the hormone that signals to the mother's endocrine system that she is pregnant. Early in pregnancy, the placenta also produces female sex hormones and replaces at the end of about six weeks the function of the mother's corpus luteum in this respect. The production of progesterone increases slowly all through pregnancy. It is this hormone that acts as the brake on uterine activity, preventing the uterus from expelling the fetus before it is mature. The placenta also produces a wide range of other hormones, some of them with feedback effects on the hypothalamus and others that appear to be identical with hormones produced by the pituitary gland.

Most Drugs Cross the Placenta to the Baby

Virtually all drugs taken by the mother cross the placenta to the fetus. There is an obvious danger that a particular drug, beneficial to the mother, may damage the fetus. Drugs that cause fetal and embryonic abnormalities are known as teratogens (Greek: *teras*, "monster," Latin: *genesis*, "birth"). The risk is greatest in the first trimester while the embryo is taking shape. But we also can take advantage of the transfer of drugs to treat a fetus prior to birth.

Beneficial Effects

Probably the first drug employed for fetal therapy was the oxygen given to the mother when slowing of the fetal heart appeared as a sign of fetal distress in labor, with the specific purpose of improving the fetal oxygen supply. This therapy is still in widespread use.

Treatment of maternal syphilis with antibiotics that cross the placenta is an example of drug therapy that affects both the mother and baby favorably. The fetus is usually also infected when the mother has active syphilis.

Abnormalities of fetal heart rate that result from improper

electrical regulation of the heart beat and not from infection or labor stress can be treated by giving cardiac drugs to the mother, who herself is normal.

Evidence exists that giving corticoids to the mother when a delivery prior to thirty-two weeks of pregnancy is anticipated reduces the difficulty that the premie has in breathing after birth. The fetus itself forms these steroid hormones from its own adrenal glands in late pregnancy. Given to the mother, they appear to speed up the maturation of the fetal lung.

Drugs Harmful to the Fetus

If anyone ever doubted that drugs taken by the mother, with trivial effect on her, could have disastrous impact on the fetus, this was dispelled by the frightening experience with thalidomide and DES (diethylstilbestrol). The former drug was introduced in Europe in the 1960's as a mild sedative to encourage peaceful sleep. Unfortunately, pregnant women often have problems staying asleep and many of them took the drug. Within a year it became obvious that a disaster had taken place. Large numbers of malformed babies were born. They had one form or another of what is technically referred to as phocomelia (Greek: *phokos*, "seal"; *melus*, "limb"). The children lacked long bones in their arms and legs and had flippers for hands and feet.

The other spectacular example of a drug effect on the fetus, which came to light in the early 1970's, is the tragic experience with DES. This artificial estrogen was given to pregnant women who had diabetes, uterine bleeding, previous spontaneous abortions, and previous unexplained second trimester losses in the mistaken expectation that it would improve the expectation for the fetus. No one has any idea how many such pregnant women were treated with varying amounts of DES for varying durations of their pregnancies during a period of well over twenty years, from the late 1940's into the 1960's. So far as we know the adverse effects were all fetal and not maternal. These effects did not make themselves obvious in most instances until the daughters were well into adolescence. For this reason there was a twenty-year delay in identifying the problems produced by DES. It took even longer to verify the less noticeable anatomical changes in the sons, who do not develop cancer but do have minor anatomical abnormalities.

The first warning consisted of the appearance in Boston of a number of cases of an unusual kind of cancer of the vagina and the cervix. (DES therapy was first employed in Boston in the 1940's.) This unusual kind of cancer had been seen frequently before and continues to be seen in rare instances, but the occurrence of a substantial number of cases in a short period of time drew the attention of investigators to the possibility of some environmental cause. The connection with DES given to the mothers was rapidly made.

The best evidence is that the cancer-causing effects of DES probably do not manifest themselves later than about twenty-five years after the daughter's birth, so that we have probably seen the last of this particular effect. The epidemic of cancer is now over. It has since been learned, however, that the DES daughters, in addition to minor nonmalignant changes in the anatomy of the vagina, cervix, and uterus—changes which are no threat to health—have relatively poor childbearing records. They have more frequent miscarriages, probably more frequent ectopic pregnancies, and certainly more frequent premature labors. The loss of wanted pregnancies among DES daughters is substantially higher than among normal women. Individual DES daughters may experience no difficulty at all.

If you think you may be a DES daughter, ask your mother whether she took any drugs during her pregnancy, but, since memory does play tricks, also ask your doctor to examine you specifically to look for the minor typical changes produced by DES.

Narcotic Drugs

Another large problem is the impact of narcotic drugs on children born to addicts. Their infants can become addicted *in utero* to such drugs as heroin, methadone, phencyclidine (angel dust), and phenobarbital. Compounding the problem, many addicted women also suffer poor nutrition, with the result that intrauterine growth of their babies is retarded for this reason as well. There is further difficulty created by the fact that so-called street drugs may be mixed with a range of impurities and pollutants. Some of these, such as amphetamines, may have effects on both mother and baby which are not obvious in the presence of other drugs.

Because the infants born to narcotic addicts may suffer from acute drug withdrawal after birth, it is important that the pediatrician be aware of the mother's addiction. This is complicated by the fact that in many communities addicted babies are subject to protection by the courts and can be taken away from their mothers. Many mothers know this and thus are motivated to conceal their addiction. The social pathology does not end with the birth of the baby, however. A substantial proportion of these infants are no longer with their mothers when they reach the age of one year.

Mind-Altering Drugs

The use of cocaine during the second half of pregnancy occasionally results in separation of the placenta, especially when it is taken in large doses. The separation results in fetal distress and may precipitate premature labor. Fetal death has been observed. Placental separation has occurred following nasal inhalation (snorting), needle injection under the skin or into a vein (skin popping or mainlining), and inhalation of the drug after it has been treated with ether (freebasing). It is understood among habitual users that they should also abstain while breast-feeding. There is growing indication that some newborns of cocaine users have difficulties similar to those seen with narcotic addiction.

We have no clear evidence at present of adverse fetal effects, beyond the indirect impact of social effects on the mother, from the use of marijuana or peyote or the like. However, in the absence of evidence, the wise thing to do is to abstain during pregnancy and nursing.

The withdrawal symptoms of an addicted newborn may appear as early as eighteen hours or as late as one week after birth. The child becomes irritable and overactive, may become tremulous, and tends to cry with a high-pitched tone. In severe cases convulsions occur, and if the problem is not recognized the infant can die. If it is known that the infant is addicted there is appropriate drug treatment to replace the addicting drug with something less harmful and allow the baby to be withdrawn gradually. The children of addicted mothers are not found to have any increased incidence of congenital abnormalities.

A final problem among babies of addicts is that acquired immune deficiency syndrome (AIDS) is commonly observed among addicts who have taken their drugs by injection. The disease can cross the placenta and be passed on to the fetus. The newborn infants then manifest very frequent infections through infancy, slow growth, and a markedly increased death rate.

The Effect of Smoking during Pregnancy

It has been shown by several investigators that babies born to smokers of one pack of cigarettes or more a day average three-quarters of a pound less at birth than the babies of nonsmokers. This lesser weight does not seem to prejudice the baby's chances for survival, unless it is also born prematurely. The infants of heavy smokers have no tendency to be born prematurely; they simply weigh less at term. There is evidence that the size of the deficit in birth weight is in proportion to the daily consumption of cigarettes. Heavy smokers do not show an increase in births associated with fetal abnormalities.

In Britain the children of three thousand heavy smokers (ten or more cigarettes daily after the fourth month) were compared at the age of seven years to fourteen thousand children of nonsmokers or light smokers. The sample comprised all the children born in the United Kingdom the week of March 3, 1958, who could be traced for the follow-up study. The children of heavy smokers averaged four months behind in reading ability and were one centimeter shorter (0.4 inch) in height compared to the controls. The findings that as a group the smoking women were poorer and older and had more children than the nonsmokers must be taken into account. The report admits these factors may have been contributory but nevertheless concludes that the cigarette smoking was of greater importance.

Cigarette smoking raises the blood level of thiocyanate, a derivative of cyanide that in large quantities is quite toxic. Trace quantities of thiocyanate can be found in the blood of fetuses whose mothers do not smoke but have been exposed to smoking by the baby's father.

Concentrations of folate, derived from the vitamin folic acid, and of carotene, the precursor of vitamin A, are both decreased in the blood of smokers. These deficiencies correlate with cleft lip in experimental animals.

For the protection of your own health as well as for the obvious benefit of the baby, give up cigarettes not only in pregnancy but for keeps. Giving up cigarettes takes conviction and the motivation to go through the discomfort of abandoning a true addiction. You can even go farther than that and avoid environments in which cigarette smoke fills the air.

Since we really do not know what specific factors are responsible for the harm done by smoking it may only be a form of self-deception to experiment with cigarette brands credited with low tar and low nicotine content.

Cigarette smoking is now at least as common among young women as among young men. Society should take steps to make sure that they are aware of the fact that they are not only incurring risks to themselves but also to their children.

The Effect of Alcohol on the Fetus

Alcoholic mothers tend to give birth to babies with a characteristic fetal alcohol syndrome. Since this syndrome was described a number of years ago, it has been possible to make the diagnosis of alcoholism in the mother by physical examination of the infant. It is not absolutely clear whether these infants are all fated to have mental retardation, although its incidence has been strikingly high among them. Whether the impairment is a consequence of receiving their care and upbringing from alcoholics, or whether such infants, given an ideal home environment, might regain the ground lost before birth is not yet established.

Effects of Other Drugs on the Fetus

The catalog of drugs that have adverse affects on the fetus is considerable and really cannot properly be covered in detail within the scope of this volume. Before you take any potent drug it would be wise to remind the prescribers that you are pregnant and to inquire whether they are certain that this is a drug that is known either to be benign or if not, that it is so essential in treatment that some risk must unavoidably be incurred. However, the following notes may be of some value if you have doubts about a drug you have been advised to take. The classes of drugs are listed in alphabetical order:

Antiacne (Accutane)
Isotretinoin (Accutane), used for severe cystic acne, has been shown to be teratogenic. It can cause shortening of the limbs of the fetus and is therefore contraindicated in pregnancy.

Antibiotics
The entire group of aminoglycosides, the principal familiar ones being streptomycin and gentamicin, can produce deafness by damaging the acoustic nerve. Since the drugs can cross the placenta, it is possible for a fetus to be similarly affected. However, the drug must be taken for a long time to cause nerve deafness in mother or fetus. This is sufficiently well known so that it is very unlikely that a pregnant woman would be treated with these drugs for long enough to produce such injury.

Tetracyclines cross the placenta and are deposited in the fetus at the growing ends of bone and in the enamel of teeth. This may delay growth of its long bones. The tetracycline in the tooth enamel is visible, when the teeth erupt in childhood, as a yellow line across the teeth. These are all baby teeth which fall out. Despite the odd appearance there is no other damage; the permanent teeth are normal.

Anticoagulants
Dicumarol (Coumadin) is a drug employed in a small number of patients with artificial heart valves and in some patients who have had repeated episodes of excessive blood clotting, sometimes called thrombophlebitis. This drug, given in early pregnancy, causes an abnormal appearance of the baby's face, which is similar to the one produced by alcohol and is diagnosable in the newborn period. There are other abnormalities of the head and the visual system and a high incidence of mental

retardation. In extreme cases there may be hemorrhage in the fetus, which can lead to death.

Anticonvulsants

These are drugs, such as Dilantin and barbiturates, which are used for epilepsy. Many abnormalities have been associated with them, but some of the defects may be related genetically to the epilepsy itself rather than the drugs. If at all possible, the doses of these drugs should be reduced in pregnancy. If it can be managed, the patient's medication probably is better switched from Dilantin to phenobarbital. Valproic acid, another antiepileptic, can cause failure of the neural tube to close when given in very early pregnancy. Tridione, also used for epilepsy, is a known teratogen and must be avoided.

Anti-inflammatory Agents

The drugs principally of interest in this group are the steroids. Used briefly to treat fetuses in anticipation of premature birth to accelerate the development of their lungs, there is no known adverse effect. When mothers are on steroids for long periods of time to treat maternal disease, the development of the fetal adrenals may be delayed. The baby may then need specific supportive therapy after birth until its adrenals recover.

Antithyroid Agents

These can cross the placenta and suppress the development of the fetal thyroid. The iodine in medications for asthma can have a similar effect. Radioactive iodine, which is used in the treatment of thyroid abnormalities in adults, readily crosses the placenta and will be accumulated by the thyroid gland of the fetus. Since it is radioactive it will have an adverse affect on the growth of that gland, and the fetus may very well be born hypothyroid. For that reason radioactive iodine should not be administered to a pregnant woman.

Cancer Chemotherapeutic Agents

Some of these, the commonest being aminopterin and meth-otrexate, cross the placenta and severely affect the fetus. There are other drugs, however, that are effective against malignant disease and do not have an adverse effect on the fetus. In individual instances, therefore, you should obtain consultation as to the safety of any particular compound proposed for cancer therapy during pregnancy.

Cardiac Drugs

Although the drugs used in cardiac therapy cross the placenta, there is no known harmful effect when they are used at ordinary dosage levels. Digitalis preparations can be used in the treatment of abnormalities of fetal heart rate; in this circumstance they are beneficial rather than harmful. This is also true of propranolol (Inderal), which has now become one of the most commonly prescribed drugs for cardiovascular disease. On occasion during pregnancy a condition technically known as paroxysmal tachycardia, in which the maternal pulse jumps from its ordinary range of about 72 to 180 or more, may occur in short bursts. This may only be a frightening nuisance. However, if it becomes persistent the pumping efficiency of the heart is reduced and the patient may develop such symptoms as faintness and dizziness. When this occurs treatment is warranted; Inderal and another drug called Verapamil have been used. They are employed briefly to treat an undesirable condition in the mother; there is no need to be concerned with the adverse fetal effects that prolonged therapy might conceivably produce.

Diuretics

"Water pills" (actually thiazide diuretics), when used in excessive doses, produce acidosis and so much loss of maternal blood volume as to interfere with blood flow through the placenta and hence fetal nutrition. Therefore, diuretics probably should not be used except for specific medical indications in pregnancy. An example of this is pulmonary edema (water in the lungs) due to heart failure, an event fortunately now quite rare. Diuretics should not be given for swelling of feet and ankles.

Hormones

The adverse effects of the estrogen DES have already been mentioned. Some of the synthetic progestogens, if given in pregnancy, can cause abnormalities of the external genitalia of female fetuses. Although readily correctable, these are certainly undesirable effects. Fortunately these hormones are rarely administered at the present time.

It has been suggested that use of oral contraceptives in the first three months of pregnancy may be responsible for fetal abnormalities but the evidence is weak and, in my opinion, not persuasive.

An antiestrogen, danazol, whose trade name is Danocrine, has been observed on rare occasions to have a virilizing effect on female fetuses when given inadvertently in early pregnancy. The administration of this drug prior to pregnancy, at which time it may be used for endometriosis, has not been observed to have any such effect. (Endometriosis is a condition in which the endometrium is found implanted in patches elsewhere than in the lining of the uterus.)

Premature Labor Drugs

The class of drugs technically known as beta-mimetics, which have general effects on the cardiovascular system, tends also to reduce uterine activity. Several of them have been used in the effort to stop premature labor. They share in common the effects of increasing the fetal heart rate and inducing abnormalities of fetal heart rhythm. This class includes such drugs as ritodrine (Yutopar), isoproterenol (Isuprel), and terbutaline (Brethine). They are ordinarily administered intravenously to hospitalized mothers and must be given with great care since they also have profound side effects on the mothers. When their desired effect is achieved, they can be continued orally. So far as is known they have no long-term adverse effects on the fetus.

Psychotropic Drugs and Sedatives

Many of these drugs, which are central nervous system depressants, have the same effect on the fetus. This may be observed in the baby at birth but disappears when the baby is able to excrete the drug. There is even some suspicion that there may be symptoms of withdrawal from some of the more potent drugs. Diazepam (Valium) can accumulate in the fetus and may produce greater depression than in the mother.

The drugs ordinarily used to improve sleep, such as barbiturates (Seconal, Nembutal) and benzodiapines (Valium, Restoril, Ativan), do not have any undesirable effects on the fetus. Alcohol in moderation probably belongs in this category. As I have mentioned, the most spectacular example of an adverse effect of a drug on the fetus is the teratogenic effect of thalidomide, an otherwise effective sleep inducer.

Bromides, which are no longer readily available as over-the-counter preparations, as they were in the days of Bromo-Seltzer, do not have any known adverse effect on the fetus.

Phenothiazines, generally regarded as tranquilizers, may produce tremors, which can continue for a number of months because the drugs are slowly excreted over a prolonged period of time.

Lithium, used for severe, recurrent, and profound depression, is one drug for which there is a consensus; it is contraindicated in pregnancy. It may be teratogenic.

Stimulants

Of all stimulants, the one most commonly blamed for undesirable fetal effects is caffeine. It is usually taken in the form of coffee. Tea does not seem to come in for criticism, although it too contains caffeine. The bad reputation of coffee is largely anecdotal. When careful studies are done, the heavy coffee drinkers are observed to deliver smaller babies than the non–coffee drinkers, but it turns out that heavy coffee users are likely also to be heavy cigarette smokers.

Coffee by itself in moderation certainly has no known adverse effect on the fetus. We have no reliable information about the effects of caffeine-containing soft drinks.

Vaccines

In principle, the use of live virus vaccines such as those against measles, mumps, German measles, and yellow fever is inadvisable, because they can cross the placenta and infect the fetus. In actual practice they are rarely dangerous. The only live virus vaccine concerning which we have much data is the rubella (German measles) vaccine Meruvax II. This has been given now to several hundred pregnant women with no evidence of any bad fetal effect. We have developed the practice of giving it just after delivery to women who are not immune; it does not appear to affect those newborns who are nursing.

The killed bacterial vaccines, such as those against cholera, typhoid, and whooping cough, can be used if necessary, but since they tend to produce fever are probably best avoided. The toxoids, such as diphtheria and tetanus, are safe. Rabies vaccine, a killed virus, is probably not unsafe, but since rabies is a rare and highly fatal disease individual evaluation is desirable.

Vitamins

The amounts of the vitamins in the usual prenatal pills are entirely safe and, indeed, for many pregnant women quite unnecessary.

But note: You can buy unlimited quantities of vitamins over the counter. You can fall into the trap of thinking that if some is good, ten times as much is better. The Food and Drug Administration has warned that excessive intake of vitamins can be harmful. Toxicity from vitamin A has been reported due to taking 25,000 international units (IU) a day. This is five times the recommended daily allowance (RDA) for men. Three-quarters of vitamin D users take more than the RDA, 200 to 400 IU a day, and can also encounter toxicity. Daily intake of more than 1,000 mg of vitamin C can interfere with tests for sugar in the urine and can cause significant acidosis in adults. A quarter of all users of vitamin E take more than ten times the RDA. However, vitamin E has no known beneficial effects in human beings; when given intravenously to premature infants, it has been responsible for fatalities.

The voice of caution must advise against overdosing with vitamins even though there are no proven adverse fetal effects. Such doses are not of any benefit to mother or fetus and should be avoided.

Over-the-Counter Drugs

Among drugs sold over the counter, aspirin and acetaminophen (Tylenol) give rise to the largest number of safety questions. At present there is no evidence that occasional use of Tylenol in ordinary quantities has any adverse effect on the fetus.

A word of caution is proper here. A statement in 1977 from the Department of Health, Education and Welfare on over-the-counter drugs described prolongation of pregnancy and of labor due to aspirin. This is based on a 1973 study of patients with arthritic diseases who took ten aspirins a day for at least six months during the pregnancy. A later study of a much larger group of patients on smaller doses found no such effect. More recent reports, however, implicate even modest aspirin doses in bleeding among premature infants and among mothers during and after childbirth. It may turn out that the best part of wisdom is to avoid any aspirin during the third trimester.

Aspartame (Nutrasweet), now widely used as an artificial sweetener, has been extensively tested and appears to be safe. It is rapidly replacing saccharin, about which questions were raised, since it can cause bladder cancer in laboratory rats. There is no evidence of such an effect in human beings.

Metabolic Diseases with Fetal Effects

Metabolic diseases are those in which there is a defect in the chemical processes essential to life. One example is diabetes mellitus (sugar diabetes), in which glucose is not efficiently used as a source of energy for the body and therefore accumulates in the blood. In early pregnancy this high blood sugar produces defects in the development of the sacrum (the rear bone of the pelvis) and the embryo's legs. In late pregnancy it results in oversized babies and fetal acidosis, which can be severe enough to cause fetal death.

Another such condition is phenylketonuria (PKU). This is routinely tested for in newborns. The metabolic defect results in an accumulation of phenylalanine, an amino acid (amino acids are the building blocks of body proteins), which poisons

the central nervous system and thereby results in mental retardation if untreated. Dietary control, when initiated early in
life, limits the effect of the disease. There are now adults with
PKU who are normal but nevertheless have an increased phenylalanine blood level. A fetus being carried by such a mother
may be at risk of nervous-system injury prior to birth even
though the fetus does not have the disease itself.

Mothers at risk of this can readily be identified by measurement of their blood phenylalanine level. If you are concerned, consult your doctor.

Environmental and Occupational Hazards

Living in an urban environment, constantly exposed to automobile exhaust, cigarette smoke, and the host of additives in
the food we eat, pregnant women always experience the theoretical risk that this exposure may result in fetal defects.
Fortunately there is no evidence that fetal abnormalities today
are any more common than a hundred years ago, and newborn
survival has vastly improved.

Let us turn our attention to specific possible hazards. Video
display terminals (VDTs) generate radiation but, as with television sets, this is almost all directed out the back of the
terminal. Studies are in progress to learn whether there is any
evidence that VDTs have a risk different from that of television
sets, other than what might result from prolonged exposure to
the VDT screen during a working day. The FDA has concluded
that if the units are in good repair there is no risk.

The screening machines for carry-on baggage at airports are
well shielded and constitute no risk in pregnancy.

Before operating rooms were properly ventilated, women
spending long hours in them experienced an increased risk of
abortion.

The automobile is a hazard, but there is no additional danger
due to driving while pregnant as long as you wear a seat belt.
The lap belt should be below the pregnant uterus. The shoulder
harness should be adjusted to rest between your breasts and
off to the side of the pregnant uterus. If late in pregnancy you

find yourself clumsy or you don't fit well under a steering wheel, turn the driving over to someone else.

The risks of sonography, X-ray, computerized axial tomography (CAT scanning), magnetic resonance imaging, and fetal monitors are considered in some detail in Chapter 16.

Factors Affecting Birth Weight

Do you want a small baby? Your chance is best if you are a Chinese peasant girl of seventeen or less, in your first pregnancy. Do you want a large baby? You are more likely to have one if you are a white woman of the upper social stratum, thirty-five years old or more, with your tenth or eleventh child.

Many factors affect the baby's size at birth. Boys, for example, are ordinarily three to four ounces heavier than girls. The child of a woman pregnant for the first time, aged sixteen or younger, usually weighs five or six ounces less than the baby born to her sister who postpones her first child until she is thirty-five or so. Mothers who themselves were large newborns tend to have large babies. Nutrition is also important. Babies of women who have eaten well before and during pregnancy are substantially larger than babies whose mothers—or whose grandmothers—had poor diets while pregnant. Birth weight also varies substantially according to race, even when the nutrition is good. For example, the diet in Japan improved remarkably following World War II, with the result that the average newborn Japanese baby one generation later weighed almost a pound more than its parents did at birth. The average Japanese baby, however, is still smaller than the average Swedish newborn.

Socioeconomic Factors

In addition, socioeconomic factors affect the weight of the newborn. Babies born to patients in the economically privileged groups average a half pound more than those born to a less-favored population sample. As brought forth in a study in Scotland, babies weighing less than 5½ pounds are far less common among the former. Their incidence in the most affluent tenth of the population was 4 percent, in contrast to 8 percent among the remaining nine-tenths. The affluent woman has relatively more rest and a superior diet, both of which probably contribute to fewer early-terminating pregnancies and fewer babies that weigh less than 5½ pounds at birth. For statistical purposes the convention is to categorize all babies weighing less than 5½ pounds at birth as premature, and those weighing more than 5½ pounds, mature, irrespective of the duration of pregnancy. This has come about because it is usually so difficult to determine exactly the date when pregnancy was initiated.

Modern studies, as we shall discuss in Chapter 6, also have revealed a number of other factors that increase a baby's chances of being born small, among them low weight of the mother and low weight gain during pregnancy.

The Role of Heredity

Heredity plays a role in fetal size. Ordinarily, parents descended from a lineage of big people breed infants of large size, and those with small parents and grandparents produce babies of less than average birth weight. In my experience the size of members of the paternal line is at least as important as of those of the maternal line. Perhaps I was overly impressed of this fact by the case of a couple whose three children I delivered. The mother was of average size, but the father was a huge fellow who had been virtually the entire right side of the scrimmage line on his college football team. His brothers also were big and powerful. Each of the three babies was over nine pounds, which made the labor difficult for the mother and me. I was very relieved when my suggestion of sterilization after the third birth was enthusiastically accepted.

Factors of Maternal Disease

Chronic maternal illnesses may affect birth weight, in general producing babies smaller than expected. Women with generalized disease affecting the smaller arteries, complicated by chronic kidney damage or chronic high blood pressure, or both, tend to deliver growth-retarded infants. The only condition associated commonly with babies of excessive size is diabetes, and even here the relationship is complex. Long-standing diabetes tends to produce kidney damage, and a patient with this condition may produce a remarkably small baby rather than a remarkably large one. As we have learned more in recent years about the importance of controlling maternal blood sugar levels, the problem of excessively large babies has declined, since the overgrowth of the baby in many instances is a response to abnormal elevations of maternal blood sugar.

All the factors listed here which affect birth weight apply to the average patient in a large series of cases; in this matter the individual is often an exception, so that the couple who, according to all rules, ought to produce a large baby may produce a small one, and vice versa. It may be said, however, that couples usually have a standard-sized term baby, so that if the first baby is large, subsequent babies are usually large, or, if the first baby is small, the second and third tend to be small.

Weight Range at Term

Babies at full term weigh between 5½ and 9½ pounds. On rare occasions babies below and above those limits are born and show no clear evidence of any sort of intrauterine or maternal disease. They function like mature babies.

Excessive Size

How common are very large babies, and what is the most a newborn infant can weigh?

One frequently hears of babies with birth weights over eleven pounds, and sometimes one hears of newborns much larger. Most of the latter reports must be considered apocryphal; in such cases careful investigation will usually show that the weight had been estimated by hefting the child with one hand, not by weighing it.

In 23,500 consecutive deliveries at the Johns Hopkins Hospital, 251 babies weighed over 10 pounds (1 in 93.6); 35 (1 in 542) weighed over 11 pounds; 8 (1 in 2,937) weighed over 12 pounds; and 2 (1 in 11,750) weighed over 13 pounds. These two were males, the smaller, who weighed 13 pounds 7 ounces, was the ninth child of a thirty-four-year-old patient; and the larger—14 pounds 4 ounces—was the seventh child of a woman of forty-four. During 1967 and 1968, Brooklyn's Kings County Hospital, which serves an economically depressed population, reported 3,232 single births. Twelve infants, nine boys and three girls, weighed over 10 pounds, 1 in 269 births. Among 30,000 deliveries in Munich, no baby weighed over 13 pounds 4 ounces, and the largest infant in 100,000 cases born at the New York Lying-In Hospital weighed 15 pounds.

World's Biggest Newborn

The world's record for the largest baby is claimed by Sale City, Georgia, where in February 1916 Dr. D. P. Belcher attended Mrs. Rowe when she bore a stillborn female weighing 25 pounds. The physician failed to stipulate the type of scale or its condition. The largest baby with carefully verified weight was delivered at a hospital in Aldershot, England, and reported in 1933 by Dr. Moss in the *British Medical Journal*. The woman, twenty-two years old, had had one previous baby, which weighed 10 pounds. Both she and her husband were six feet tall. In this pregnancy, five days before the calculated confinement date, she gave birth to a baby weighing 24 pounds 2 ounces. The newborn was thirty-five inches long—heavier and taller than the average child at one year. It was stillborn. The largest surviving infant, weighing 22 pounds 8 ounces, was born in Italy in 1955.

We are interested in excessive birth weight because babies of more than 10 pounds may have difficult births. As mentioned earlier, a baby of 11½ pounds can be born normally, without injury to either infant or mother. However, these large infants often have broad shoulders so that even after the head has been born, there may still be serious difficulty with the delivery. It is clear though that fetuses over 12 pounds are so bulky that unmistakable delay in the descent of the head usually occurs and eventually recourse is had to cesarean.

By sonography it may be possible to identify massive fetuses so that we need not wait for obstructed labor to make the diagnosis clear. As recourse to cesarean rather than a difficult vaginal birth increases, more babies of great size are likely to survive.

One memorable couple came to my attention because of my interest in assisting mothers in vaginal birth following a previous section. This young woman in her first labor had failed to move the baby's head down into the pelvis. When the cesarean section was carried out it produced a wee tyke of 15 pounds. When the patient became pregnant again I had to tell her that if her second baby was even larger than the first, as could be expected, that of course she would have another cesarean. After an uneventful pregnancy she fell into labor with what seemed to be a baby of large but not extraordinary size. She readily delivered an infant who weighed 11½ pounds, itself something of an achievement.

Ordinarily in such cases, as will be discussed later, one suspects an abnormality to the mother's sugar metabolism, but we were unable to demonstrate any such phenomenon. What was really crucial was that this woman's husband was six foot five and weighed approximately 250 pounds, most of it bone and muscle.

World's Smallest Newborn

I have had the rare opportunity to see the newborn baby girl who is probably the smallest fetus ever to survive the neonatal period. At birth she weighed 390 grams—just about 13 ounces. She did remarkably well and required a minimum amount of assistance, in part due to the fact that she was probably born at about twenty-eight weeks of pregnancy instead of the twenty-three weeks her weight would suggest. Now, at the age of five, she is intellectually and neurologically normal but very tiny— literally one of the little people. The children in her kindergarten class treat her like a doll, much to her annoyance. Her four-year-old sister is of normal size, but her two-year-old brother, who weighed 7 pounds at birth, now also is very small for his age.

The Sex of the Fetus

Whether the baby will be a boy or girl is determined approximately eight and one-half months before birth, at the critical second of fertilization. The mother's egg has nothing whatever to do with determining the sex of her offspring. The father ejaculates two types of spermatozoa in apparently equal numbers. The two types differ from each other to a minor degree, yet this small variation makes a major difference—the sex of the individual. Every spermatozoon contains the same twenty-two chromosomes (autosomes) which affect the inheritance of all bodily structures and functions except the sex of the fetus and some associated characteristics. The twenty-third chromosome, the sex chromosome, is very different in the two kinds of spermatozoa. In half, the sex chromosome of the sperm cell is relatively large, a replica of the twenty-third or sex chromosome of the egg, and is called the "X chromosome." In half of the sperm cells the sex chromosome is much smaller and very different in appearance; it is called the "Y chromosome." When an ovum is fertilized by an X-bearing sperm cell, a female fetus is created; when it is fertilized by a Y-bearing sperm cell, a male results.

Is Sex Inherited?

There is a popular fallacy that the tendency to produce a preponderance of males runs in some families and an equally strong tendency toward the creation of girls in other families. This concept has been repeatedly investigated by geneticists and statisticians, and each study leaves no doubt that the production of a child of one sex or the other is not affected by heredity; the sex of an infant is purely a matter of chance, as exemplified by the old coin-tossing experiment. Once in 128 tosses there will be seven tails or seven heads in succession.

Your chances for having a boy in the next pregnancy are precisely the same whether you have already had six daughters in six pregnancies, or six sons.

Sex Ratio

Sex ratio, by definition, is the number of males to every hundred females. There are several kinds of sex ratio: primary, which is the number of male embryos conceived per hundred female embryos; secondary, the ratio at birth; and tertiary, the number of living males at any time during the postnatal period per hundred females.

A careful recent study from Finland based on abortions by choice seems to indicate a sex ratio from the first five to seven weeks of pregnancy (by ovulation age) of 164. This is far higher than previous figures. The same authors found a ratio of 112 from eight to ten weeks, still in the first trimester, and 102 from eleven to fifteen weeks. How can we account for this tremendous preponderance of male embryos at the start of pregnancy? One explanation is that their sample of very early embryos is smaller than for the later weeks and hence may be misleading. Another possibility is that there are many more male-producing sperms than female-producing sperms but that is not the case. As stated before, X-bearing and Y-bearing spermatozoa are produced in approximately equal numbers. It has been supposed that the Y-bearing spermatozoa, being slightly lighter, may travel up the reproductive tract faster than their X-bearing sisters, but the difference in weight is hardly adequate to account for the marked disproportions between male and female embryos. At the moment, we really do not have a satisfactory explanation for this observation.

In the same Finnish study, the ratio in fetal life, at about the eighteenth to twentieth weeks, was found to be 111. The authors of the paper suggest that the loss of male fetuses takes place during the period in which organs are forming, in the first trimester of pregnancy.

This is not the end of the story. The sex ratio at birth, the secondary sex ratio, is uniformly between 105 and 106 in almost all populations that have been studied. We do know that the death rate among male newborns is somewhat higher than the death rate among females. Among stillborn infants, the ratio of males to females is 3 to 2.

Can Fetal Sex Be Diagnosed?

The answer is an unequivocal yes. The present techniques for doing this in the first and second trimesters, chorionic villus biopsy and amniocentesis, each incur a risk of abortion. For genetic counseling of families who have an inherited disease that appears only in males, determination of fetal sex is essential. Curiosity as to fetal sex in normal families is hardly a sufficient reason for testing.

There are two basic diagnoses possible. One is that of genetic sex, based on the information encoded in the sex chromosomes that direct the formation of male or female gonads. The gonads in turn determine the development of male and female genitalia. The other diagnosis is that of anatomic sex, that is, the apperance of the external and internal genitalia.

Genetic Tests for Sex

The diagnosis of genetic sex is based on two kinds of examination of cell nuclei. The first is the study of the nuclei for the presence of the Barr body, a structure named after Murray Barr, a Canadian anatomist. Barr noted that a high proportion of the nuclei of female fetuses has a small spherical structure attached to the outer shell of the nucleus. This structure is rare or absent among male fetuses. It was subsequently learned that one of the two X sex chromosomes present in all female nuclei is inactive and forms the Barr body. This inactive X becomes adherent to the nuclear membrane. Under the microscope it is seen as a one-micron (4/10,000 of an inch) structure along the nuclear edge. Since male fetuses have only one X chromosome, this is not inactivated and the Barr body is therefore rarely seen in males.

The other examination of nuclei, more specific than the observation of the Barr body, is the identification of the chromosomes of the nucleus. These separate from one another when the cells undergo division. With luck they can be observed under the microscope in fresh preparations of actively dividing cells. More commonly, however, the harvested cells from the embryo are grown in tissue culture and then later treated chemically to arrest cell division at a point where the chromosomes are separated. These nuclear spreads are next examined under the microscope. The chromosomes are photographed, identified, and rearranged in an agreed-upon order. In either case it is possible to decide whether the embryo or fetus is of 46XX or 46XY constitution, that is, whether it is genetically female or male.

Chorionic Villus Biopsy

Chorionic villus biopsy is being perfected for the harvesting of embryonic cells as early as the ninth or tenth week of pregnancy. Preliminary sonographic examination is desirable to be certain that the pregnancy is normal, since it would be pointless to perform a biopsy on an embryo destined to abort spontaneously.

The doctor uses an ordinary speculum to visualize the cervix while performing the biopsy. A fine catheter is passed under local anesthesia through the cervical canal up to the embryo. Early in pregnancy almost the entire surface of the embryo is covered by primitive villi, the fetal structures through which exchange between mother and fetus takes place. The villi eventually grow to form the placenta. Tiny samples can be removed quite safely by suction. The biopsy is continuously monitored by sonography to be sure that the biopsy catheter does not damage the embryo. At present the loss of pregnancies with this new technique due to the procedure itself appears to be about 2 percent. There is every reason to expect that the loss rate will drop further with greater experience.

The cells harvested in this manner can be studied immediately for the distribution of Barr bodies and, with some luck in finding dividing cells, for the appearance of the chromosomes. The cells are also suitable for culture. In either event it is possible to make diagnoses of fetal sex and of abnormalities of chromosome number (see Chapter 20).

Amniocentesis for Diagnosis

At the sixteenth week or later amniocentesis can be carried out. The technique for this is described in Chapter 20. Suffice it to say at this point that the needle, similar to that used for drawing blood but longer, is introduced into a pocket of fluid that has been identified by sonography. Some of the fluid is removed; it always has floating in it cells shed from skin of the fetus. These can also be examined immediately for the presence of Barr bodies or grown in tissue culture for a subsequent mapping of their chromosomes.

The External Genitalia of the Fetus

The other basic method of sex identification depends upon visualization of the external genitalia of the fetus. A report by Dr. Eiichi Natsuyama of Kyoto, Japan, describes his study of fetal sex, by high resolution sonography, of 1,879 fetuses ranging in age from twelve to forty weeks. He was successful in visualizing the external genitalia in 97 percent of the fetuses. Near term he made a correct diagnosis in 100 percent of the males and 99.8 percent of the females. However, between the twelfth and eighteenth week his rate of correct diagnosis of sex was just below 90 percent.

Sonography has the advantage of being noninvasive. However, if a decision on abortion for genetic reasons is at stake, a 10 percent error rate in sex diagnosis, which is what obtains up to the eighteenth week of pregnancy, seriously limits its usefulness.

Fetal sex can be diagnosed in the second trimester by fetoscopy. In this method a needle like the one used for amniocentesis but larger in diameter is placed into the amniotic cavity. An optical instrument is passed through the needle, making it possible to see the fetus. Only small areas can be seen at a time. The risks of fetal injury are considerable and failure to see the genitalia frequent, so that the method is not useful in the diagnosis of sex.

The rate of correct diagnosis of genetic sex by study of the chromosomes is close to 100 percent, however. Additional studies can be done to corroborate the diagnosis if there is any doubt about the chromosomes. The diagnosis of anatomic sex on the basis of genetic sex cannot be 100 percent, since there are rare instances which the anatomic and genetic sex are not identical.

Can We Control the Sex?

Chance controls the sex of the fetus, and by definition we cannot affect chance. But there now appear to be methods to separate X and Y sperm from each other *in vitro*. Semen is exposed in the laboratory to either of the two processes, one for the X and the other for Y sperm, that take advantage of minute differences in the motion of the two kinds of spermatozoa. The proportion of X to Y sperm is thus altered. The product is then used for artificial insemination. In either case, the sex ratio of the resulting newborn is markedly changed in the desired direction.

Chorionic villus biopsy has become a reliable method for the identification of the sex of an embryo in the first trimester. Combined with the availability of safe abortion, it would be possible then to continue to carry only a baby of the desired sex. The same degree of safety of abortion for the mother is of course not present later in pregnancy, when determination of fetal sex must be made by amniocentesis or sonography. The noninvasive Japanese studies described above are not reliable enough prior to the eighteenth week to serve as a basis for selective abortion.

Students of population trends have gone to some pains to point out that in the absence of severe limitation in the number of children, the availability of choice of sex by abortion would in all likelihood not greatly alter the sex ratio of the population. The matter of sex selection is most dramatic in China, where concern over an immense population on an underdeveloped industrial economy base has motivated delay in marriage and limitation of family size to one child. This is achieved by programmed social pressure in the workplace and by restrictions on social benefits for child rearing. There are intense government campaigns to persuade couples to use effective birth control. Women are urged to abort later pregnancies. The difficulty is that for thousands of years Chinese tradition has dictated that old people be cared for by their sons. Thus, every couple wants to have at least one male child. And with the government endorsing only one child per couple, there is suspicion that female infanticide has become frequent in many parts of China.

The Fetal Position in the Uterus

In the earlier works on obstetrics it was taught that the fetus might assume any position in the uterus, the number of positions being limited solely by an author's imagination. Accurate observations gradually eliminated the more fanciful.

The positions which the child assumes *in utero* may be divided into two general classes—longitudinal and transverse. In the longitudinal the spinal column of the child is parallel to the spinal column of the mother; in the transverse it is at right angles to that of the mother, forming a cross with it. The former is normal, accounting for more than 99 percent; while the transverse position is rare, occurring in less than 0.5 percent.

These two general classifications of fetal positions may be subdivided into more exact groups. We term these more specific positions "presentations"; this refers to the precise part of the fetus which presents over the bone-surrounded birth passage, the pelvis. At term, 96 percent of fetuses present by the head (cephalic presentation); 3.5 percent by the buttocks (breech presentation); and in less than 0.5 percent the child lies transversely with a shoulder presenting.

Cephalic Presentations

If, during labor, the head presents, it ordinarily flexes, so that the infant's chin rests on its breastbone. When this occurs, the crown of the head first enters the mother's pelvis and is the part of the fetus earliest visible as the birth takes place. This is the common variety of cephalic presentation, accounting for almost 99 percent of the cases in which the head presents. Such babies frequently are born with a temporary swelling over the area which the hair whorl will later occupy; the swelling is caused by pressure, since this area is the lead point in the birth process.

Occasionally, instead of being flexed, the head of the fetus is extended during labor, and the infant delivers with the face presenting. Under such conditions the features may appear as swollen as those of a badly mauled prizefighter, but within forty-eight hours the contusions and swellings have disappeared. If the head is only partially extended, the baby's brow is the lead point.

In a cephalic presentation, the back is convex, the thighs flexed over the abdomen, the legs bent at the knee joints, and the feet crossed so that the toes point toward the opposite armpit. The arms are either crossed over the chest or straight and parallel to the sides. The umbilical cord nestles looped in the abdominal space between the arms and legs.

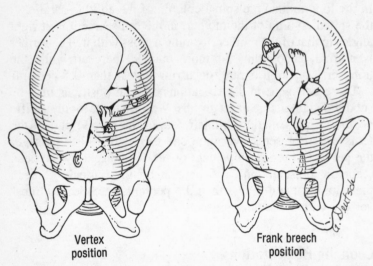

Vertex
position

Frank breech
position

On the left, a fetus near term, lying with its spinal column parallel to its mother's, head down, in the mother's pelvis. On the right, also lying parallel, the fetus has its buttocks down into the pelvis—a frank breech presentation. The legs of the fetus are extended.

Breech Presentations

A breech presentation and even a transverse lie are relatively common during the earlier months of pregnancy, when the volume of amniotic fluid may be greater than the volume of the baby, so that the shape of the uterus places no restraint on fetal position. Indeed, babies have even been observed to rotate 180 degrees from breech to head down right up to the onset of labor. One would expect from these facts, and indeed it is the case, that breech presentation is more common in premature labors than at term.

There are three types of breech presentation—frank, footling, and full. In a frank breech, much the commonest, the legs of the baby are flexed up over the abdomen, with the knees straight so that the toes touch the shoulders and the two buttocks present over the pelvis. If it were not for the very loose joints of the fetus, this position would be almost unattainable and, to say the least, uncomfortable. After delivery it is not uncommon for the baby who delivered as a frank breech to keep its legs flexed at the hip and straight at the knee for several hours. Since the buttocks and genital area are the lead points in the birth of a frank breech, they are often swollen and discolored black and blue at delivery. This clears up rapidly without permanent damage. In a footling breech one or both legs are held straight, as in the standing position, and act as the lead point in labor and delivery. The full breech is rare; in it the fetus sits cross-legged in the mother's pelvis, like a tailor on his sewing bench. Breech presentations have a slight tendency to recur in subsequent labors.

Presentation of Twins

In twins the ordinary proportion of the various presentations is greatly altered. Both children present by the head in 39 percent of the cases, one by the head and the other by the breech in 36 percent, both by the breech in 11 percent, and one or both transversely in 14 percent.

Determination of Fetal Position

The position of the fetus is usually determined by feeling or palpating the abdomen. From the thirtieth week on, the physician can usually identify the fetal head, back, and extremities without great difficulty.

The position of the fetus is ordinarily not fixed until somewhere about the thirty-fourth or thirty-fifth week of pregnancy. There has been recent revival of interest in external version to convert breeches to head down presentations. The fetus is manipulated through the mother's abdominal wall. If this is done early enough in pregnancy it's really rather easy and probably also unnecessary, since the great majority of babies who present by the breech prior to the thirty-third or thirty-fourth week convert spontaneously to head down presentations anyway. Fetuses who present by the breech at term usually persist in this presentation and are correspondingly much more difficult to turn by external version.

Transverse Presentations

As labor starts, once in two hundred pregnancies the fetus lies transversely, with the long axis of its spinal column at right angles to the long axis of the mother's spinal column. In this case a shoulder or hand may enter the pelvis or the baby may be lying back down and the only part that can be reached through the mother's vagina is the baby's back. Normal birth under these circumstances is impossible and a cesarean is done.

Recently there has been some interest in suitable cases in treating the mother with drugs which cause the uterus to relax and then, by external manipulation, turning the baby to a longitudinal lie. Probably the minimum necessary conditions for this is that the patient be quite early in labor, that the membranes be intact, and that the baby be of ordinary or small size.

Activity of the Fetus in the Uterus

Obviously we lack subjective observations of intrauterine life, but many objective data have been obtained. I have already mentioned the fact that the fetal kidneys function *in utero* and the fetus voids into the amniotic fluid. The fetus also swallows amniotic fluid, whether or not to quench its thirst will never be known. The intestines are also active, and a thick, viscid, tarlike excrement (meconium) is found in the lower bowel. Under normal conditions meconium is not excreted until after delivery. The fetal heart and some phases of fetal movements have already been discussed; there are several additional facts about intrauterine activity which merit discussion.

The fetal movements felt by patient and doctor are usually the thrusting and bending of arms and legs. The motion of the legs is more extensive than that of the arms, and therefore if movements appear most active in the upper abdomen it is likely that the fetus presents by the head. If late in labor, in a breech presentation with membranes ruptured, a foot protrudes from the vagina its movements can be seen some time before birth. If the foot is pinched the child attempts to withdraw it, and if the sole is scratched the toes bend wildly. Occasionally a hand may present along with the head (compound presentation) during labor, and if on vaginal examination the obstetrician should shake hands with the unborn patient, the baby's fingers squirm. In face presentations sucking movements are produced if the examiner inserts a finger into the child's mouth.

Dr. Friedrich Ahlfeld, a German scientist, was the first to claim that the fetus sucks its fingers *in utero*. He reported the case of a child born with a swollen thumb; immediately after birth it put the swollen member into its mouth and sucked. Now that we have been able to watch babies with real-time sonography, all such activity has been recorded on movie film and videotape.

Fetal hiccups have been repeatedly observed by both physician and patient. The movements are short, quick, regular jerks of the child's shoulders and trunk, fifteen to twenty a minute. They can be seen, as well as felt, by movements of the mother's abdomen. They resemble ordinary hiccups except for the absence of the stridor, the harsh noise. An attack of intrauterine hiccups usually lasts about fifteen minutes and may recur several times before delivery.

In the very strictest sense the fetus does not breathe *in utero* simply because there is no air inside the uterus. However, steady chest movements by the infant clearly play a role in the development of the lungs. Exchange of gases between the mother and the baby and therefore between the baby and the outside environment is carried on by the placenta and the maternal circulation.

Respiratory movements of the fetal thorax were first observed over one hundred years ago by noting a rhythmic rising and falling of the abdominal wall of the mother near the navel. On one occasion with a patient in very early labor I observed this phenomenon and showed it to a group of medical students. The rate of movement was about fifty times to the minute and was quite unmistakable. Since the mother's pulse was 70, the fetal heart rate about 140, and the mother's respiratory rate 20, the movement could only be attributed to *in utero* rhythmic thoracic activity. On the rare occasions when air has entered the uterus and replaced the amniotic fluid, the fetus has been heard to cry (*vagitus uterinus*)!

A baby that is badly stressed *in utero* may very well gasp. Since breathing movements can be readily observed by sonography, studies are underway in an effort to correlate abnormalities of fetal breathing with the condition of the fetus. Up to now, however, the relationships are not sufficiently sharp to be a solid basis of obstetrical treatment.

Fetal Sensibility and Learning

In recent years we have accumulated an astonishing variety of evidence of fetal sensibility and learning in the uterus. These phenomena are apparently limited to late pregnancy. For one thing, the fetus has brisk responses to light. If a real-time sonography unit is focused on the fetus's face and a bright light flashed at the baby, through the mother's abdominal wall and uterus, the baby can be seen to blink. We do know that babies have reasonably well-developed visual acuity at term birth. This is discussed further in Chapter 23.

That babies are able to hear *in utero* at term has been known for several decades. It was noted that their heartbeats accelerate in response to the sound of an ordinary tuning fork at 120 cycles per second. In a fascinating study reported in 1984, however, this was carried a good deal further. The experimenters, psychologists at the University of North Carolina, discovered that a baby sucked on a pacifier in one way when it heard its own mother's voice and in a different pattern when it heard a strange voice. It didn't seem to matter whether the babies were breast-fed or bottle-fed or indeed even how young the babies happened to be. The researchers did find that the babies had to be at least a few weeks old before they had a clear preference for their fathers' voices.

The next question that the researchers wondered about was

whether the babies did any of this learning in the uterus, since they manifested a preference at a very early age. They played tape recordings of a maternal heartbeat and a male voice for the newborns and were able to demonstrate that the babies sucked considerably more often in order to hear the heartbeat than the male voice. The North Carolinians then carried the test an ingenious step further. A group of women in the last seven weeks of pregnancy read Dr. Seuss's children's book *The Cat In The Hat* aloud in a voice directed at their pregnant abdomens twice a day every day. By the time the babies were born it was calculated that each had heard the story for about five hours. After birth the babies were tested with a tape recording of their mothers' reading of *The Cat In The Hat* or of another children's book by Dr. Seuss, which was also a poem but had a very different meter. The babies showed a clear preference for *The Cat In The Hat*. This is scientific proof of what we have known about prenatal impression, on a casual and unverified basis, for many years.

It is also abundantly clear that a newborn has a cry that is quite readily identified by the baby's mother. Indeed, the baby itself can tell its mother's voice and smell from that of other women.

The Fetal Heart

Contractions of the heart muscle of the fetus begin about a month following conception. The motion of the tiny heart can be demonstrated by sonography when the embryo is only a few weeks old. As early as the ninth week of pregnancy, counting from the first day of the last period, it is possible to hear it with an ultrasound device (commonly called a Doptone) in the lowermost portion of the mother's abdomen. This depends on the mother being slender and the uterus in a forward position, so that the distance from the fetus's heart to the microphone is minimal. For that reason, inability to pick up the fetal heart by Doptone is not really meaningful until about the twelfth week. For parents, hearing the baby's heartbeat gives the pregnancy a reality that it would not otherwise have until several months later when the mother begins to feel the baby move. A few years ago one of my sons and his wife came in with tape-recording equipment and made a record of the fetal heart of what later turned out to be my fourth granddaughter; this was when she had been in existence only about eight weeks.

It is my preference to use the Doptone only very briefly to listen to the fetal heart, and to do so only if the mother wishes to have it done. During prenatal examinations with the mother recumbent, a jellylike contact material is placed on the hand-held device and the unit is pressed against the mother's abdominal wall. The fetal heart rate normally is between 120 and 160 beats per minute throughout pregnancy. This rate is substantially greater than that of the mother's pulse. It is absolute proof of pregnancy.

The fetal heart can be heard with a stethoscope at about the twentieth week of pregnancy. It is simply astonishing that this was not realized until early in the nineteenth century—one would think that curiosity would have led people to put their ears to the abdomen millennia earlier. The fetal heart has a double beat like the tick of a watch and it has a soft nonmetallic pitch.

A curious but common misconception is that a pregnant woman occasionally can feel the baby's heart pulsate as she lies on her back. Actually she may be sensing any of several other phenomena. Most commonly she is noticing the pulsations of her own aorta, the large main artery in the trunk, as the pregnant uterus rests upon it. When the uterus contracts the uterus itself can transmit the pumping of the artery to the abdominal wall. This rate, being synchronous with the mother's heartbeat, is easily recognizable as her pulse. Occasionally too, late in pregnancy the baby will have a substantial run of hiccups. These are also transmitted to the abdominal wall and could, except for their slower rate, be mistaken for a heartbeat. Finally, slender women occasionally are able to see, though not to feel, the baby's breathing movements in the uterus. The woman may see the skin around her belly button moving up and down rhythmically about fifty times a minute.

Late in pregnancy our ability to record the fetal heart by ultrasound becomes a means of testing the baby's state of health. When the baby is in good health in the last couple of months of pregnancy, its heart rate fluctuates, the extent depending on whether it is asleep or active. In abnormal circumstances, if the uterine blood flow and the placental circulation have begun to fail, these fluctuations no longer occur. This is called loss of variability. Such a loss may also be a response to sedative drugs taken by the mother and to anesthetic agents used for pain relief in labor.

A severely stressed baby will respond to the stress by slowing down its heartbeat from time to time, usually in response to the decrease in maternal blood flow in the placenta that results from uterine contraction. These are referred to as decelerations. They may, of course, simply result from pressure on the baby's head from the contraction, or may have a more ominous significance.

These changes can give early warning of fetal distress. Fetal heart rate recording prior to labor (NST) and during labor has therefore become a common practice.

It is also possible to detect some of these changes simply by listening with a stethoscope. We are not absolutely certain that ultrasound monitoring of the fetal heart for long periods of time is completely safe. My preference among low-risk patients in normal labor is to use the stethoscope or intermittent Doptone to record heart rates every fifteen minutes. Continuous ultrasound monitoring is limited to patients at high risk for fetal problems in labor.

When the patient is in labor, direct recording can also be done from a fine electrode passed through the mother's dilated cervix and attached to the skin of the baby's head or buttocks.

Fetal Heart Rate Does Not Indicate Sex

The superstition still exists that it is possible to diagnose the sex of the fetus by counting the fetal heart rate. This is simply not so. We can now identify fetal sex by chorionic villi biopsy at ten weeks of pregnancy, by amniocentesis at sixteen weeks, and by sonography after twenty weeks, all with considerable accuracy. But fetal heart rate counting will not tell the story any more precisely than tossing a coin.

Disorders of Heart Rate and Rhythm

Even in the absence of distress, abnomalities of fetal heart rate and rhythm can occur. A rate as high as 220 beats per minute may be picked up on a routine prenatal visit by Doptone, although it has not produced symptoms in the mother. A rate this fast cannot be counted by listening with a stethoscope. The aberration, called tachycardia (Greek: *takhus*, "swift"; *kardia*, "heart"), is due to an overreactive electrical system in the heart. Since, if it persists for several days, the fetus can suffer heart failure, it must be treated by cardiac drugs given to the mother, unless the fetus can be easily and safely delivered.

A very slow rate, down to 50 beats per minute, is the result of incomplete conduction of electrical signals and may reflect anatomic defects in the fetal heart. Other defects in conduction may cause the fetal heart to be markedly irregular.

In each of these cases, echocardiography— a special form of sonography—should be used to study the muscle and valves of the fetal heart to establish an exact diagnosis to form the basis for proper treatment.

Sonography, X-ray, and MRI

Sonography makes use of very-high-frequency sound beams that are reflected to different degrees by soft tissues, bone, air, and fluid. Most of the sound beam is scattered as it passes through the body, but some is reflected directly back and picked up by a microphone. These echoes also can be translated electronically into images and displayed on TV screens, or photographed or taped, either in one or two dimensions.

Two basic sonography techniques are in daily use in obstetrics. The first employs the small hand-held device, the Doptone, which can be placed against the mother's abdomen during prenatal visits. It gives the parents an audible reassurance that their baby is alive and ticking. It can be adapted to a larger apparatus with several microphones, used in late pregnancy to make continuous records of fetal heart rate for periods of from a few minutes to many hours. The rate is printed on a moving strip of paper as part of the evaluation of fetal well-being late in pregnancy and in labor. Both of these Doppler devices take advantage of the fact that sound waves change in frequency when they echo from a moving target. The change in the echoes from a beating heart is converted electronically to an audible and recordable heartbeat.

The ultrasound generator in all devices based on the Doppler effect is continuously on at a frequency of 2 million cycles per second. This contrasts with the audible frequency range, which runs from about 30 cycles to 12,000 cycles per second. The ultrasound generator delivers energy at 10 to 15 milliwatts per square centimeter. This is not very much energy—a 100-watt light bulb produces 10,000 times as much. The beam generates so little heat in tissues that it cannot be recorded, not even if the detector is kept in place for eight hours of labor.

Sonographic Images

In order to obtain images from sonography we employ sound frequencies of about 3.5 million cycles per second. Each pulse lasts for 1.5 millionths of a second. These pulses occur every thousandth of a second, so that the sound beam is on for 0.15 percent of the time, the rest of the time being used to receive and convert the echo to a picture on a video screen. This produces a fetal exposure to ultrasound that ranges from 0.1 to as much as 60 milliwatts per square centimeter; the latter occurs with prolonged monitoring over a period of many hours. The heat thus produced is still below what can be measured.

Sonography has developed a wide range of uses. It is possible to visualize the fetus in the uterus at about the seventh week after the last period. If the fetus is not in the uterus and the woman's pregnancy has been proven by a measurement of the hCG, one must search sonographically for the fetus even at this early stage, thus demonstrating the pregnancy to be ectopic.

There is a rare abnormality of pregnancy in which only a placenta forms; there is no fetus and the placenta under these circumstances may exhibit excessive growth. This is a hydatidiform mole (Greek: *hydatid*, "watery vesicle"; Latin: *mola*, millstone; *mole* is a tumor in the uterus). This is easily diagnosed by sonography, which displays a mass of small round images without an embryonic sac.

The remarkable degree of accuracy with which the fetus can be displayed by sonography allows us to measure the increasing size of the head of the fetus, as well as its trunk and long bones, from an early stage of gestation. This keeps us in constant touch with the rate at which the baby is growing. Sometimes the head grows slower than the rest of the infant, on other occasions the head grows faster. When either of these observations is made it is possible by sonography to visualize the brain and learn whether the cause of these deviations is an abnormality of the brain itself.

When there is doubt as to the duration of pregnancy, examination of the width of the skull just above the ears (biparietal diameter, BPD) will help to indicate the duration of pregnancy. This estimate will be correct within two weeks either way. Ninety-one percent of the infants with BPDs of 8.5 centimeters or more will be mature and will weigh more than five and a half pounds. When the BPD exceeds 9 centimeters, 98 percent of the infants are at term and will be mature. These measurements can be supplemented for greater accuracy by measurements of the length of the femur, the long bone in the thigh, and the circumference of the abdomen. By these techniques reliable estimates of fetal size and age are possible.

Sampling of amniotic fluid by amniocentesis and study of this fluid for the presence of certain phospholipids (chemical substances, related to fat, which indicate the maturity of the lungs) has been used for a number of years to gather evidence of the maturity of the fetal lung. In most instances, however, this procedure can be replaced by a reasonably accurate menstrual history together with an ultrasound measurement of the fetus done at about the twentieth week and a later determination of the BPD by sonography. The invasive technique of amniocentesis to determine maturity need only be applied when the other evidence is conflicting. The frequency of amniocentesis except for genetic studies and for maternal sensitization to Rh is steadily declining.

Multiple pregnancy is readily diagnosed by sonography earlier than by any other diagnostic method. It can also be employed in identifying the location of the placenta and is therefore useful in the diagnosis of patients who may have placenta previa, the condition in which the placenta is found low in the uterus ahead of the baby's head.

The excellent images of the fetus make it possible to diagnose major congenital anomalies and fetal sex with reasonable accuracy. The diagnosis of sex becomes quite reliable past the twenty-second week of pregnancy, but is a time-consuming examination.

Sonography is of help in the sometimes very difficult determination of whether a fetus is alive or dead. Demonstration of a beating fetal heart is conclusive.

Ultrasound examination of the ovaries is now being used extensively for the timing of ovulation in connection with *in vitro* fertilization and embryo transfer. The details of this will be discussed further below.

Finally, sonography is used to guide the needles employed for amniocentesis into pockets of amniotic fluid. Chorionic villus sampling as has been described also makes use of sonographic guidance.

Risks of Ultrasound

At present there is no clear scientific evidence that ultrasound is in any way damaging to either fetuses or adults when employed for diagnosis as described above. In laboratory tests, ultrasound has caused some changes when directed at thin layers of cells in tissue culture, but it is not known whether this happens to cells in the living body. Following an intense study of this subject, the National Institutes of Health wisely took the position in 1984 that it was not possible to say that sonography was completely safe. Therefore, ultrasound studies should be used only for a clearly defined medical reason.

X-Rays

X-rays are only slightly impeded in their passage through soft tissue and fluid but are obstructed by bones and metal objects. They are not blocked at all by air, so it is possible to get excellent X-ray pictures of soft-tissue structures in the chest where the lungs are ordinarily air filled. Images of the intestinal tract, which contains a good deal of swallowed air, are also readily obtained and quite clear. Maternal and fetal bones are easily seen, but the soft tissues of pregnancy are much more difficult to identify.

As the X-rays pass through the body, they can be directed

into a X-ray-sensitive TV camera from which a TV image is made. They can also be recorded on film and tape. The X-rays may also be directed at a sensitive screen, which gives off visible light where the X-rays hit. The images thus created can be looked at directly as in a fluoroscope, or registered on sensitive photographic film. This last technique produces the familiar X-ray pictures.

At present X-ray has very limited use in obstetrics. It will produce excellent images of the maternal pelvis, of value when a decision has to be made whether the available space in the pelvis is adequate for the delivery of the head of the breech baby. A dermoid cyst of the ovary—a benign tumor commonly observed in young women—often includes skin structures, other internal tissues, and primitive jawbone and teeth. The latter are very well demonstrated by X-ray, providing unmistakable diagnosis.

CAT Scan

Computerized axial tomography—CAT scan or CT scan—produces brilliant still pictures, but requires a radiation dose to the abdomen and fetus too large for safety in obstetrics.

Risks of X-Ray Diagnosis

Several kinds of risks are known to be associated with radiation. For example, the very large doses of radiation used in treating cancer can destroy a fetus early in pregnancy and cause major damage to a fetus's nervous system later in pregnancy. Unfortunately, much of our early knowledge in this area was learned through radiation accidents under poorly defined conditions. The extreme risks mentioned above do not occur with diagnostic radiation, the doses of which are about one-thousandth the dose of radiation for cancer.

Radiation of the teeth, the head, the extremities, and the chest—all areas remote from the abdomen—with modern X-ray equipment does not expose the fetus to any more radiation than would be encountered in daily living. It is worthwhile to mention that X-rays are not transported around the body in the bloodstream, so that their effects are felt only in the areas where they actually hit.

X-rays directed at the gonads of mother or fetus do have potential genetic effects. They can cause changes in the DNA which carries the genetic information on the chromosomes. This kind of damage to the DNA cannot be demonstrated by looking at the chromosomes but can be detected in laboratory animals by very careful observations of a decrease in the number of normal offspring over a number of generations.

Among the children of human beings whose gonads have been exposed to diagnostic radiation there are known to be no visible immediate effects. The theoretical increase in the number of stillbirths among grandchildren and great-grandchildren of such irradiated individuals is sufficiently small so that we will probably never have proof that this theoretical risk is real.

The amount of radiation delivered to fetuses by X-ray examination of the pregnant abdomen in the 1940's and 1950's was responsible for an increase in childhood leukemia among the infants born of these pregnancies. Having learned that, we have cut down the number of abdominal X-rays among pregnant women. At the same time the radiation dose for each X-ray examination has also been substantially reduced by technical improvements in X-ray machines and X-ray film. The incidence of known effects has dropped markedly since these changes.

The studies of the outcomes of pregnancy among those women pregnant in Hiroshima at the time of the nuclear bombing make clear that radiation dosage measured in hundreds of rads are needed to produce unmistakable fetal effects. Present diagnostic studies involve less than 4 rads at the very most.

X-rays now are of use in hospitals that do not have suitable sonographic equipment available twenty-four hours a day, seven days a week.

If the pregnant woman has an abdominal condition not readily diagnosable by ultrasound techniques then X-rays may have to be done, but their number will be limited. This may occasionally be necessary in a mother who has had previous bowel surgery and who is now thought perhaps to have a mechanical obstruction of the bowel. Fortunately, there is only minimal fetal risk incurred by obtaining such X-rays, and it may be life-saving for the mother.

Magnetic Resonance Imaging (MRI)

This technique of producing images by using a very intense magnetic field is so new that we do not know of what value it may be or whether it is harmful in pregnancy. It is probably safe, but it may be of limited use in clinical diagnosis.

6

Care during Pregnancy

Before discussing the care of the woman already pregnant, it is well to point out the desirability of care before pregnancy has begun. Conditions such as anemia, undetected diabetes, underweight, high blood pressure, and a pelvic tumor can complicate pregnancy without producing any warning symptoms. Ideally they should be corrected or controlled before you start a pregnancy. Your regular health care providers can screen you for their presence and institute the necessary care. Also, if you have never had German measles (rubella), the vaccine to prevent it should be given before pregnancy. Finally, if you know of a disorder that runs in your family, the time to secure genetic counselling is before the pregnancy starts.

Predelivery medical care has greatly changed in the last half century. Until the late 1920's or early 1930's physicians felt their task to be wholly a technical one. Their goal was simple, to conduct pregnancy so that it ended with a healthy mother and a perfect infant. The concept that the process of having a baby in itself could and should be a full, happy experience, bereft of fear and anxiety, was virtually nonexistent. In their attitude toward pregnancy and labor, doctors were as well starched intellectually as they were externally. They conducted prenatal care with the viewpoint, "Don't bother your pretty young head about pregnancy and labor; expunge them from your thoughts; this is an area of my concern, not yours. And as for my answering your questions, a little knowledge is a dangerous thing." Obstetric hospitals thought along the same lines; the concept of giving patients emotional support or confidence through prenatal instruction was foreign to their responsibilities.

Today both physician and hospital have executed an about-face. Recognizing the immense value of knowledge in the eradication of fear, we are attempting to deprive reproduction of its mystery through instruction in the facts of conception, pregnancy, labor, and infant care. This effort to replace ignorance with understanding has been waged with the help of the printed page, motion pictures, mothers' classes, radio, television, lay tours of hospital obstetric facilities, and discussions between the doctor and patient. The discussions have become so frank that there is no question which the pregnant woman and her partner may not ask.

Prenatal Care: An Overview

This is a relatively new concept in the history of medicine. The first clinic in the United States to give periodic care to pregnant women who had no symptoms, were not ill, and were not in labor was established in Boston in 1909. Its main concern was the early detection of toxemia of pregnancy by routine blood pressure measurements, regular weighing, and tests of urine for protein among women who appeared healthy. The concept of preventive care in pregnancy has grown impressively since.

Problems such as tuberculosis and syphilis, common in 1909, have been solved by antibiotics. Toxemia today is a less serious disease and our treatment of it is much improved. But there remain problems with diabetes, high blood pressure, and prematurity that can be minimized by early and continuous prenatal care. An important function of that care is to establish a confident personal relationship between you and those providing it.

Books to Read

Many books for pregnant women are available besides this one, including volumes on such specific topics as pregnancy for the working woman, preparation for childbirth for women over thirty-five, general and special diets for pregnancy, exercises to prepare for and recover from delivery, and care of the newborn, including breast-feeding. You can find books outlining each of the several approaches to psychological and physical support for the woman in labor. Books for pregnant diabetics and for women who have had cesarean deliveries are available. If you think you might have a cesarean, there are books describing what such an experience is like. There are even books for the partner of the pregnant woman. As the Bible says, "Of making many books there is no end." And, remember, it also warns that "much study is a weariness of the flesh." In any event, if you are a reader, you will not be at a loss for material.

I have appended a short list of books in particular areas of interest, along with brief comments about each.

The American College of Obstetricians and Gynecologists publishes a series of informative pamphlets about pregnancy. You can get them by writing to the College at 600 Maryland Avenue SW, Suite 300 East, Washington, DC 20024. The March of Dimes also has a fine series of brochures which can be obtained from the National Office, March of Dimes, 1275 Mamaroneck Avenue, White Plains, NY 10605. An excellent source of information is the International Childbirth Education Association, PO Box 20048, Minneapolis, MN 55420, which will forward your request to the local chapter.

Your local bookstore and public library most likely have shelves set aside for books on pregnancy, breast-feeding, and baby care, which will be of help in finding information suited to your needs. They and childbirth education groups in your own community may also be able to supply you with audio tapes, video tapes, and movies to add to your education.

A Personal Tape of Instructions

All this is in addition to the information that you get directly from the people who provide you with care. For years I have sat down with my patients at the end of the initial prenatal visit and reviewed for them my attitudes on patient care and specific instructions in regard to diet, clothing, activity, medications, and the comforts and discomforts they might anticipate. Over the years, after repeating this time and time again, I became somewhat jaded and began to worry that I might be omitting items from the monologue. I also became concerned that, because of the almost unavoidable barriers to communication between woman and doctor (consumers of health care are taught not to take up the time of the busy doctor) that patients might be failing to interrupt my speech with questions that occurred to them.

With all this in mind I decided to make a tape recording of what I thought of as patient instructions. I made one tape for women having their first baby and a somewhat different tape for women having a second baby. I introduced the tapes by explaining why I had made them and encouraging the listeners to replay anything that wasn't clear. I also encouraged them to take a pencil and make notes of what I was saying, something I found that most patients were reluctant to do in my presence. Included on the tapes are the telephone numbers that the patient can use to get in touch with me or the physicians and midwives who provide my backup at odd hours.

There are concerns of individual patients which need to be explained further. Furthermore, a tape of instructions is not the ideal technique for everybody. I therefore include a statement telling the patients that if they are not comfortable with the tape they can turn off the recorder and meet with me directly.

Patients seem to find the tapes supportive and informative. Any doctors or midwives who are reading this book might consider this a helpful approach, too.

Prenatal Visits

Whether you receive your care from physicians or from midwives, the first thing we do is to obtain your medical and social history. You may be asked to fill out a form or you may be personally interviewed by a member of the team providing care. The questions will start with data such as your date of birth and the nature of your occupation and that of the baby's father. If you have had previous pregnancies a detailed record will be obtained. If you have had an abnormal pregnancy or labor and delivery elsewhere there will probably be a request made for a detailed report from your previous care providers. If you have had an infertility problem this will also be noted. Any medical conditions or surgical operations that you have had will be recorded and you will be asked whether you are taking any medicine or what are commonly called drugs. An inquiry will be made about the family history of such conditions as high blood pressure and diabetes, since both complications are more common in women who have close relatives with these conditions. Exposure to infectious childhood diseases will also be recorded. It is important to note any familial diseases as part of the genetic background. You may also be asked to provide information as to your ethnic background as a simple screen for some genetic conditions. For example, Tay-Sachs disease is common among Eastern European Jews, whereas neural tube defects are common among the Scotch and the Irish. Anemias tend to be more common among people whose families come from the shores of the Mediterranean. Sickle-cell trait, which has clear genetic implications, should be noted.

The presence of fraternal twins in the family is important to note since this type of twinning runs in families, through the maternal line.

In regard to the duration of the pregnancy, it is important to record the date of the last menstrual period, particularly if you have made a written record. If the pregnancy is fairly well along, a record of such symptoms as nausea and vomiting, with the dates on which they began and when they disappeared, is made at the initial visit, and helps to establish the expected date of confinement (EDC).

In addition to the history taking and physical and pelvic examination on this first visit, there is a battery of laboratory tests. There is a count of red and white blood cells and blood platelets. The major (ABO) and Rh type of the red blood cells is determined. The fluid portion of the blood is studied for antibodies to red blood cells, the so-called antibody screen. In many jurisdictions, a serologic test for syphilis is also done and there is the option of testing for prior exposure to rubella and to toxoplasmosis. It may be that we will soon add screening for herpes. It has also been suggested that testing for alpha-fetoprotein also be carried out at about the sixteenth or eighteenth week. Some laboratories, particularly those that are fully automated, also carry out determinations of a number of chemical substances normally present in the blood, simply on the ground that this is now an inexpensive screen for abnormality.

Another step in the laboratory is a complete examination of the urine, looking for such things as protein, which may indicate high blood pressure or kidney disease, and sugar (glucose), a clue to the presence of diabetes.

The physical and pelvic examinations are described on page 40. These are ordinarily completed on the first prenatal visit.

Subsequent Prenatal Visits

You will be asked to come in for further visits once a month through approximately the thirtieth week of pregnancy. Following this, a two- or three-week interval is used up to the thirty-sixth week. Thereafter you are seen once a week. On these visits you are weighed and your blood pressure and growth of the fetus and uterus recorded. As noted elsewhere, unusual weight gain was used in the past as an excuse for chastisement, but we seem to have emerged from that unnecessarily parentalistic approach. The weight record is now principally regarded as a general reflection of the woman's well-being.

At each visit there is a brief interview carried out to find out how you feel. For many women, especially with first pregnancies, it is reassuring for the abdomen to be examined, to know that the uterus is growing at the appropriate pace. Now that the Doptone is in common use, you may request a brief run to allow you to hear the fetal heartbeat.

Since the equipment has become available in doctors' offices, sonographic visualization of the fetus at each visit has also been added to prenatal care by some providers. I have not done this because I am concerned that we do not know with certainty how much exposure to sonography is safe. I have discussed this in greater detail in Chapter 5.

At prenatal visits beyond the thirty-eighth week, women frequently will request an abdominal examination to reassure them of the normality of the fetal lie, and they commonly ask whether the head is or is not engaged. Engagement prior to labor makes little difference in the management of the labor but if this is reassuring to the patient I don't hesitate to determine it. Some women will ask to have a pelvic examination. These can be done safely in the office or clinic. I have found this to yield useful information only in women who have had prior pregnancies and who might be expected to have rapid labors. I have on occasion been able to predict labors of less than an hour in duration simply by finding that the baby's head is deep in the pelvis and the cervix already thinned out and substantially dilated. But for the great majority of women this kind of prediction is neither available nor reliable and for that reason I do not insist on doing a pelvic examination late in pregnancy. I do it without hesitation for those who request it but emphasize that for the most part there is not much to be learned. In the event of an abnormal presentation found by abdominal examination, pelvic examination late in pregnancy is of value to confirm it, because the patient with a transverse lie or a breech merits special attention early in labor.

For the most part, the subsequent prenatal visits after the first one can be perfunctory, particularly with normal healthy patients who have had babies before and who are therefore alert to the possible danger signs.

An Adult Approach to Prenatal Care

When I learned obstetrics some forty-five years ago, the doctor's attitude to prenatal care was paternalistic. The pregnant woman was expected to place herself in the hands of the doctor, to ask a minimum of questions, and to leave decisions entirely up to the physician. This was an epoch when women were given large quantities of drugs during labor with the goal of obliterating the memory of the event. They were very likely to be delivered under general anesthesia.

The changes in obstetrics during and immediately after World War II have reeducated us to the point where books on preparation for childbirth are published under such titles as *Awake and Aware*. The women's health movement has assured women that it is proper for them to participate in their own care and to learn as much as possible about it.

This has created a problem of vocabulary. Competent health care during pregnancy and delivery is provided in the United States by family doctors, by midwives, and by obstetricians. No single word identifies all these people. "Midwife" has traditional but outmoded meanings. "Obstetrician" is properly limited to people with medical degrees and specialty training. The French word "accoucheur" suggests that the activity is limited to the time of delivery. A term that has come into some currency, "care provider," is comprehensive but I find it clumsy and vague. I am also reluctant to perpetuate the era of professional exclusivity by using only the term "obstetrician." At the moment I have no solution for the semantic difficulty, but in a real sense the argument is academic.

Carrying a pregnancy and going through labor and delivery is inevitably the task of the mother. It is she who delivers the baby. In this, she should have the aid of a group of people, each contributing a certain competence and a certain function. This includes the pregnant woman's partner, her medical attendants, her family, her other children, and her friends. We are in the process of re-creating the extended family, which once took for granted that the pregnant woman would be supported, especially in labor, by other women who had experience with childbirth. An instance of this is the example of the Mormon pioneers in Utah in the mid-nineteenth century. When they experienced a shortage of physicians they decided to send church members back to the East for medical education. Despite the complete male domination of their society, they preferentially chose mothers for this mission, knowing that a large fraction of the new doctors' future practice was to be the care of women in childbirth.

Now, in the 1980's, we are experiencing a steady growth in the care in labor provided by midwives, a group that is overwhelmingly female. Furthermore, for the past decade there has been a continuing increase in the proportion of women in training as specialists in obstetrics; by now about one-third of such trainees are women.

Prepared Childbirth

Childbirth is a life crisis, and for many women it is a period of discomfort in addition to being a period of hard work. In the 1940's the realization belatedly dawned that specific preparation for this event would help in its successful completion. Grantly Dick Read in Britain concluded that the ill-defined fears of labor were an obstacle to many women, and he proposed techniques to minimize that fear by education and by suggesting exercises to pregnant women that they could practice to prepare themselves for the inevitable effort of labor. Elsewhere in Europe obstetricians used the Russian physiologist Pavlov's concepts concerning conditioned reflexes to prepare patients to tolerate the pain of labor without altering the physiological process.

Later, Fernand Lamaze, a French obstetrician, combined these two concepts into a program of childbirth preparation that included education and a series of programmed and, one might even say, choreographed breathing techniques, taught to patients in group classes prior to labor. The babies' fathers were brought into the classes and the exercises. This preparation, the Lamaze method, is probably the most widely used technique for preparation for childbirth in the western world today. As could reasonably be expected, it has since been modified, particularly with the recognition that some of the techniques that are part of the orthodox Lamaze preparation do not work for all, and that women should have the chance to substitute other procedures that work better for them. Thus, whereas the vogue in the 1930's and 1940's was to have a baby under some variant of twilight sleep, which provided for sedation and amnesia, the style in the 1970's became rejection of any drugs and strict adherence to the precepts of a specific routine for the conduct of labor.

There are several other methods of preparation. One of them, which briefly enjoyed a considerable vogue, was introduced by another French obstetrician, Frédérick Leboyer. It emphasized reducing the stimuli that could affect the baby by turning down the lights, speaking quietly in the delivery room, and stressing gentleness in the management of the delivery. Leboyer's focus was principally on the baby. He recommended that the newborn be placed in a tub of warm water, which has the unhappy effect of separating the baby from the mother and clearly interfering with early bonding. It gives the accoucheur a role more important than that of the mother.

Another method, introduced by an American obstetrician, Robert Bradley, has gone under the title of "husband-coached childbirth." For my tastes this places the woman's partner in too prominent a position in the process. Long before it was fashionable or even in accordance with hospital rules, I stayed with my wife during several of her labors, although I took no responsibility for her care. This seemed to both of us to be the obvious way to do it, rather than submit to the separation that had been imposed on us by hospital policy for her deliveries in the 1940's. Nevertheless, I think it would have been presumptuous of me to claim any credit for her accomplishments in labor.

All of these methods, and the list is by no means complete, are of value if they work well for the patient. They are negative if they give the women a sense of failure if she does not meet the expectations of the method. The patient and her support system must do what works well for her and must avoid attempting to fit her into a system which does not meet her needs at the moment. Nora Ephron pointed out, in an essay reflecting on her own first delivery, that the tyranny of the doctor had now been replaced by the tyranny of the method. I personally am an eclectic in this regard.

Childbirth Education

There has also been the development of formal classes for patient education for childbirth. Classes are conducted under a large number of auspices: hospitals, the American Red Cross, childbirth education groups, midwifery groups, doctors' offices, college- and university-sponsored graduate education, churches, and visiting nurses services. National organizations such as the International Childbirth Education Association (ICEA) have set up specific outlines for these courses and training courses for the childbirth educators themselves. If you intend to take one of these classes, check on the preparation and the qualifications of the people teaching them.

If the classes are taught by individuals, you can check with the ICEA to learn whether the teachers have met its standards. The qualifications of midwives can be learned from the American College of Nurse Midwives, at the address on page 123. You can and should check with your doctor or midwife for help in finding the course that is best for your needs. Remember that good intentions and personal experience with labor are not sufficient to make a capable or a safe teacher.

Classes in preparation for childbirth should probably be started somewhere about the twenty-eighth week; you may wish to set this up for your own needs with your own childbirth educator. I think all methods emphasize, quite properly, the need for others than the "care provider" to help the patient in labor. This can be the woman's partner (husband, boyfriend, lesbian lover), who will stay with her for the duration of the childbirth process, however long it may be. In some circumstances it may be appropriate to include her mother, her mother-in-law, or sister. In still other situations, unrelated coaches with whom the patient has worked in the preparation for the birth may be part of the team.

In recent years, in addition to preparing women for their experiences during late pregnancy and labor, there are also classes devoted to the care of the newborn. Indeed, hospitals often offer such teaching sessions to patients following delivery. These include the obvious features, such as diapering and feeding a newborn baby, the basic pattern of urination, the appearance of the stools of the newborn, and the advantages and disadvantages of breast- and bottle-feeding. It may seem strange to the experienced, but women who are mothers for the first time sometimes are quite unsure of how to respond to a crying baby. They may be hesitant to follow their instincts, which usually direct them toward bonding to the baby.

Some childbirth classes devote considerable attention to nutrition during pregnancy. Women who regularly eat a well-balanced diet do not need this instruction because their habits are sufficient to keep them and their babies in good health. However, instruction in the principles of good nutrition is essential for pregnant women who have not been following an adequate diet.

Exercise is another subject that may be stressed in classes in preparation for childbirth, not necessarily as part of a "method" but under the general heading of physical fitness. The mothers who are motivated to do these exercises seem to benefit from them. Those who are not so motivated do not seem to suffer particularly from their absence. The studies that have been done on the effect of exercise on the fetus indicate that if a woman is accustomed to strenuous exercise it will harm neither her nor her baby if she continues to practice it during her pregnancy. Accustomed jogging, running, and swimming are completely benign.

Apart from the subjects usually covered in these classes, two other matters deserve mention. First, rooming-in (see page 552 in Chapter 23). This has become part of the present style of postpartum care. I believe it is a very effective way for a new mother to learn to know her baby before they both go home. I like to urge my patients to room-in with their babies. One difference this practice has made for me is a marked reduction in anxious telephone calls in the first few weeks about minor complaints, which often serve as an acceptable reason to call and talk about problems in adjustment to the new baby. Second, circumcision (see page 560). This is not a medical procedure, but rather a social custom. It is not needed for either the health or cleanliness of the infant. It is no more a medical procedure than piercing earlobes.

Unsolicited Amateur Advice

A pregnant woman is a ready target for a wide range of well-meant but unasked-for amateur instruction. Much of this consists of personal reminiscence and superstition, often serving no function other than to please the persons making the remarks or provide them an opportunity to ventilate grievances. I remember a nurse who presented a woman in hard labor with an account of how useless the nurse's husband had been when she was having her baby and how she told him in no uncertain terms that the next time he could have the baby. There are books that are little more than expressions of anger against one aspect or another of the author's pregnancy, labor, and early experiences with motherhood. Few pregnant women have escaped the warnings of well-wishers who caution them against going swimming, reaching up to high shelves, wearing high heels, indulging in intercourse, eating certain foods, and so on. The list is apparently endless. Some self-constituted authorities purport to be able to predict the sex of the fetus by gazing into the eyes of the mother-to-be or by looking at the shape of the bulge. They do not hesitate even momentarily to communicate their prediction to the mother. Of course they are correct about 50 percent of the time.

The best way to handle advice of this sort—which you will probably readily recognize in most cases as pure superstition—is to listen to it politely and then follow the dictates of your own common sense. When in doubt consult the person who is giving you prenatal care.

A word is in order, though, on the subject of prenatal influence on the fetus, a matter on which many people have opinions. There is no truth to the old wives' tale that port wine stains or that strawberry marks, which are actually diffuse collections of blood vessels within the skin, are produced by experiences of the mother during pregnancy. But it has been scientifically proven that the baby does experience events in the world outside the uterus and can remember after birth sights and especially sounds that it experienced in the late months before it was born. A baby may be born knowing the rhythm of its mother's voice through hearing it repeatedly while *in utero*. Sensitive fetuses can even learn a melody in this way. There is evidence that the higher centers of the fetal brain are working in the last trimester of pregnancy. There is no evidence, however, that visual, auditory, or other sensory stimuli received by the mother during pregnancy can cause any physical changes in the fetus.

The Environment for the Conduct of Labor

Along with the changes in patient care and in patient education has come a change in concepts of what labor facilities should look like. I recall visiting the labor room of a major university hospital in the Midwest in the late 1940's. It consisted of a rather large room done in gray ceramic tile. A low bedspring, coming to about eighteen inches off the floor, stood in the middle of the room. The bed had neither headboard nor foot-board; nor was it in any way adjustable, and it was covered by a thin mattress. The only other furniture in the room was a bedside table. The windows were barred by heavy wire.mesh, and the room looked for all the world like the isolation room in a psychiatric hospital.

In the thirty-five years since, we have changed to labor beds with ample springs and innerspring mattresses, and sometimes with bolsters and all the other appurtenances of bedroom lux-ury. Floors may be carpeted and comfortable overstuffed fur-niture provided for both the woman in labor and her support team. The electronic gear that we have come to employ so extensively can be stored inconspicuously and everything done to attempt to simulate a comforting home environment. Music is occasionally piped into the room, illumination is indirect and soft, curtains are provided for the windows, and it is taken for granted that a maximum of privacy will be provided.

Not every hospital is able to provide environments as pleas-ant as this, but more and more the effort is being made in modern obstetrical facilities to make the surroundings homelike and comfortable.

How to Choose Your Support System

More than 90 percent of the births in the United States are presently being managed by specialists in obstetrics. About

8½ percent of pregnant women are cared for by family physicians. Approximately 1½ percent receive their assistance in labor from nurse midwives.

How are these care providers prepared for their work? Obstetricians will have graduated from medical school and then undertaken four or more years of training in obstetrics and gynecology. At the conclusion of this training program they are authorized to take a more than three-hour written exam on the factual basis of the practice of this specialty. Those who pass the examination may then represent themselves as Board-eligible. After two or more years of practice in the specialty the candidates submit to the American Board of Obstetrics and Gynecology a list of all the patients they have cared for during the last full year of practice for review by the Board. If this review indicates that the quality and quantity of practice are sufficient to meet the standards of the Board, the individuals are invited for a three-hour oral examination. This is intended to scrutinize the level of their knowledge and the style of their practice. If all this is successfully completed, the individuals are authorized to identify themselves as Diplomates of the American Board of Obstetrics and Gynecology. At present, there are about twenty-one thousand Diplomates. Most Diplomates are required to be recertified by examination at regular intervals so that the Board can be certain that they have kept themselves up-to-date with the changing standards of practice.

You can find out whether the doctor that you intend to go to is Board-eligible or a Diplomate by consulting the local medical society, the local medical library, or the office of the administrator of the hospital where your doctor practices. The doctor's office can also give you this information. The directories that list those doctors who are Board-certified also list their age, where they went to medical school, and where they took their training. You can always reinforce the available information by consulting people in your own community whose opinion you value, including doctors in other fields. There is no need when seeking medical care to accept a pig in a poke.

Doctors in general practice have not spent nearly as much time on their education in obstetrics, although they have done work in the field in the course of their training. The American Academy of General Practice conducts qualifying examinations and certifies practitioners much as does the American Board. The Academy also requires regular attendance at refresher courses. Most hospitals that are accredited by the Joint Committee on the Accreditation of Hospitals authorize such general practitioners to take care of normal patients, specifying only that major problems and operative obstetrics be referred to doctors with obstetrical qualifications. Once again, local sources of information can be used to indicate a particular doctor's experience and certifications.

Incidentally, you should be warned that the Yellow Pages of the telephone directory are not a solid reference for doctors' qualifications. Many local telephone companies will list as an obstetrician any physician who claims to be one. Since there are many Diplomates of the American Board of Obstetrics and Gynecology, however, if you live in an urban or suburban area, there is little doubt that you can find a person fully qualified to provide your care.

Nurse Midwives

The traditional image of a midwife was established by two models. One was portrayed by Charles Dickens in his novel, *Martin Chuzzlewit*. Sairey Gamp is a prominent character in this novel. Shortly after she is introduced, Dickens describes her place of residence with "her sign board boldly headed, midwife." He then goes on at some length to describe her as sloppy, alcoholic, exploitative, and actively manipulative of other characters.

The other model of the midwife in the United States is a composite of two types: the granny-midwife, found mostly in the Deep South, and the midwife who came from Europe to the United States in the second half of the nineteenth century with the poor immigrants of that epoch, who had been her patients in the "old country." Both of these types of midwife were mostly self-trained, had learned their skills by trial and error, and were without any formal training in medicine or midwifery.

These midwives attended patients in the poor rural areas of the South or the overcrowded urban ghettos of the North. They commonly first saw a patient when she went into labor. The patients themselves had had no prenatal care. They were often undernourished. If they were city dwellers, many of them had tuberculosis and rickets and suffered the stress of repeated pregnancies, relying only on breast-feeding the last baby as a means of preventing the conception of the next one.

The inevitably poor maternal and newborn outcomes were blamed entirely on the midwives rather than in large measure on the situation the midwives encountered. Determined efforts were therefore made early in the twentieth century to eliminate midwives from the care of women in the United States. Licensure and certification of midwives was of some assistance in improving their standards of practice. Indeed, midwifery schools were established in the early decades of the century, but they were ahead of their time and failed to thrive.

Since World War II, a new concept of nurse midwifery has come into existence, borrowed in large measure from the experience in Scandinavia, the Netherlands, Britain, and France, where trained midwives have accounted for the greatest proportion of care during childbirth. I remember my surprise in Sweden in 1958 when I learned that the wife of an obstetrical colleague of mine, who was expecting twins, was under the care of a midwife and that an obstetrician would be involved only in the event of difficulty.

In the United States there are now university training programs for nurse midwifery. The prerequisite for admission to the programs is completion of nurses' training; most of the programs are directed toward advanced degrees in nursing. The American College of Nurse Midwifery has established high standards for certification of its members. You should find out whether the midwife of your choosing is a certified nurse midwife and whether she has appropriate arrangements for hospital and physician backup in the event of problems in labor or delivery. This information is probably available in your community from the midwives themselves, or from the American College of Nurse Midwives, at 1522 K Street NW, Suite 1120, Washington, DC 20005. There are now a few men who are certified nurse midwives.

One brief word about the lay midwife. There are a few jurisdictions where lay midwives are tolerated despite the fact that these individuals are self-trained and that there is no supervisory body. There is simply no way of telling what standards these unschooled midwives are prepared to meet.

Be Comfortable with Those Who Give You Care

It seems to me most important that you be comfortable with the thought of working with whatever provider of care you choose. You must have confidence in the individual or individuals, and this in itself is a good reason for looking into their qualifications and attitudes before making a commitment to them. If, for example, you have a strong feelings that you wish to breast-feed, it is not good for you to get your care from someone who is cool to the idea.

The same goes for the style of conduct of labor. If you have attitudes about or experience with fetal monitoring, you should find out whether it is the practice where you intend to deliver to require it or to limit its use. If you have had a previous birth by cesarean and wish to undertake a normal birth, you should find out, early on, the attitudes toward such care on the part of those you choose to assist you in labor. I experience great difficulty in dealing with the problems of a woman who learns at the thirty-eighth week that she and her doctor have serious disagreement about her care in labor, and who then asks me to take over her care.

The fact that you have gone to a care facility does not mean that you are contracted to stay with it, if it turns out in the course of prenatal care that you are not at ease. If necessary, discuss this candidly with the people who have been providing your care so some resolution of the problem can be worked out amicably. Most of us who practice obstetrics take prenatal care as a commitment to follow through. Furthermore, we are usually aware of the women who are not comfortable in our care; I would prefer that such patients transfer themselves elsewhere. When this is done belatedly and in anger, it does not go well.

Obstetrical Fees

The obstetrical fee is ordinarily an inclusive fee for prenatal care, care during labor and delivery, and the period up to eight weeks postpartum. This allows the patient to seek prenatal visits as often as she deems appropriate. It also allows the attendant to ask the patient to come in more frequently without the suspicion that an attempt is being made to affect the fee, as might be the case with a fee per visit arrangement.

There are generally well-known community standards as to what constitutes a reasonable fee for care. More and more, insurance policies tend to reflect these standards. If there is any question in your mind about the reasonableness of an obstetrical fee, probably the simplest thing to do is to speak to the local medical society.

Recently, as a part of the discussion of obstetricians' concern about the relentlessly increasing rate of cesarean section, it was suggested that it might be in the interests of society and the patients to reverse present practice and begin paying a higher fee for normal birth than for surgical abdominal delivery. I share the opinion of many obstetricians that when we have spent many hours with a patient in labor and eventually have succeeded in assisting her to a normal birth, we could reasonably receive a larger fee than when we spend approximately seventy-five minutes doing an abdominal delivery.

It appears to me that if there is any real chance of altering the fee schedules for obstetrics it ought to be in the direction of establishing a flat fee for support and assistance during pregnancy and labor and delivery. This would eliminate the premium for doing a cesarean section, which in the final analysis would balance out against the number of occasions in which labor is rapid and uneventful.

7

The Pregnant Months

I wish to make the clear-cut, unqualified statement that the comments included here are intended in no way to displace or alter those of the reader's physician or midwife. There are great differences of informed opinion on the lesser details of the conduct of normal pregnancy. Further, every obstetrician's treatment will vary in detail to suit variations in individual patients. No matter how carefully a pregnant woman may study this or any other book, she will not obviate the necessity of paying an early visit for prenatal care.

It is remarkable how life during pregnancy has been simplified in recent years. With the observation of large numbers of healthy women—previous to the eighteenth century midwives cared for all normal cases, and doctors had the opportunity to see only ill pregnant women—the medical attitude toward pregnancy has changed. Since in the past pregnancy was treated as an illness from its very inception, it was deemed imperative to employ the most complicated measures to prevent dangerous complications. We now realize that pregnancy is a normal physiologic state, and ordinarily all that need be done is to maintain the woman in good physical condition by an uncomplicated, common-sense regimen. If an abnormality develops, then of course the doctor must step in and aid nature to correct it.

The Declining Risk

Until 1930 the maternal mortality in the United States (all deaths occurring during pregnancy, delivery, and the first six weeks following delivery, in which the state of being pregnant or having been pregnant plays the primary role, conditions such as hemorrhage, or infection arising from the reproductive tract) was high and stationary. Maternal mortality is expressed in terms of the number of women who die per 100,000 babies born alive. In 1930 the rate was 67; then it began to decline, slowly at first, later swiftly. It dropped to 37 in 1959, 28 in 1967, and in 1982, the last year for which complete data from the National Center for Health Statistics are currently available, to 7.9. The number of women who died as the direct result of pregnancy and childbearing in 1982 was 292 in the course of 3,680, 537 live births. In 1930 one woman died from obstetric causes in every 1,492 live births; in 1982 one in every 12,605. In other words, in five decades, childbirth in the United States became eight times as safe. I am convinced that, given ideal care, the risk of death in pregnancy in the mid-1980's need be no more than 3 deaths in every 100,000 live births, or about 1 maternal death in every 33,000 live births.

This achievement in obstetrics has few, if any, parallels in the whole field of modern medicine.

Factors Affecting the Risk

The risk of childbirth is not uniform; it is sensitive to various factors. If one examines the matter superficially he will come up with the conclusion that the most important factor in this country is the race to which one is born, because statistics show a maternal mortality for United States whites of 5.8 per 100,000 live births and for nonwhites of 18.2. Therefore one may assume that the nonwhite woman is less sturdy and has some inborn defect which makes childbirth less safe. This is not true. The difference in mortality rate derives from social and economic factors such as paucity of available facilities for prenatal care and failure to make use of them, lifelong inadequate nutrition dating back to the mother's own prenatal experience during her mother's pregnancy, improper living conditions associated with poor hygiene, a high frequency of adolescent pregnancy and excessive childbearing related to limited contraceptive services, and poor health education in general. Two decades ago it was thought that the high nonwhite mortality was due to lack of hospitalization for delivery. Seven percent of nonwhite mothers were not hospitalized. In three of the states with the worst maternal mortality records—Mississippi, Alabama, and Arkansas—nearly a quarter of births took place outside hospitals. This has now changed: 99.1 percent of all births in the United States by 1978 were in a hospital, and in the three states mentioned nearly 99 percent. The poor nonwhite mortality rate persists nonetheless to the present.

The chief causes of maternal death continue to be toxemia (high blood pressure with kidney and liver complications), hemorrhage, and infection. The last has diminished greatly since the near disappearance of illegal abortion, a principal cause of death through infection. The startling recent change has been a great increase in the incidence of ectopic pregnancy and in maternal death due to it.

The Birth Rate

The birth rate is the number of births for every 1,000 people in the population in a year. In 1915, the first year for which figures are available, it was 25. It declined steadily thereafter until it reached a low of 16.6 in the midst of the Great Depression. This rate remained unchanged until World War II.

During that war, the rate rose somewhat, but, understandably, the extent and speed of the rise were affected by the disruption and postponement of marriages and family formation caused by the entry of large numbers of young men and young women into military service. At the end of the war in 1945 the young people were able to go back to civilian life, get married, and start having children. By 1947, the birth rate rose to 25.8, where it remained until the early 1960's. This was the baby boom. A steady downturn then began, arriving at a rate of 18.4 in 1970 and of 14.6 in 1975. By this time the children born in the late 1940's and the 1950's had achieved reproductive age. The birth rate subsequently rose again, to 15.9 in 1980, and has remained there since.

Like the stock market, the birth rate is affected by a number of factors, economic and social, that interact in ways that appear baffling. I make no attempt to explain how these things work, but simply note a number of circumstances that seem to have influenced or accompanied the changes described above. For example, in 1957, the average number of children per family was 3.8, reflecting the baby boom that began in 1946. In 1965, women in their twenties expected to have a total of 3 children, but in 1970, they expected only 2.5. Actually, in 1971, the average number of children per woman dropped to 2.2 and in 1980 was only 1.9. Another way of saying this is that, as reported by Census Bureau statistics, there has been a substantial decrease in the rates of birth of second, third, fourth, and higher order babies.

Throughout the 1970's the population of women aged thirty to thirty-four, born in the baby boom, grew rapidly, but the fraction of them that was childless grew even faster. For thirty-year-old white women the rate of childlessness was nearly 30 percent in 1980. For twenty-five-year-old women the rate was 35 percent in 1970 and 52 percent in 1979. These phenomena are related to the steady increase in the average age of marriage and the average age at which women had their first child.

The availability of effective measures of birth control and of abortion by choice has had a major impact on these figures.

The Fertility Rate

Trends in the fertility rate also illustrate the same phenomena. The fertility rate is the number of births per 1,000 women in the age group from fifteen to forty-four. It is sensitive to the relative numbers of men and women and the changing proportions of childbearing and nonreproducing women. The fertility rate was 118 in 1960, 96 in 1965, 88 in 1970, and fell to 66 in 1975. It has remained stationary since.

Rate of First Births

In the latest figures available from the National Center for Health Statistics, between 1979 and 1982 the number of first births increased 3.7 percent among women aged fifteen to twenty-four and 11 percent among those from twenty-five to twenty-nine. But for women thirty to thirty-four, the increase was 44 percent and from thirty-five to thirty-nine 62 percent. Above forty the rise was 33 percent. These increases are far greater than the percentage increase in the number of women in these older age groups.

Rate of First Births

Age Group	Year 1979	1982
15–19	39.7	41.0
20–24	52.6	54.7
25–29	34.5	38.4
30–34	10.1	14.6
35–39	2.1	3.3
40–44	0.3	0.4

Rate of All Births

The number of women per 1,000 who gave birth to any baby in the same years was as follows.

Rate of All Births

Age Group	Year 1979	1982
15–19	53.4	52.9
20–24	115.7	111.3
25–29	115.6	111.0
30–34	61.8	64.2
35–39	19.4	21.1
40–44	3.9	3.9

Summarizing these tables, I can say that it is a simple fact that at present there are more older women having first and later babies than a decade ago. It is no accident that there are now several books of special advice for new mothers over thirty-five years of age.

Population Impact of Birth Rates

The baby boom began in the late 1940's and continued into the 1950's. These children are now all in their reproductive years and the youngest of them are in their late twenties and early thirties. Some of the children of the babies in the baby boom have now begun to swell the ranks of the fifteen to nineteen age group. Because the baby boom increased the absolute number of young women who were able to reproduce between 1979 and 1982, the absolute number of babies born during that time increased overall, although there was no change in the birth rate as I have defined it above. The figures show a slight difference in distribution, however: a decline in the rate of babies born to younger women aged fifteen to twenty-nine from 285 to 275 per 1,000; and in the older age groups an increase from 85 to 89 per 1000 of first and later children. There were 3,681,000 babies born in the U.S. in 1982; 3,618,000 in 1983; and 3,690,000 in 1984.

The present and projected distribution of women aged fifteen to forty-four according to the Census Bureau is as follows.

Age Group	1980	1990	2000	2010
15–19	10,381,000	8,294,000	9,262,000	9,343,000
20–24	10,699,000	9,134,000	8,416,000	9,744,000
25–29	9,905,000	10,647,000	8,589,000	9,554,000
30–34	8,975,000	10,992,000	9,438,000	8,733,000
35–39	7,160,000	10,071,000	10,834,000	8,797,000
40–44	5,993,000	9,048,000	11,051,000	9,522,000
Total	53,113,000	58,186,000	57,589,000	54,693,000

If the present trends continue, the shift of births into the older age groups will help to maintain the number of births until the end of the century. Predictions of this sort are obviously hazardous in view of the multitude of social factors that affect human behavior in large groups. It is nevertheless reasonable to expect a decline in the number of births as the number of reproducing women decreases after the year 2000.

At present, if current fertility rates continue, the estimate of the total fertility rate for those women now fifteen to forty-four years of age for their entire reproductive lifetimes is 1,819 births per 1,000, or less than 2 children per woman. This is below the number needed for replacement of the population. If there is to be any increase in the total U.S. population, under these circumstances it will have to come from immigration and from an increase, if any, in life expectancy. This predicts a continually aging population.

Subjects You May Be Wondering About

Exercise

Before offering advice about activities during pregnancy, I once again stress the point that if the words printed here are at variance with those given you by your physician or midwife, pay heed only to those instructions, not mine.

The long-held conviction of yesteryear that practically anything except lying alone in bed might bring on abortion or premature labor must have been devastating to both mind and conscience. Until very recently, whenever a woman miscarried she searched her life for the cause and with no difficulty discovered it either in some minor accident or in the simple exertions of her everyday existence. With advances in knowledge concerning the real causes of abortion, our attitude toward exercise during pregnancy has changed. We realize that the majority of miscarriages are blessed acts on the part of nature to terminate further development of an abnormal ovum.

Some lingering concern has been expressed about possible adverse effects of exercise late in pregnancy. This is undoubtedly related to the popularity of such activities as jogging, bicycling, and aerobics. The evidence is satisfactory that accustomed and moderate exercise in no way damages the fetus at any stage of pregnancy. The fetal heart rate increases if the mother engages in exercises that approach the limits of her tolerance, but this is a transitory change.

It goes without saying that late in your first pregnancy is not the ideal time to learn downhill skiing. On the other hand, if you are an experienced skier and familiar with your own exercise tolerance and limits of safety, there is no risk specific to pregnancy to be attributed to a slalom course. It *is* unhandy to delivery with your leg in a cast!

Women often ask if there is a minimum amount of exercise required in a normal pregnancy. The answer is that it depends on you. It is an entirely individual decision related to what you are accustomed to and comfortable with. It makes no difference to the fetus.

There has been a proliferation of books recommending particular exercises for childbirth and for recovery from the delivery. Insofar as exercises assist the pregnant woman in maintaining a positive body image, I am sure they are all to the good. They may also play a significant role in some of the methods for pain relief in labor.

Sexual intercourse, a special kind of exercise, is also not harmful to mother or baby. Nor is there any evidence that orgasm has anything other than transitory effects on uterine contractions and fetal heart rate. However, an increase in uterine activity may be undesirable in patients who have a risk of premature delivery.

Employment

You need not change or stop your ordinary work just because you are pregnant. My observation has been that if a pregnant woman finds her work satisfying or if her family needs the money she earns, she is better off both physically and psychologically if she continues working. It is desirable that the employer accept the fact that a pregnant woman is subject to fatigue, especially late in pregnancy. She may have to take additional rest and indeed may occasionally have to be absent without being truly sick. Your own frame of mind and the state of your discomfort are the critical issues that determine when to stop working.

In the Soviet Union, China, and Cuba for example, pregnant

women are given a six-week leave with pay both before and after delivery. Pregnant professionals in those countries, however, do not hesitate to make exceptions for themselves from this regulation.

I have known several young doctors in this country who worked right up until the time of delivery. They certainly were more tired than their nonpregnant colleagues, but I have seen no evidence that this did them or their babies any harm.

For the sake of a quiet recovery and for convenience in breast-feeding, you may very well decide to stay away from work for many weeks after delivery. This is not to suggest, however, that the postpartum period—even if the birth was by cesarean—is one of illness or disability. Cesareans are now performed so efficiently that the woman whose baby is delivered in this way need not contemplate a long or difficult convalescence. Neither she nor the woman who has delivered vaginally need consider herself sick at all, but both are entitled to take time to become acquainted with their babies, and, if they are breast-feeding, to see that the process is well established and that the baby is thriving.

Travel

There are only two arguments against travel during pregnancy:

1. Abortion or labor can happen at any hour on any day, and it is nearly always impossible to predict the occurrence. If the pregnant woman happens to be traveling at the time of such an emergency, or is residing in a community other than her own, it is both inconvenient and frightening. One way to lessen the difficulty is to obtain the name of an obstetric facility in the area you plan to visit. Put the memorandum in your wallet and expect not to need it—almost certainly you will not.

2. Traveling can be fatiguing and uncomfortable, especially in late pregnancy. This is particularly true of automobile travel. The only antidote is to break up the trip every two to three hours, get out of the car, void, and walk about for a few minutes. It is probably unwise for you to sit in a cramped position for several hours. The real limit is fatigue.

There is no qualified evidence that traveling by any means of locomotion brings on labor, abortion, or any complication of pregnancy. Naturally, if a thousand women who are eight to twelve weeks pregnant travel, a certain small percentage will miscarry; or if a thousand are thirty-four to thirty-five weeks pregnant, a certain proportion will go into premature labor. However, the same thing is almost certain to happen to the same women if they stay home in bed. Carefully balanced studies of the pregnant wives of armed-services personnel in World War II, those who traveled about with their husbands and those who remained at one post, showed no significant difference in the incidence of abortion, premature labor, or any other obstetric complication.

Travel in the third trimester (the last thirteen weeks) of pregnancy is inadvisable for a women with a history of premature labor or the diagnosis of multiple pregnancy. During her last month, the patient should stay within easy reach of a hospital.

It is not injurious for the pregnant woman to drive a car herself, and she may continue to do so as long as she can sit comfortably behind the wheel. During the last trimester it is inadvisable that she drive alone at night, or on little-frequented roads, because of the potential problems that might arise from a flat tire or other automotive emergencies. Unless a car is equipped with power steering, urban parking may be very exhausting, and this should be taken into account during the late months of pregnancy.

Decisions as to mode of travel during pregnancy should be governed mainly by common-sense considerations. For example, if the woman is prone to motion sickness, the train is probably best. Long distances are usually accomplished with least fatigue and discomfort by air. Air travel during the first three months has been subjected to discussion on the basis that lessened oxygen at this critical, formative period of the fetus's development might in rare cases cause a fetal abnormality. There is no grounds for such apprehension if the cabin is pressurized, as it always is in commercial planes. The equipment used by security personnel at airports to screen passengers and baggage poses no danger to mother or fetus.

Sleep

In early pregnancy the average woman requires an unusually large amount of sleep; this need disappears between the twelfth and sixteenth weeks. The last months are marked by sleeplessness, mainly due to difficulty in finding a comfortable position. Frequently I am asked if it is harmful to sleep on the back or stomach. No possible harm can result from any position, since the fetus is so well protected that pressure on the pregnant woman's body does not affect it. Pregnant women often observe that the fetus is nocturnal in its habits and chooses nighttime to cut capers. As there is no way to diminish fetal movements, the remedy is anything that will make the woman relax and sleep despite them. The amount of sleep should be governed by habit and desire, the safest rule being to sleep enough to awake well rested.

Care of the Breasts

The breasts require no special care during pregnancy. There is so far as I know no benefit to massaging them with or without ointments or to attempts to initiate lactation by manipulating the areola and the nipple.

Whether it is necessary to wear a brassiere during pregnancy is a matter of your personal comfort. The breasts do become heavier and comfort may be enhanced by wearing brassiere cups sufficient in size to contain all the breast tissue, especially the breast tissue which extends out to the armpit. The shoulder straps should be wide enough not to cut into the shoulder.

Manipulating your nipples or your breasts as a preparation for breast-feeding can stimulate uterine contractions. Signals go via the nervous system to the hypothalamus, which reacts by releasing oxytocin from the pituitary. The oxytocin in turn causes uterine contractions. This response is probably best avoided by patients who have a history of previous premature labors, by those who have had any treatment for the incompetent cervical os syndrome, and by women who have threatened premature labor in the present pregnancy. The same may be true for orgasm, which also releases oxytocin and results in contractions.

Even educated, motivated women may have irrational anxieties about their ability to breast-feed, often based on their own body image and the size of their natural equipment. This was dramatized for me one day when I saw two women for initial prenatal visits, one a head nurse of a maternity unit, and the other the nurse in charge of a newborn nursery. One was tall and thin and could be described as flat-chested; the other was short and stocky with relatively large breasts. At the end of the postexamination discussion, I asked each—as I always do—whether she had any questions to ask. And each of them, visibly nervous and with quivering lips, asked whether I thought she could nurse successfully. Knowing that breast size has virtually no effect on a woman's ability to breast-feed, I assured each that she would have no trouble at all. Nor did they, to everyone's delight.

If you plan to nurse, your nipples may require special care. Nipples which project normally require no preparation. To test this, pinch the areola, the pigmented circular zone around the nipple, between your fingers and see what happens. If the nipple projects you have no problem. If the nipple appears to remain flat or even turns inward, you may have permanently inverted nipples. In four out of five cases, however, the condition corrects itself during pregnancy, and by term the nipple can be erected. Recalcitrant inverted nipples may be made erect by a process called nipple rolling, which should be started two months before term and done twice daily. Support the breast with one hand and grasp the nipple at its base between the thumb and first finger of the other hand. Pull the nipple out gently and roll it between the fingers. Even if this fails to cure inversion there still may be a chance that you can nurse successfully. Many a strong, hungry baby has made an inverted nipple erect by sucking.

There is no approved technique for toughening nipples to prevent the development of cracks or soreness while nursing. Scrubbing them with a nail brush or applying alcohol has been proven harmful.

Normal nipple secretion helps prepare them for sucking and should not be washed off with soap. During the last six weeks, wash the breasts with plain water.

Breast Asymmetry

It is not unusual to observe that one breast is larger than the other; this difference in size may become accentuated as pregnancy progresses. Some asymmetry between anatomic structures on opposite sides of the body is common and normal.

The Sagging Abdomen

The retention of youthful shapeliness has been one of the main concerns of womankind probably since the days of Eve. Therefore, in all ages remedies have been employed to prevent the belly from sagging after delivery. The preventives were most elaborate and consisted of two types: the wearing of an abdominal support and the anointment of the abdomen with some greasy medicament. The supports were of two varieties: either a specially treated animal skin, or a broad linen swath "made fit for the purpose to support her Belly." The rubbing ointments were legion, and each author seems to have had several of his own special concoction; the very number leads one to suspect their efficacy.

Today some people still retain this partiality for rubbing the abdomen. Most doctors are skeptical of the value of this undertaking. However, if the patient enjoys doing it, for whatever reason, there is no objection, provided she uses a noninjurious substance such as cocoa butter, cold cream, or Eucerin, a waxy proprietary emulsion for dry skin.

No method is known for preserving the tone and integrity of the skin and abdominal musculature during pregnancy. Their preservation depends on the sinewy strength of the abdominal wall before pregnancy, the relative length of the abdomen, its capacity, and the degree of distention during pregnancy. The latter is increased by multiple pregnancy, excessive amniotic fluid, or a single oversized fetus.

Even if the abdominal wall bulges and sags immediately after delivery, it will spontaneously regain much of the tone it previously possessed within the first six to ten postpartum weeks.

Bathing

Today both showers and tub baths are safe throughout pregnancy. The only time that tub baths are taboo is after the membranes have ruptured. Pregnancy makes no special requirements as far as the temperature of the bath or shower is concerned.

Care of the Genitals

No special hygiene of the genitals is recommended. They should be carefully cleansed with a soft washcloth and soap and water as usual.

Vaginal douching is unnecessary during pregnancy or at any other time. Women have been taught since childhood and are now encouraged by television commercials to think of their genitalia as dirty and requiring frequent cleansing. The vagina is really a self-cleaning structure, dealing with its problems of cleanliness quite efficiently unless it becomes infected. Infection requires specific therapy. Douching is unquestionably hazardous for a pregnant woman who has vaginal bleeding or whose membranes have ruptured. Deodorant douches and deodorant perineal sprays are quite unnecessary. A surprising number of patients are allergic to some of the chemicals in these preparations and can do themselves harm, however minor, by using a procedure that has no medical benefit.

Clothing

We have already considered the matter of brassieres. Clothing should in general be loose and comfortable, and, if possible, hung from the shoulders to prevent constriction of the waist. The weight of clothing and underclothing should be the same as usual. Circular garters should not be worn; they act as tourniquets and serve to increase the likelihood of varicose veins, which are common in pregnancy because of the normally increased pressure in the veins of the pelvis and legs. Pantyhose are therefore to be worn instead. Shoes with broad toes and low, flat, rubber heels are usually more comfortable at this time. The extra weight that the woman carries in front tends to disturb her sense of balance, and she is liable to trip and fall forward; low heels help to prevent this. However, if balance remains undisturbed and ordinary shoes with ordinary heels are comfortable, continue to use them.

Teeth

"For each child a tooth" was one of the commonest aphorisms about pregnancy. It is certainly no longer necessary, however, to consider teeth as coin in exchange for babies. The damage women suffered to their dentition with repeated pregnancy was almost certainly a consequence of nutritional inadequacy; if you eat adequate balanced meals you need have no concern.

It is wise to use pregnancy as an occasion for securing good dental care. I think you should go to the dentist early in pregnancy to find out whether there is any maintenance called for. Attention to small cavities at this time can very well save teeth. Since the enamel on the teeth is laid down long before pregnancy and is not part of the mobile body store of calcium, the calcium content of the diet is of no direct importance in the integrity of the teeth. It is, however, significant in the integrity of the cement substances that hold the teeth in place.

The gums in some patients have a tendency to overgrow in the presence of pregnancy; they become spongy in texture and bleed readily when the teeth are brushed. If you notice this change, you might try massaging the gums twice a day with dry sodium perborate or dry sodium bicarbonate (baking soda) liberally sprinkled on a finger. If this does not bring the bleeding under control you should consult your dentist.

Modern dental X-ray machines, combined with the extremely fast films that are used for dental X-rays, expose the patient's teeth to very small radiation doses. The radiation dose to the baby and reproductive organs a foot or more away is probably not even measurable. Your dentist will want to throw a lead apron over your abdomen for greater safety. There is certainly no harm from having dental X-rays taken under these circumstances. Furthermore, as far as I know, there is no problem with the use of local anesthesia for such dental surgery as may be necessary. If for some reason your dentist wishes to work under general anesthesia, it probably would be wise for you to request hospitalization and that the anesthetic be given by an accredited anesthesiologist.

Sexual Intercourse

The desire for intercourse, the libido, varies greatly from one woman to another in pregnancy. In most women it's unchanged, while some who have regarded intercourse only as a way of becoming pregnant and not as a source of love or gratification may have a marked drop in their libidinous drives. On the other hand, both sex interest and response may be markedly increased for those patients for whom contraception was a great nuisance. Occasionally, a pregnant woman develops an aversion to intercourse, perhaps because of some unexpressed fear that sexual activity might adversely affect the fetus. These reactions are by no means fixed and may be present at one stage of pregnancy and disappear in another.

So far as we know, orgasm during pregnancy has no adverse effects on either the mother or the fetus, although the induction of uterine contractions by orgasm may have transitory effects on fetal heart rate. However, there is concern about the hazard of such induced contractions in women who have a history of incompetent cervix or of premature labors.

In the absence of vaginal bleeding, ruptured membranes, or a history of repeated miscarriage, sexual intercourse is safe at any stage of pregnancy. Bleeding following coitus calls for examination. Unless some abnormality exists, abstinence during pregnancy is entirely a matter of choice by the partners.

Almost no information is available about the effects, if any, of masturbation or fellatio. Cunnilingus is dangerous if it is associated with blowing air into the vagina.

The positions of the couple during coitus may have to be modified on simple physical grounds as pregnancy progresses. There is no reason not to experiment with new positions. The vagina is ordinarily quite well lubricated during pregnancy; if there is difficulty or discomfort on penile entry, it would be well to consult professional advice.

Drugs

The best general rule is not to medicate yourself with potent drugs during pregnancy. A few common over-the-counter preparations are probably safe; these include mild analgesics, drugs for indigestion and heartburn, preparations for constipation, and for the relief of mild insomnia. The use of aspirin and acetaminophen (Tylenol) is discussed on page 78.

8

Diet during Pregnancy

Because most middle-class Americans consume a rich and wholesome diet, it may seem unnecessary for me to advise you on nutrition. Yet experience has taught me that the demands of pregnancy are not always met by a continuation of a woman's prepregnant diet. Furthermore, some patients will probably rely on multivitamins to make up for dietary inadequacies, when they should be relearning and practicing good eating habits. In addition, as I will discuss below, the latest thinking is to discard the emphasis that used to be placed on severely limiting weight gain during pregnancy and instead to advise ample nutrition and nearly complete disregard for limits of weight. So I have presumed to write a relatively brief essay on nutrition in pregnancy—introductory, elementary and, I hope, reassuring.

In the course of pregnancy you will be building another human being—on some occasions even more than one. To equip your body to do that, to nurture and deliver the baby and to feed it months thereafter, it is necessary to add new tissue. The first new additions are the tissues of the baby itself, the umbilical cord, the placenta, and the amniotic fluid. Second, there is the growth of those maternal organs directly involved in pregnancy, specifically the growth of the uterus, the enlargement of the breasts, and the addition of new breast tissue, and a considerable increase in the solid and fluid elements of the circulating blood. Besides all of this, there is the

143

fact that most pregnant women retain additional water in their tissues along with the necessary mineral salts. The addition of fat is a frequent but not a necessary part of the process.

The average weight gain during pregnancy over the whole period is in the neighborhood of twenty-four pounds. This is distributed as follows:

Baby	8.0 lbs.
Placenta	1.0 lb.
Amniotic fluid	2.0 lbs.
Growth of the uterus	2.0 lbs.
Growth of the breasts	1.5 lbs.
Increase in blood and fluid	3.5 lbs.
Total	18.0 lbs.

The additional six pounds consist of the retained fluid outside the circulating blood, and the stored body fat. The greatest portion of the body fat settles down in the lower abdomen, the hips, and the thighs.

Weight Gain in Pregnancy

Although it is possible to say that there is an average weight gain of twenty-four pounds, there is a tremendous range of gains among pregnant women. For one thing, among normal women the weight gain is proportional to the nonpregnant weight. Those with small frames can expect to gain less weight than women with large frames. Women with a personal or family tendency to put on fat readily are likely to do so in pregnancy. Women who have been slender all their lives can expect to maintain that pattern in pregnancy. For that reason, within the range of normal, we find women who have gained nothing or even lost a little weight during pregnancy, on up to women with amazingly large weight gains, without evidence of any long-range impact on their health. These changes may influence the weight of the newborn since, on the average, that weight is proportional to maternal weight gain. Also, we know that the outlook for a newborn infant is to an extent related to its birth weight and therefore maternal weight gain is directly correlated with newborn outcome. This is an oversimplification but a good guide as a general rule. The way in which this information is applied must be individualized but, put directly, the more weight you gain, the larger and healthier your newborn will be.

For most of the present century, especially in the United States, obstetricians believed that limitation of weight gain had two major benefits in pregnancy. One was that the newborns were smaller than they would otherwise be and therefore allowed an easier delivery. The other was the conclusion that restriction of weight gain reduced the incidence of hypertensive complications of pregnancy. The upshot of this was that for decades obstetricians in this country harassed patients about their gain in weight. I recall a woman in Baltimore in the 1940's in a clinic where the patients were weighed as they entered. Their weights were recorded on slips of paper which they then handed to the doctor who saw them for the prenatal visit. One of my junior staff members consulted me, very puzzled about a patient who had become so swollen late in pregnancy that her ankles had disappeared completely. She could no longer wear her shoes and her hands and face were puffed up; nevertheless her reported weight had not changed. I was just as puzzled about this as he was but then, on a hunch, I escorted the patient back to the scale and weighed her myself. It turned out that she weighed twenty-eight pounds more than what was written on the slip of paper. Confronted with this she readily confessed that it upset her a great deal to be chastised about her weight gain at every prenatal visit. She therefore came to the clinic with a slip of paper already prepared with a weight that seemed to her to be entirely reasonable.

The fallacy of the old weight-gain concepts has now been pretty effectively demonstrated. We know that the increase in fetal weight with increased maternal gain is not large enough to make a meaningful difference in the outcome of labor. But, more significantly, it is an abnormal accumulation of fluid and not an increase in body tissue that is the cause of weight gain related to pregnancy toxemia. Nevertheless, the impression in the public mind is not as yet entirely dissipated. I believe that some pregnant women are still being advised that it is proper that they gain a certain theoretical amount of weight, no more and no less.

Underweight and Obesity

It is clear that the chronically undernourished woman who has suffered a lifelong pattern of nutritional deprivation often delivers a relatively small baby that does not thrive as well as its appropriately nourished contemporary. I emphasize lifelong dietary deficiency. Apparently the pregnant woman carries the imprint of malnutrition experienced while she herself was a fetus, infant, and a child. The deficit persists through the present pregnancy and cannot be fully corrected by changes in her food intake at this time. In addition, this disadvantaged group of women carries the burden of other diseases of social deprivation such as an increased incidence of urinary tract infection and of toxemia of pregnancy. The conclusion from all this is that the weight gain for a particular pregnant woman relates to a number of factors: her prepregnant weight, her family history of weight gain, and her general state of health and well-being, to name a few.

The best evidence at present in regard to young people is that obesity by itself is not a health problem though it certainly may be a cosmetic issue. Women who start pregnancy substantially overweight have a tendency toward exaggerated weight gains during pregnancy, making their cosmetic problems even more severe. It seems to be reasonable to discuss appropriate diet plans for pregnancy with such patients and to explain to them that if they wish they can limit their weight gain during pregnancy without exposing their babies or themselves to harm. It is probably not wise to undertake strenuous dieting intended to achieve material weight reduction. It may be appropriate for obese women instead to restrict weight *gain*, which, in view of the inevitable increases in fetus, fluid, and uterus, may result in a net loss of maternal weight.

The rate of weight gain varies greatly from woman to woman. Because of the change in appetite combined with queasiness in early pregnancy, some women gain little weight in the first three or four months and then take off beautifully to get back to the average well before term. Other patients have a sense of euphoria in early pregnancy, gain a great deal of weight, and then level off. These variations are individual and personal and do not call for any particular changes in diet or nutrition.

The one thing that needs to be looked out for is sudden weight gain toward the end of pregnancy, since this generally represents abnormal accumulation of water, possibly heralding the appearance of pregnancy toxemia. This is a medical and not a nutritional problem. For a long time it was thought that such accumulation resulted from an excessive intake of salt in the diet. A number of well-done clinical experiments have demonstrated that this in fact is not the case and that pregnant women do not have any abnormality of their ability to dispose of extra salt. Indeed, clinical studies have been done in which pregnant women were deliberately fed excessive salt without the production of any pathological process. Their kidneys, being normal, managed to excrete the excessive salt gram for gram and their body economy was not altered.

Salt in the Diet

Eating an ordinary and not a specially prepared experimental diet, it is impossible for a pregnant woman to reduce her salt intake below what her body can retain. There is a considerable depot of salt in the water of the body, and the tissues are so arranged as to maintain a normal salt concentration. If you cut down your salt intake your kidneys will retain salt almost completely. The usual loss of salt in the urine comes to an end and thereafter salt can only be lost in perspiration. When a woman tries her best to eliminate salt from her diet, she ends up with food that is so terribly unpalatable that her caloric intake inevitably drops. This results in weight loss for the wrong reasons. Fortunately, most patients are unable to comply with significant salt reduction.

Except in a few serious metabolic disorders in which there is an abnormality of the kidneys or of the steroid hormones involved in salt metabolism, and in the rare patients in heart failure, restriction of dietary salt makes no difference in medical conditions in pregnancy.

Failure to Gain Weight

Four particular groups of patients require special attention in regard to failure to gain weight. One category includes depressed women who are simply not eating enough. If this cannot be solved by ordinary efforts at support, psychiatric attention is needed. Some of them are actually battered women, many of whom are reluctant or unable to deal with the reality of their situation.

A second group consists of women acutely malnourished in early pregnancy due to nausea and vomiting. This problem usually corrects itself without harm to mother or fetus.

Pregnant adolescents, perhaps accustomed to a diet of fast and junk food of little caloric merit, are a third group. For a while I taught prenatal care to a group of pregnant, single, high-school students in the Bronx. It was so arranged that this was an informal talk during their lunch hour. I was astonished to see what these students brought to eat—primarily snack foods and diet sodas. Clearly these young women needed more than an academic education if they were to be brought to a state of reasonably normal nutrition.

The final group consists of those mothers who, late in pregnancy, fail to gain the expected amount of weight. In the absence of incidental illness, this may reflect intrauterine delay of fetal growth. This calls for intensified study of fetal welfare to detect a cause and, if possible, to initiate corrective measures.

Elements of Nutrition

For a successful pregnancy, you will need to add calories to your diet. For the typical patient with average activity, this calls for a total intake of 2,200 to 2,400 calories. You can distribute these during the day in almost any way you find comfortable and convenient. If you are working vigorously out of doors, or exercising regularly, you will need a larger allotment. You can use the curve of your weight gain as a guide to whether or not your diet is adequate.

In addition, you need a distribution of the calorie sources among proteins, carbohydrates, and fats to be certain that you take in the full range of amino acids, minerals, and liquids on which proper nutrition depends. The animal protein group of foods—meat, fish, poultry, eggs, cheese, and milk—should supply three to four portions a day, and give you the full range of amino acids and minerals. You certainly do not need each kind of protein source each day; the attractiveness of the diet is enhanced by mixing them up.

A word of caution about cow's milk. Many adults lack the digestive enzyme (lactase) that converts lactose to simpler sugars, which are then easier to digest. When they drink milk these lactase-deficient people develop upper abdominal distress, gassiness, and ulcerations in the intestines. This not only interferes with their food intake but results in blood-loss anemia. These women are ill served by campaigns to persuade them to drink milk. The problem can be minimized by taking milk in fermented dairy products such as yogurt, cottage cheese, and sour cream. There is ample calcium in these foods as well as in meats in general, so that a pregnant woman need not drink milk except as a beverage. (I like to drink it myself.) One of the advantages of breast milk for babies is that it virtually never is a cause of the bad effects of lactose intolerance.

Next, you can enliven your diet with fruits and vegetables, which are the main natural source for most vitamins—certainly A, the B group, and C. Vitamin D comes principally from sunshine and fortified milk. E has no proven value in human nutrition. Vitamin K is given to us by our intestinal bacteria. Four to five servings in the fruit and vegetable group a day add calories and variety to the diet. During winter months, it is well to reinforce your diet with fruit juices, especially citrus, and with carrots and oranges.

The third and last general nutritional group includes cereals and bread and such farinaceous foods as noodles, rice, and spaghetti. These are also good calorie sources and provide a wide but incomplete range of amino acids. Several servings a day from this group are in order. They have the virtue of being more filling than the foods in the other two major groups. They do traditionally get the blame for unwanted weight gain, but in truth, they will add to your weight only what they add in calories.

If there is any question in your mind about the adequacy of your diet, probably the thing to do is write down everything you eat over three-day period, and the amount of each, and then compare your list with general recommendations such as those above or the much more detailed recommendation in books specifically on nutrition.

Many patients have been comfortable for years on a diet that does not include animal protein other than that provided by milk and eggs. They have no difficulty in meeting their need for an appropriate range of amino acids and remain very well nourished.

Problems occasionally arise among strict vegetarians who do not consume milk, milk products, or eggs. The legumes in this diet—mainly dried beans, peas, and lentils—are deficient in a number of amino acids, principally tryptophane and the amino acids containing sulphur. The nuts and seeds such as sunflower seeds, peanuts, and sesame seeds have substantial amounts of these amino acids but are deficient in lysine and isoleucine. It is therefore important for people on strict vegetarian diets to mix between these two groups in order to avoid developing serious amino acid deficiencies. Such patients might wish to consult the advice for such dietary control in a book entitled *Diet For a Small Planet* by Francis Moore Lappé.

Vitamins

Nutritional supplements have become a fixed feature of prenatal care in the United States. I myself am convinced that the ample middle-class American diet is so richly supplied in vitamins that it makes absolutely no sense for a middle-class woman to take vitamin supplements. Some researchers have even questioned whether taking excessive amounts of the fat-soluble vitamins A and D may not cause congenital anomalies. The kidneys can excrete excessive amounts of the water-soluble vitamins B, C, and K, but the immense overdoses of vitamin C urged by some of its enthusiasts have resulted in development of kidney stones and a tendency toward metabolic acidosis.

In any event, vitamin deficiency in pregnant women is almost unheard of as a separate condition and occurs only with dietary distortion of a considerable degree. I have seen one patient on a bizarre vegetarian diet, characterized by a huge excess of carrots, prescribed by a "naturopathic nutritional adviser." This woman had a strange discoloration of her skin, resulting from a combination of carotenemia, due to the carrots, and severe swelling, due to edema from marked protein deficiency. When we were able to persuade this woman to bring her diet closer to what was required for a normal pregnant adult these conditions rapidly cleared up. The only other vitamin-deficient patient I can recall was a farm wife in Minnesota. She was a patient who had had a long series of closely spaced pregnancies and whose diet during the entire winter, as she approached term again, consisted of small amounts of milk and meat, along with large quantities of home-canned vegetables. She was concerned about the safety of these vegetables and so she overheated her canning and completely destroyed the vitamin C. All this combined to give her a special kind of anemia associated with combined vitamin C and folic acid deficiency; this responded very rapidly to diagnosis and appropriate vitamin supplements. These exceptional cases are the only ones I have ever seen who had any verifiable need for vitamin medications.

Iron

On the other hand, most pregnant women require supplementary iron in the diet. There is a steady loss of iron in menstrual blood every month. When menses cease with the beginning of pregnancy, iron stores are often low. The pregnant woman's ability to absorb iron increases under the influence of hormones and she may be able to reestablish her iron stores to a normal level. If everything is ideal, this is probably sufficient. However, reliance on the body's ability—with normal nutrition—to replenish iron stores is not adequate for women who have had excess bleeding prior to pregnancy nor for the patients who have had a number of pregnancies close together. It is therefore appropriate to supplement the diet with iron. Certainly, in the second half of pregnancy when the fetal demands for iron have increased, this is essential.

The absorption of iron from the diet is enhanced by an adequate intake of vitamin C. This need not be in the form of ascorbic acid tablets but can be in the form of orange juice, grapefruit juice, and tomato juice. The amounts of iron that are included in multiple vitamin tablets are generally not sufficient to meet the needs of late pregnancy and I therefore advise patients to take iron as separate tablets. These come in several forms—ferrous sulfate, ferrous gluconate, and ferrous fumarate—and under various trade names. In some tablets these are combined with other dietary elements such as other minerals and folic acid. These additions probably are unnecessary and only help inflate the cost of the tablet. Since many patients develop distress after taking iron on an empty stomach, it is advisable that iron tablets be taken with meals. Many patients find that iron causes constipation. The goal is to take just enough iron to change the color of the stool. Excessive iron intake tends to make the stools dry and excessively firm. An occasional patient responds to iron with diarrhea, and under those circumstances the dietary intake should be reduced. What this amounts to is that you have to test yourself to see how much iron you can take comfortably.

It is important to remember to keep your iron tablets where small children cannot get them. One of the common forms of poisoning seen in pediatric emergency rooms comes from children eating their mothers' iron tablets.

Calcium

If you feel you need a calcium supplement, take it by chewing one or two Tums a day—the least expensive readily available form. This antacid consists entirely of calcium carbonate.

Avoidable Dietary Hazards

Some dietary elements probably should be avoided in pregnancy. These include food additives such as the nitrates and nitrites which are used for treating meat, and monosodium glutamate, which can produce what has been called Chineserestaurant disease. Some of the preservatives that are put into food products have unknown effects on the fetus and are best omitted from the diet. Ideally, if you have the time and can afford it, it is best to prepare your own fresh foods. You should read the label on the prepared foods so that you can reduce the number of possibly harmful artificial substances that you consume.

Caffeine has been incriminated in a number of adverse effects in pregnancy. When the studies have been carefully analyzed, however, it has turned out that the problems are due more to smoking. People who take in large quantities of caffeine tend also to be smokers and, when the data are corrected for smoking, the adverse effects attributed to the caffeine are reduced markedly. At the very least, however, caffeine is a stimulant and you might reflect on the extent to which you want to load your body with it. Caffeine also turns up in tea, chocolate, and cocoa; in some soda pop, and in such combined analgesic preparations as APCs, a mixture of aspirin, phenacetin, and caffeine.

Alcohol has been discussed elsewhere. At present, we simply do not know what constitutes a safe intake in pregnancy. Low levels of alcohol are almost certainly not harmful. The fluid intake of pregnant women in many of the nations of Western Europe includes modest quantities of alcohol, in the form of beer and wine.

Special Problems

Pica is the name for the craving for bizarre and unusual foods, some of which are not foods at all, but are nevertheless eaten by pregnant women afflicted with these strange appetites. The condition has often been made the subject of jokes about the yearning for odd combinations of foods, such as pickles and ice cream. In fact, however, pica usually goes along with severe iron deficiency in women with chronic malnutrition. These women eat substances like clay, laundry starch, or ashes in an attempt to fill their nutritional needs, and also—because they are constantly hungry—to take in enough bulk to fill their stomachs. It is a self-defeating effort, because filling the stomach with nonfoods both creates a physical obstacle to the ingestion of wholesome nutritious foods and interferes with their absorption.

Nausea and vomiting in early pregnancy may cause dehydration. Taking tea and fruit juices will replace the lost fluids. Small frequent meals of high protein content and a substantial amount of carbohydrates will help maintain caloric balance. You will find that it usually helps to avoid foods that are high in fats and which have strong odors. If these measures do not suffice, seek professional help.

Lactose intolerance already has been described. There are now available such preparations as Lactaid, which artificially provide the missing enzymes to convert lactose to readily absorbable breakdown products. It is probably better for patients who have lactose intolerance to avoid milk and milk products.

Constipation, a not infrequent complication of pregnancy, is sometimes alleviated by increased intake of liquids as well as bulk materials such as bran. Some preparations add bulk to the stools, a familiar one being Metamucil; they produce soft, bulky stools and thus alleviate the constipation. It is also likely to help if you increase the amount of raw fruits and vegetables in your diet. Chemical stool softeners are probably best avoided.

Specific Details and Special Diets

Many fine books on diet in pregnancy have been published in the last decade. *Eating For Two* by Isaac Cronin and Gail S. Brewer, is a good example. I suggest that you refer to one of these books if you wish to look further into more specific details on diet.

9

Complaints and Complications of Pregnancy

Minor Complaints

A pregnant woman is more prone to physical discomforts than the nonpregnant. Some of these are occasioned by pregnancy, others exaggerated by it.

Nausea and Vomiting

Since nausea and vomiting are usually mild, confined to the first few waking hours, and self-limited to six or eight weeks, they rarely require specific medication. Nevertheless, there are a few hints that may prove valuable even for those mildly affected.

Before going to bed, place a couple of dry, crisp crackers in a tin box on the bedside table. Upon awakening, eat the crackers without raising your head from the pillow and continue lying on your back for twenty minutes, then get up.

If washing your teeth on arising induces or exaggerates the queasiness, postpone that ritual until later in the day when your stomach feels settled; in the interim simply rinse your mouth.

If the nausea persists after the dry-cracker routine, ignore temporarily the diet rules in Chapter 8 and eat the following:

1. A light breakfast—for example, oatmeal (or a poached

or boiled egg); unbuttered toast with marmalade, jelly, or honey; and a cup of coffee or tea.

2. At midmorning, crackers, cake, or toast with a glass of milk or a cup of cocoa.

3. Luncheon, some broth or soup with crackers or toast; rice or a baked potato sprinkled with salt; a salad without oily dressing; and a roll or slice of toast.

4. Midafternoon, crackers, zweiback, or toast with a glass of fruit juice.

5. Dinner, lean meat or sea food; a green vegetable; baked, mashed, or boiled potato; salad; a dessert of ice cream, sherbet, or any other sweet you feel confident you can keep down; plus bread, toast, or crackers according to taste.

6. Before bed, crackers, cake, or toast with a glass of milk, a cup of cocoa, or a malted milkshake.

Additional fluids should be taken throughout the twenty-four hours. Over a short period fluids are more important to health than solids. Very often iced liquids are best tolerated. Many women in early pregnancy find plain water nauseating, but if a little lemon or orange juice is added it becomes drinkable. Almost all patients, no matter how nauseated, can take teaspoons of crushed ice flavored by fruit juice, which is a splendid source of fluids. The same may be said for sherbet or water ice, which makes an excellent midafternoon supplement; ginger ale and *non*-diet soft drinks are valuable drinks since they are rich in carbohydrates.

There are other aids besides diet. Your physician may prescribe a mild sedative such as phenobarbital, 30 mg three or four times a day, or 10 mg of Compazine in the same frequency. A difficulty with most medications for nausea is that some patients experience great relief and others note no effect at all. Going out into the air frequently makes you feel better. Don't feel sorry for yourself, keep occupied, and remember the condition is self-limited in duration and almost always a memory by the twelfth week. Keep going; if you have a job, continue working if possible. Carry some crisp salt crackers, graham crackers, or zweiback to munch if a wave of nausea strikes you while en route or on the job. Eat small amounts often, not much at one time, to prevent your stomach from becoming empty.

The nausea and vomiting of pregnancy usually do not clear up dramatically. Improvement is gradual, with the appearance of good days which soon gain the ascendancy over bad days, and then the bad days become fewer and fewer and finally disappear.

Sometimes, though rarely, a pregnant woman vomits severely enough to become seriously dehydrated and acidotic. The treatment for this is intravenous fluids: salts and glucose in water, given in amounts sufficient to restore body fluids. Sometimes this can be done on an ambulatory basis, but if facilities for out-patient treatment do not exist, the patient is hospitalized for the therapy. One indication for hospitalization is a marked concentration of the urine, together with a decrease in its amount. The patient will notice a deepening of the urine's usual yellow color and a stronger odor; laboratory tests will show the presence of acid bodies, formed when the body uses up its own fat to provide the calories that are not eaten or not retained.

The salts and glucose in intravenous feedings protect the liver and kidneys and provide calories. Water-soluble vitamins B_1, B_6, B_{12}, and C are added to the fluids to correct vitamin deficiencies. As soon as the patient feels equal to it, she can resume regular eating. Mild sedatives such as phenobarbital or Valium may be helpful in restoring appetite. Patients whose vomiting fails to respond to these simple measures and those who have suffered severe weight loss or stubborn acidosis will often benefit from psychiatric help in addition to the medical measures.

Heartburn

Heartburn, a fiery burning sensation in the chest, is frequently associated with the belching of small amounts of bitter, sour fluid. The name given to the disorder is a partial misnomer because the condition has nothing to do with the heart but results from a reflux of acid stomach juices into the lower esophagus. It may occur in anyone but is more common during pregnancy because of the upward displacement and compression of the stomach by the enlarged uterus and delayed emptying of the stomach. It is a type of indigestion. The omission from the diet of rich, greasy foods, such as mayonnaise, cream, and fried foods, or, in fact, any food that the woman learns by her own experience to associate with heartburn, helps, as do smaller and less hurried meals. Relief from heartburn may be gotten by taking a level teaspoonful of milk of magnesia or a milk of magnesia tablet after each meal and again whenever heartburn occurs. If this should cause loose stools substitute other antacids such as Amphojel, Gelusil, Rolaids, Tums, or Maalox. Some are in tablet or liquid form, others in both. Chewing gum after meals lessens heartburn for some.

Excessive Salivation (Ptyalism)

This uncommon complaint, caused by excessive secretion of the salivary glands, is very annoying and difficult to cure. The secretion of saliva virtually floods the mouth and is so profuse that the woman cannot manage to swallow all of it, so she must continually expectorate. Ptyalism is often accompanied by a foul taste, which some patients find can be relieved by sucking peppermints or chewing gum. Small daily doses of a mild sedative such as phenobarbital may diminish the ptyalism. The condition, which frequently persists throughout pregnancy, tends to diminish in its latter half and always disappears promptly with delivery.

Constipation

Some women become constipated only when pregnant, and others prone to constipation find that pregnancy increases the difficulty. The condition results from physiologic changes occurring normally as the effect of pregnancy: decreased contractions of the intestinal tract and diminished expulsive ability of the overstretched abdominal muscles. The hazards of constipation are greatly overrated in the public mind, probably in part from the emphasis on a daily bowel movement in pharmaceutical advertising in all popular media of communication. There is no evidence of harm resulting to the patient who does not have a daily movement, except the harm which her propaganda-fixed mind imagines.

The following regimen will minimize constipation.

1. Take a moderate amount of physical exercise.

2. Keep up your fluid intake.

3. Eat a coarse cereal such as oatmeal for breakfast, and have whole-wheat bread in place of white bread. Also eat freely of salads and leafy vegetables.

4. Take some fruit at night before going to bed. Certain fruits are especially efficacious, notably prunes, apples, figs, dates, and raisins.

5. Licorice candy has a mild cathartic action; take advantage of this property.

6. Try to develop the habit of a regular visit to the bathroom at the same hour each day, preferably after breakfast. This is the best preventative against constipation in pregnancy. A stool reflex should be established on the basis of habit.

7. Refrain from excessive straining while at stool.

If necessary a mild laxative such as milk of magnesia, which is not absorbed from the intestinal tract, may be employed. Dulcolax is another safe contact laxative, taken either as oral pills or as a rectal suppository. Medications such as Colace and Doxinate, which cause the stool to absorb water and therefore to remain softer, may be taken daily. Rectal suppositories of glycerine can also be used freely. Occasional small enemas may be helpful, particularly when the stools are very hard and dry, but it would be wise to get professional advice before taking enemas. Another useful method is to take one of the natural-fiber laxatives such as psyllium hydrophilic mucilloid, marketed as Metamucil and under other trade names. It is not absorbed from the large intestine but retains a good deal of water, so that the stools become soft and bulky and are readily defecated.

Flatulence

Distention of the stomach and intestines by gas, resulting in a bloated feeling and the frequent need to pass flatus, is a common complaint during pregnancy. Avoidance of gas-producing foods such as beans, parsnips, corn, onions, cabbage, fried foods, and sweet desserts may help, but this condition is more a nuisance than a real disease.

Hemorrhoids (Piles)

As pregnancy advances, the veins at the anal opening become enlarged by the gradually increasing pressure within the venous system of the lower half of the body. Hard bowel movements and straining at stool have a tendency to cause these veins to protrude through the anal opening and to cause local pain, bleeding, and itching. The best treatment is the prevention of constipation through employment of the measures listed under that heading. If there is slight rectal bleeding without pain or a bulging lump, it is usually sufficient to apply cold cream to the anus with the finger on arising, before bedtime, and after each defecation. If this does not cause the rectal bleeding to stop within forty-eight hours, notify your medical attendant.

If there is a tender, swollen mass protruding through the anus, you should attempt to reduce it with a well-lubricated finger after sitting for several minutes in a tub of comfortably warm water. When this is unsuccessful, lie on your back with the hips slightly elevated and apply to the anal region a wash-cloth or piece of cotton that has been soaked in iced water— or, better yet, iced witch hazel. Change the dressing frequently so that it remains moist and cold. This may shrink the hemorrhoidal mass sufficiently to permit its reposition. If the pain does not subside with this regimen, an anesthetic ointment such as Nupercainal can be applied to the area, or medicated suppositories such as Anusol may be inserted.

Occasionally a painful clot occurs in one of the protruding small branches of the hemorrhoidal vein (thrombosed hemorrhoid). Immediate relief follows incision under local anesthesia and evacuation of the small clot. It is inadvisable to undergo a radical operation for hemorrhoids either during pregnancy or at the time of delivery, since even the severe ones may disappear soon after labor.

Varicose Veins

Varicose veins are common during pregnancy because of normal physiological effects that cannot be controlled. Heredity also plays a role; there is a familial tendency toward the occurrence of varicosities that may be inherited from either parent. According to two different studies varicosities were present in 11 percent of pregnant women in one group and 20 percent in the other. Varicose veins first appeared as early as the second month in one-fourth of the cases and as late as the fifth month in one-fifth of those developing them.

In susceptible women varicosities are likely to be noted in a first or second pregnancy and tend to reappear earlier in the next pregnancy. Each succeeding pregnancy makes them worse. Fortunately the enlarged veins regress between pregnancies; with the first few pregnancies, after their initial appearance, almost completely, but only partially after later pregnancies. The vessels first involved are most frequently on the inner aspect of the calf, but the process may begin in the space behind the knee or on the thigh, and may involve one leg or both. In the early stages the veins may appear as a spidery network of superficial blood vessels, but when more advanced they stand out as straight, tortuous, or knotted, soft blue cords just beneath the skin. A less common site is the outer vaginal region.

Varicose veins may cause either no symptoms or considerable discomfort. Once the veins become large, a feeling of "heaviness" and fatigue may occur. A dull ache is not infrequent. True pain is only met if the vein becomes inflamed.

If varicose veins develop during pregnancy, several measures may help:

1. Do not stand if you can sit and, when you sit, sit with your legs elevated so that your heels are above the level of the hips. Do not sit if you can lie down, and, when you lie, lie with your legs raised on a pillow.

2. Elastic Ace bandages can be used to compress all varices from the time they appear until several days after delivery. They are worn from the toe to the knee for varices involving the lower leg. With enlarged thigh veins a second elastic ban-

dage is wound from the knee upward. If there is swelling of the leg the elastic bandage is applied in the morning before arising. This will necessitate bathing or showering the night before. If there is no swelling the bandage can be applied in the sitting position.

Elastic stockings are probably preferable to even the four-inch elastic bandage. Two available types are marketed over the counter, in a variety of lengths and sizes, as Teds and as Bauer and Black therapeutic hosiery. Shorter stockings can be used for varicosities limited to the calf, and longer ones are used if the varicosities extend up into the thigh. A more effective type of stocking is sold under the name of Jobst. This stocking requires individual measurements and construction and is substantially more expensive. The amount of bother and expense you wish to go to obviously will be related to the severity of your symptoms. The varicose veins themselves are no material threat to health.

3. Every few hours the pregnant woman with leg varicosities should elevate her legs for several minutes while sitting or lying down, if possible. When standing she should encourage the blood flow by rising up on her tiptoes frequently. When sitting, if it is impossible to elevate the legs, the feet and toes should be flexed and extended frequently for the same reason.

Sometimes there are large varicosities in the labia of the vulva. These may give sensations of fullness or heaviness in this area, but once again are no threat to health. I once encountered a tear in such a vein at the time of delivery. It bled profusely, but as the disrupted area was on the surface of the vulva it was the matter of but a moment to clamp it and sew it closed.

Varicose veins can be treated by injections and surgical removal, but it is inadvisable to undertake such therapy during pregnancy. Varicosities almost always recede dramatically after delivery and may not need further care.

Nosebleeds and Nasal Congestion

Nosebleeds are common during pregnancy, particularly during the winter months. Since ordinarily they are brief, they rarely present a serious problem. Usually they result from a drying and crusting of the membrane lining the nasal cavity, a membrane that temporarily has a greatly increased blood supply. If you have nosebleeds, lubricate the nasal cavity by instilling night and morning a few drops of a .25-percent solution of menthol in white oil, with an eyedropper, in both nostrils. Then tip your head back so the medicine runs into your throat, and spit it out. Almost certainly this will stop the nosebleeds; if not, notify your medical attendant.

Frequently, throughout pregnancy, the pregnant woman feels as though her nose is swollen by a perpetual cold which interferes with breathing. Doctors have a specific name for it, allergic rhinitis of pregnancy, but they do not have an equally specific cure. Vasoconstrictor nose drops such as Neosynephrine or Privine, sprays, and inhalers or Sudafed tablets produce temporary relief but should be used seldom and sparingly; their excessive use succeeds in making the condition worse. As with almost all the evils mentioned in this chapter, there is a cheerful addendum; allergic rhinitis clears up with delivery.

Leg Cramps

Spasm of the calf muscles and muscles of the foot is a common and painful nuisance during pregnancy. The condition is likely to begin about mid-pregnancy, but is usually less frequent the last month. It comes unannounced; most often the patient is aroused from her sleep to find the calf muscles of one leg knotted into a painful, firm ball. The best treatment is local massage, a kneading of the muscle until it relaxes.

The area may remain tender for several hours thereafter. Such muscle spasm is not damaging, nor does it denote any abnormality of health. It is not related to milk or calcium intake in any direct way.

Swelling of the Ankles and Legs

About one-quarter of the normal weight gain during pregnancy results from an increase in the amount of water held by the tissues. This excess fluid tends to pool into the dependent part of the body, so that the feet and ankles first show evidence of it. Many normal pregnant patients complain of swelling of the ankles, the lower legs, and the feet toward the end of the day. This is aggravated by periods of standing and is materially worse in warm weather. A patient with these symptoms should elevate her feet whenever possible during the day—prop them on a chair or bench, or stretch out on the bed or sofa. Larger shoes may have to be worn in late pregnancy to allow for the swelling of the feet. If the feet have a tight feeling and burn, immersing them in cold water gives relief. Ordinarily the swelling of the leg and foot subsides during the night, and by morning the normal contours of the ankle are visible once again.

The fingers are the next commonest site of pregnancy tissue swelling, which causes them to feel stiff. Frequently the puffiness of the fingers makes rings uncomfortably tight, and they may be difficult to remove. If so, soak the hand in cold water; then hold the finger pointing upward and soap the finger and ring before attempting to remove it.

Swelling of the face may normally occur to a limited extent, causing features to look relatively thick and gross. If, however, there is marked accumulation of fluid in the face, particularly around the eyes, so that they become puffy and the eyelids only open with difficulty, this is probably an early sign of toxemia of pregnancy. It must be brought to the attention of the professionals who are helping you in pregnancy care.

Frequency of Urination

Many patients experience increased frequency of the urge to urinate both at the beginning and the end of pregnancy. The sensation in early pregnancy most likely results from the hormone-induced increase in local blood flow in the pelvis. The perceived fullness results in the sensation of needing to empty the bladder.

The cause toward the end of pregnancy is somewhat different, being related to the marked increase in the circulating blood volume that occurs as pregnancy proceeds. Thanks to gravity, fluid accumulates in the legs during the day. The enlarging uterine mass tends to increase the blood pressure in the veins below the waist even further. When you lie down, putting your legs at approximately the same level as your heart, the gravitational effect is reversed. Water flows back out of the legs into the general circulation. If, in addition, you rest on one side or the other, so that the weight of the uterus on the abdominal blood vessels is removed, movement of water out of the lower half of the body will be even greater. The kidneys promptly respond by increasing the rate at which they form urine and therefore, some hours after you have stretched out, you may find that your bladder is filling up rapidly. Consequently, when you get up in the morning your ankles will have reappeared, the water having run out of your legs much as it pours out of a pitcher when the pitcher is tipped.

You may be able to reduce the number of times you have to get up at night by limiting fluid intake after the late afternoon and by lying down while you are still awake in the early evening, so that you can eliminate some of the extra water before going to bed.

Painful Contractions

The uterus, like all smooth muscle structures, is constantly alternating between a phase of contraction and a phase of relaxation. This begins before you are born, but is not noticeable to you until the middle of pregnancy, when you may feel a hard lump in your lower abdomen which remains for thirty seconds and disappears, to reappear ten or fifteen minutes later. Such contractions ordinarily are not painful. However, in some women—rarely in a first pregnancy—these contractions become painful at times during the late months. Such painful contractions, false pains, are difficult to differentiate from true labor. We have noted that a change of position often stops the false type of painful contractions, so, if you are lying down, stand and walk about; if you are standing or sitting, lie down. Also, true labor pains gradually get closer together and harder. Then, too, true labor pains may or may not be accompanied by a show of blood, whereas false pains never are. If a bout of painful contractions begins during the night and you think this may not be true labor, take a teaspoonful of paregoric; if the pains are false, you will probably soon drop back to sleep, but if they are the contractions of true labor, the teaspoon of paregoric will not stop them. In many states paregoric is a prescription drug and therefore if you don't have it in your medicine chest you will have to get your doctor to prescribe it.

Faintness

A tendency to light-headedness and even fainting may occur at any time during pregnancy. Sitting, standing, or lying flat on your back for too long may result in a drop in the return of blood to the heart and therefore a period of inadequate supply of blood to the brain. This accounts for brief periods of dizziness when you sit up suddenly from lying down flat.

I recall one pregnant woman who did a great deal of desk work and frequently felt faint. She eventually realized that this happened when she sat at her desk in one position for long periods of time. She learned to correct this by getting up briefly, walking around, and doing a few deep knee bends at regular intervals. At any time when you feel faint during pregnancy the ideal thing to do is either to sit down with your head between your knees or to stretch out on your side. As a backup, in case you cannot do either of these things, you might want to carry a small bottle of smelling salts with you and employ it as soon as you feel the faintness coming on.

Backache

Increased production of the hormone relaxin, now pretty well shown to occur in normal pregnancy, may have some connection with backache. In pregnant laboratory animals, relaxin causes a loosening of the joints of the pelvis, providing additional space for the birth of the young. In pregnant women there may be, on rare occasions, a loosening of the pubic joint, at the place where the bones of the pelvis join together in the region behind the sexual hair. When this happens, the patient feels discomfort at the joint and in the low back, and may have to walk with a waddling gait.

Backache itself is a very common complaint, however. The most likely explanation for this is the usual posture in pregnancy, with the woman leaning backward to counterbalance the weight of her pregnant uterus up front. This puts an unaccustomed strain on muscles and produces a sense of fatigue and a discomfort on the low back. Women who are accustomed to moderate physical exercise and therefore have good muscle tone are less likely to experience this discomfort.

Massage and heat often provide welcome relief for the tired or aching back of pregnancy. Rubbing liniment applied with the palm of the hand to the back is particularly excellent, but one must be careful not to apply heat over freshly applied liniment lest it blister the skin. Pain from a herniated disc occurs in pregnant women with about the same frequency as in the nonpregnant.

Insomnia

Despite the increasing fatigue and the desire for additional rest that most women experience in the last trimester, sleep may be seriously disturbed by the nocturnal athletic pursuits of the fetus, plus inability of the mother to get into a comfortable position. This is particularly distressing in the heat of midsummer and may be aided by an air-conditioned bedroom. A relaxing bath before bed may be helpful. If the insomnia is severe and causes you concern, discuss it with your physician or midwife.

A sleep-producing medicine may be prescribed. When my patients have trouble falling asleep I advise them to take the sleeping medicine about an hour before they are ready to go to bed. On the other hand if they find that they can fall asleep easily but wake up after a few hours and then cannot resume sleeping I suggest that they take the sleep medicine just before going to bed.

Many patients ask if sleep medicines will affect the baby. All these drugs cross the placenta and have a tendency to quiet the baby as well as the mother. They do not alter placental efficiency, however, and thus have no lasting effect. Examples of drugs that are frequently used to produce sleep are barbiturates (Seconal and Nembutal) and benzodiazapines (Dalmane, Ativan, and Restoril); this does not exhaust the list.

If a patient seems to be having difficulty sleeping principally because she is tense, I am inclined to recommend some wine or a glass of sherry in the late evening to take advantage of the soporific effect of small doses of alcohol. I do warn patients not to take any drugs uninterruptedly, simply because it is possible to develop a dependence on them for sleeping and in that event they are likely to diminish rapidly in their effectiveness.

Vaginal Discharge (Leukorrhea)

A certain amount of pale yellow, thin vaginal discharge is normal for pregnancy, resulting from the increased activity of the cervical glands. Usually bathing with the liberal use of a soft washcloth is sufficient to take care of the problem. If the discharge becomes very profuse and thick and is associated with vaginal itching, consult your doctor promptly. Occasionally the leukorrhea is the result of a vaginal infection with a troublesome parasite called a trichomonad, or with a yeastlike fungus that has the poetic-sounding name of *Candida albicans*.

The trichomonads may enter the vagina from the patient's own intestinal tract or be transmitted to her by her sexual partner. The diagnosis can be readily made by a pelvic examination. Trichomonas vaginitis has a characteristic appearance and when a drop of the vaginal discharge is looked at under the microscope it is possible to see the helter-skelter movement of this protozoan. The treatment for this is metronidazole (Flagyl, Protostat) in a dose of two grams, to be taken by mouth in a single day. Since it is common for a couple to pass this infestation back and forth between them it is advisable for the patient's partner to be treated at the same time. The use of a condom is also helpful. A follow-up examination at an appropriate interval is desirable even if symptoms have subsided, to be certain that the parasite is gone.

Like most effective drugs, metronidazole can have side effects. It may, for example, be associated with abdominal discomfort after drinking alcoholic beverages. Concern that it might cause congenital anomalies has been expressed, but there is no acceptable evidence for this, and, in any event, this cannot occur past the end of the first trimester. The drug has been shown to produce mutations in bacteria and cancer in mice if given to the mice over long periods in large doses. We have no evidence of such effects in humans, to whom the drug is given in much smaller doses for brief periods. As metronidazole is overwhelmingly the most effective treatment for trichomoniasis, it may be prescribed when the diagnosis is confirmed; of course the patient should be informed of the possibility of annoying side effects.

In pregnancy the vagina offers an unusually hospitable environment for the yeast monilia (*Candida albicans*). Throughout pregnancy the vagina is rich in glycogen, on which the Candida readily thrive. The discharge with moniliasis (*Candidiasis*) is generally found in clumps, sitting on somewhat inflamed areas of vaginal mucosa and looking a bit like cottage cheese. The clumps can be also studied under the microscope and a diagnosis made. It is also possible to grow the organisms on suitable culture media to get absolute proof. If such investigation shows Candida to be the cause of the vaginal discharge, a fungicide such as nystatin (Mycostatin), miconazole (Monistat) or clotrinazole (Lotrimin) can be prescribed for vaginal insertion at bedtime for several days. Candidiasis has a tendency to recur during pregnancy and therefore treatment may have to be repeated on several occasions. When the pregnancy ends, the chemical environment of the vagina changes and the complaint tends to subside. If no diagnosis is obvious when the patient is seen, immediate relief of the itching can often be obtained by the application of plain yogurt to the labia and lower vagina, thereby giving the patient some respite while awaiting specific diagnosis.

Shortness of Breath

In part because of the raised diaphragm from heightened pressure within the abdomen, and in part because of increased weight, shortness of breath is common in pregnancy, especially during the last two months. In many, particularly in those with first pregnancies, decided relief may occur a few weeks before confinement, when the summit of the uterus drops two or three inches as the baby's head descends part way into the opening of the bony pelvis. If the shortness of breath interferes with sleep, the head and shoulders should be propped up by several pillows to a semisitting posture. If you find that you are markedly short of breath in climbing stairs and have to stop several times before getting to the top, or if sleep is difficult no matter how high you are propped up, you should report it promptly to your obstetrical attendant.

Skin Rash

Pregnant women are subject to the same kind of annoying but trivial skin rashes as anyone else. They are generally of no significance. Some may be due to mechanical problems. Stout women with heavy breasts tend to develop skin rashes beneath the breasts or in the groins. This is particularly common in warm humid weather, and is caused by an accumulation of perspiration. The best treatment for this is cleansing and drying the area by dusting it with cornstarch.

In the last few years, a new condition has been described, with the extraordinary name of PUPPP. These initials stand for Pruritic Urticarial Papules and Plaques of Pregnancy. PUPPP occurs predominantly among women having their first children. Small red elevated patches appear and tend to run together to form larger itching areas. Surprisingly, although patients have difficulty refraining from scratching, loss of the top layers of the skin is unusual. The plaques begin ordinarily on the skin of the abdomen and in about half the cases are limited to the area directly around the navel. They may also be distributed over the buttocks, the hips, the thighs, and the upper inner arms. The face is ordinarily spared. There are no known maternal or fetal complications from PUPPP. It has not tended to recur in women in a follow-up of at least six years, nor has it reappeared in later pregnancies or when the patients take oral contraceptives. The syndrome is only a nuisance as far as we know. It responds to the local administration of corticoids, the drugs which are related to the hormonal secretions of the adrenal cortex. With severe symptoms the systemic administration of corticoids has been tried, with relief in a limited number of patients.

There are other diffuse rashes that occur in pregnancy, but they are in no way different from those occurring in the non-pregnant state.

Pregnancy Moods

Any pregnancy is a major event in the life of a woman. The problems and rewards are well known. You may experience wide mood swings, ranging from depression to euphoria. Most of these are temporary; if they persist you may need help. Generally it is best to share your concern with the members of your personal support system. Professional assistance is as rule not necessary unless a mood becomes fixed. It is comforting, however, to exchange experiences with other pregnant women as you will be able to do in childbirth education classes or even sitting in the office of your doctor, midwife, or clinic.

What to Do in Case of a Fall or Accident

First discover whether you have injured yourself. Determining this does not differ from doing so when you are not pregnant. Do you hurt? Are you bleeding from any wounds? Are your movements restricted? If these three questions are answered in the negative, you are probably uninjured—yet if you are in doubt, seek professional advice at once. Next, turn your attention to the pregnancy. If there is no vaginal bleeding and the fetus continues to move, pregnancy was unaffected. If you are too early in pregnancy to have felt fetal movements, the only criterion regarding the status of the pregnancy will be vaginal bleeding. The fetus is so perfectly protected by the cushioning fluid surrounding it and the veritable shock absorbers built in the uterus that only rarely does even the most direct blow disturb either the infant or the fortress in which it is ensconced.

Occasional Complications

Complications may arise during pregnancy that are peculiar and specific to the pregnant state. They are uncommon, and your mathematical chances of developing any one are slim—in fact, so slim that the odds are better than you would get on a long shot at the race track. Be additionally reassured by the knowledge that by now, there are very few obstetrical problems that we cannot safely resolve.

Pregnancy in the Tube (Ectopic)

There is much concern over the striking increase in the past few years in the incidence of pregnancies outside the uterus. All these are referred to as ectopic, which means that the pregnancy is not in the uterine cavity. Most such pregnancies occur in the fallopian tubes, and are therefore referred to as tubal pregnancies, but they can also occur in the ovary and the peritoneal cavity.

The increased incidence has been noted all over the United States and apparently in all social groups. We do not know why this is the case. Can it be that there has been an increase in pelvic inflammatory disease, one of the known causes of tubal pregnancy? Can it be due to the late aftereffects of the subtle pelvic infections related to intrauterine devices? Is it in some way related to the increased average age of pregnant women? The facts are not yet in.

At present, among women twenty-five to thirty-four years old, the annual rate of ectopic pregnancies is 10.3 per 10,000. For those between fifteen and twenty-four the rate is 5.2, and for women over thirty-five, 2.8. However, after correcting for the known differences in fertility rates among these age groups, we find that for women over thirty-five there are 15.2 ectopics for every 1,000 pregnancies; the rate from twenty-five to thirty-four is 9.7, and from fifteen to twenty-four, 4.5 The overall rate in the population is 6.4 ectopic pregnancies for every 1,000 pregnancies among white women and 10.1 for every 1,000 among black women. As will be described later, ectopic pregnancy can be a catastrophic event associated with massive hemorrhage. Improvement in care has reduced the mortality rate to less than 1 death for every 1,000 cases of ectopic pregnancy. Nevertheless, in recent statistics from New York City, ectopic pregnancy accounts for somewhere between 12 and 15 percent of all deaths of women due to pregnancy. The death rate among black women is disproportionately greater than among white women.

How does ectopic pregnancy come about? The sperm meets the egg and formation of an embryo proceeds to the point where it is a tiny hollowed-out ball of cells. This growth takes place in the fallopian tube. The interior of the tube is a complex labyrinth with many folds in its lining. It is not surprising that an occasional embryo loses its way, becomes stuck in the maze, and makes efforts to implant there. However, the association of ectopic pregnancy with previous tubal infection makes it likely that adhesions among the folds of the lining of the tube, due to the infection, create pockets in which the embryo is trapped. It may also be that patches of endometriosis (cells that normally form the lining of the uterus but growing in other locations) in the lining of the tube provide an attractive area for premature implantation during the normal passage of the embryo through the tube.

Whatever the reason, the embryo tries to implant in this unsuitable location. It immediately begins to form hCG (see page 11), which gets into the mother's circulation and signals to the ovary that a pregnancy is under way. At the site of implantation the embryo produces estrogen and progesterone, which together cause an increase in the local blood supply. As the placenta burrows into the tubal wall, it seeks and invades these blood vessels, causing local hemorrhage, and the placenta itself frequently is thereby damaged and dislodged. Neither the lining of the tube nor its muscular wall is adapted for maintaining a pregnancy. The blood supply is inadequate and the wall too thin. As a consequence, an occasional tubal pregnancy will burst through the wall of the tube and implant itself secondarily elsewhere on a surface within the peritoneal cavity. These surfaces are also ill suited for maintenance of a normal pregnancy.

Ectopic pregnancies are thus not normally supplied with blood or placental exchange, and there is a very high incidence of embryonic defect and consequent death of the embryo. There is reason to believe that some ectopic pregnancies actually cure themselves as a consequence of such embryonic death. It is the rarest of the rare for an ectopic pregnancy to continue to the point at which the fetus might survive.

There are no early symptoms of ectopic pregnancy, with the possible exception that there may be irregular bleeding rather than the complete cessation of menses noted with a normal pregnancy. A number of ectopic pregnancies are now being diagnosed at the time of elective early abortion when it is noted that the material removed from the uterus does not contain any embryonic tissue.

As the ectopic pregnancy grows and distends the tube or bleeds into its walls, the patient may have discomfort on one side of the lower abdomen, along with some of the vague sensations of early pregnancy. If the process continues these discomforts become greater, though they are not necessarily constant. During episodes of internal bleeding from the tube there may be severe cramping pain. If any substantial amount of blood gets into the peritoneal cavity the patient may notice urgency to urinate or defecate due to irritation of the rectum and the bladder by the blood on their internal walls. This much bleeding is ordinarily associated with dizziness and fainting, symptoms that are frequently seen in advanced ectopic pregnancies.

Diagnosis of Ectopic Pregnancy

The diagnosis of ectopic pregnancy has been immensely improved in the past decade by the combination of the blood test for hCG with early pelvic sonography. As has been mentioned, the early embryo can be seen by sonography. If it is found outside the uterus at the same time that the uterus is seen to be empty, a presumptive diagnosis of ectopic pregnancy can be made.

Because ectopic implantation is in tissues unsuited for a pregnancy, the concentration of hCG does not rise at the rate anticipated with a normal pregnancy. The hormone is then found in the mother's blood at a lower concentration than the duration of pregnancy would suggest. When there is bleeding into the peritoneal cavity from tubal abortion, this can be demonstrated by what is known as culdocentesis. The corner of the vagina behind the cervix is directly opposite a pouch of the peritoneal cavity, which comes down behind the uterus and in front of the rectum. This is known as the cul-de-sac, and also as the pouch of Douglas. Using a needle similar to the one used to draw blood from the arm, it is possible to puncture this corner of the vagina and attempt to suck fluid up out of the cul-de-sac. If one obtains free-flowing nonclotting blood, the diagnosis of intraperitoneal hemorrhage is established. This, combined with other compatible findings, will make clear that the correct diagnosis is ectopic pregnancy. The proper management is surgical exploration to find the source, stop the internal bleeding, and remove the embryo.

If the findings are not quite so clear-cut, it is possible to view the pelvic structures by laparoscopy unless the patient has adhesions caused by severe prior infections. Using laparoscopy, ectopic pregnancy can then usually be ruled in or out by direct vision.

The great advantage of combining a determination of serum hCG and sonography is that it allows the diagnosis of the majority of cases of ectopic pregnancy by noninvasive means, that is, without laparoscopy.

Treatment of Ectopic Pregnancy

As has been stated, the treatment of ectopic pregnancy is surgical. If there has been severe hemorrhage into the peritoneal cavity the surgeon must first clamp off the blood vessels leading to the area of the ectopic pregnancy to stop the blood loss. This involves at least removing some or all of the fallopian tube and, if the ovary is involved in the process, perhaps the ovary on that side as well.

If the pregnancy is found quite early and is out in the tip of the tube, it is sometimes possible to milk the embryo out of the tube without disrupting the tube itself. There is not as yet complete agreement as to what to do if an unruptured ectopic pregnancy is found along the course of the tube. Some surgeons recommend that the involved segment of tube be removed and that the two cut ends of the tube be immediately rejoined. Others recommend either splitting the tube lengthwise to remove the embryo, or removing the involved segment of the tube, leaving the cut ends free for a later operation intended to reunite them to reestablish continuity (known as tubal reanastomosis).

When hemorrhage has been quite severe it is ordinarily necessary also to treat the patient with blood transfusion.

What of the future? Approximately 15 percent of subsequent pregnancies in women who have had ectopics are again ectopic. This is true whether they have had the previously affected tube repaired or removed. We are more successful at restoring tubal continuity than in achieving term pregnancies. When a patient has had two or more ectopic pregnancies her chances of ever having a term pregnancy are less than 50 percent no matter what efforts have been made to retain tubal continuity.

With a high index of suspicion and early diagnosis, the risks to the patient, should a repetition of ectopic pregnancy occur, are not very great. The decision whether to risk another pregnancy after an ectopic has to be personal. At present, patients with destruction of both tubes, for whatever reason, can only turn to *in vitro* fertilization or embryo donation.

Placenta Previa and Premature Separation of the Placenta (Abruptio)

These conditions are relatively infrequent, and each happens about once in two hundred pregnancies. They usually occur in the last trimester, and the predominant symptom in both is vaginal hemorrhage. In placenta previa, the placenta, instead of being at the top of the uterus, is situated low down, and part of it overlaps the mouth of the womb (internal os). The uterus is shaped like a large inverted bottle, and ordinarily the placenta is implanted high up inside the bottle, usually on the back of the bottle, less often on the front. In the case of placenta previa, however, it is situated so low down that part, or all, of the round opening from which the cervix arises is covered by it. Late in pregnancy, preparatory to the onset of labor, the cervix expands slightly and any placental tissue that overlies it is torn loose from that part of the uterine lining to which it is attached, leaving a raw area from which the patient bleeds. The more completely the cervix is covered, the earlier in pregnancy is the bleeding likely to commence. There are three types of placenta previa, depending on whether the placenta covers all of the cervical opening in the lowermost part of the uterus (central placenta previa), only a part of the opening (partial placenta previa), or only the edge (marginal placenta previa). The relative frequency of the three is 20 percent, 25 percent, and 55 percent respectively. Placenta previa is uncommon in a first pregnancy and increasingly more common with additional gestations, the rate rising from 2.5 per 1,000 first births to 8 per 1,000 for eighth births. As women grow older they are more likely to have a placenta previa, not solely due to the fact that they are likely to have had a larger number of children. Placenta previa is also more common in women who have had a previous cesarean.

Every patient who bleeds in the latter half of pregnancy merits prompt hospitalization. If this bleeding is simply staining and if, for example, it follows intercourse, then no more need be done than a speculum examination. Late in pregnancy, a small amount of bleeding associated with mucus is more likely to be the bloody show of the onset of labor than anything of serious consequence. However, if the patient has painless bleeding that produces clots, it is very likely that she should be hospitalized.

The first step after hospitalization consists of accurate recording of the amount of bleeding and a careful estimate of the state of the patient's circulation. The circulating blood volume in a pregnant woman is considerably increased and she will therefore tolerate amounts of bleeding that would produce serious difficulty in a nonpregnant adult. If signs of hypovolemia (insufficient blood in the vascular system) are present, it is important immediately to start intravenous fluid administration with the expectation of adding blood transfusion. The patient should also be put to bed, so as to decrease the blood pressure at the placental site. It is the mother and not the fetus who is bleeding. Fetal welfare therefore depends on the efficiency of the mother's circulation.

If bleeding persists at a rapid rate, steps must be taken to deliver the fetus so as to protect it and the mother. If, on the other hand, the bleeding slows down there is time to locate the placenta with sonography. Under the circumstances described this will ordinarily very rapidly confirm the diagnosis of placenta previa. In the rare instances when the placenta is found to be in the upper uterus it is necessary to reconsider the diagnosis.

Neonatal loss of babies associated with placenta previa is almost always due to prematurity. We have therefore learned to try to carry such pregnancies as far as possible with bed rest, transfusion, and avoidance of pelvic examination. If, in the effort to establish the diagnosis, the doctor feels inside the cervix, this may separate the placenta still further and aggravate the bleeding.

If hemorrhage is persistent or if labor ensues, intervention can no longer be postponed. Many obstetricians, and I am one of them, feel that at this time the patient should have a pelvic examination in an operating room that is fully prepared to carry out a cesarean section. Digital examination may make clear that the placenta is off to one side and that it is possible, especially in women who have had previous vaginal deliveries, to rupture membranes and induce labor. If labor has already begun, the cervix may be dilated and the baby's presenting part may be well down the pelvis. In either case vaginal delivery may be expected. However, with first pregnancies, with babies in an abnormal presentation (which occurs more frequently in placenta previa), or when the placenta completely covers the cervix, there is no choice but the decision to deliver the baby abdominally. Approximately six out of every ten women with placenta previa deliver by cesarean. As we are becoming increasingly skilled with expectant treatment, the neonatal loss from placenta previa has dropped well under 5 percent and maternal mortality is rare.

Abruptio Placentae

Premature separation of the placenta, also referred to by its technical name, *abruptio placentae*, is the disruption of a part or all of the placenta from its normal attachment in the body of the uterus, prior to the birth of the child. It is also a cause of vaginal bleeding. This separation is the same process by which the placenta separates and delivers after birth but, since it cuts the placenta off from the maternal blood supply before the baby is born and breathing, it is extraordinarily hazardous to the unborn fetus.

In approximately one case in five, a limited hemorrhage occurs in the plane between the placenta and the uterine wall. The blood becomes trapped there and does not come through the cervix into the vagina, so that there is no visible bleeding. In such cases, pain and faintness are variable, but in every instance the uterus, instead of being soft, is tense and irritable; it may be rigid and tender to touch on examination.

In some instances the separation and bleeding coincide with

the onset of labor. The diagnosis of abruption may then only be made because there is otherwise unexplained evidence of fetal distress.

The underlying mechanism of this abruption appears to be abnormality of maternal arteries serving the placental site; the reasons for the rupture of these vessels is not quite understood. Associated with *abruptio placentae* is an appearance of protein in the urine and occasional elevation of blood pressure. Since these are also features of toxemia of pregnancy it is not absolutely clear whether the separation of the placenta causes an acute toxemia or the acute toxemia causes the separation. In unusual circumstances the placenta may be jarred loose by severe abdominal trauma such as might be incurred in an automobile accident.

There is a clear relationship between repeated pregnancy and abruption, the incidence being about three times as great in women who have had more than five children than it is in first pregnancies. Age does not seem to be significant. There is also a tendency toward recurrence, which takes place in approximately 10 percent of subsequent pregnancies.

The treatment of the woman thought to have a placental abruption begins with admission to the hospital. Administration of intravenous fluids and preparation for blood transfusion are begun at once. Fetal monitoring is established.

The next step is ordinarily a pelvic examination, at which time the appropriate measure, if feasible, is to rupture the membranes. This seems to bring the active process of separation to a halt. Provided that the patient can be kept in good circulatory condition by the use of intravenous fluids, including blood replacement, it is possible then to await the onset of labor or follow its continuation to a vaginal delivery.

Since abruption of the placenta is frequently accompanied by an abnormality of blood clotting, cesarean is fraught with danger to the mother and should only be undertaken if there is clear evidence of fetal distress or if, with the baby in good condition, there is an inordinate delay in the onset of labor. In many of the severe instances of this syndrome, where separation of the placenta has been extensive, the baby has already died when the patient first reports for care. At one time it was thought necessary to deliver all these women very rapidly in order to prevent maternal kidney injury, but we have learned that this is best prevented by maintaining an adequate maternal circulation.

Large doses of cocaine, by any route, are now recognized as a cause of otherwise unexplained placental abruption.

In summary then, if the fetus is alive and labor is well underway, vaginal delivery may be anticipated. If the fetus is alive and shows evidence of distress, abdominal delivery is appropriate. If the fetus is no longer alive, it is reasonable to await a normal birth. This may be hastened by the appropriate use of oxytocin to stimulate the labor.

The prognosis for the mother with abruption is quite good: the mortality rate is substantially less than half a percent. The fetal loss is unfortunately much greater than this, probably in the vicinity of 25 percent of all cases of severe abruption.

Toxemia of Pregnancy

Toxemia of pregnancy includes high blood pressure or an increase in an already elevated blood pressure in the latter half of pregnancy, accompanied by the appearance of protein in the urine and excess water in the tissues. When it worsens, convulsions and coma ensue and death may occur. It is then called eclampsia (from the Greek *eklampsis*, "a shining forth," in reference to its sudden onset).

The word "toxemia," derived from Greek roots meaning poison and blood, suggests that this is a kind of poisoning that arises in some way from the pregnancy itself. We have been searching for well over a hundred years for some firm evidence that such a poison exists. No toxic substance has ever been identified, despite all sorts of studies. Abnormal amounts of some normal components appear in the blood of women with toxemia, but no new ones have ever been found. In the search in the circulating blood for a substance that can cause the condition, blood and blood plasma have been transfused into volunteers and into experimental animals but nothing resembling human toxemia has been produced. A whole host of substances has been suspected but the evidence for any one of them is unfortunately very weak. Toxemia thus remains a disease of theories. We are able to diagnose it, but the treatment and cure are still on shaky ground because we do not really know its cause.

That convulsions and death could occur in pregnancy was known to the ancients. It is only in the last hundred years that it has been recognized that these are the end stages of a process that shows itself earlier by increase in blood pressure, protein in the urine, and waterlogging of the tissues. This condition, which may be accompanied by headache or persistent pain in the pit of the stomach, is now known as preeclampsia. When the only evidence of trouble is elevation of blood pressure, the condition is referred to as pregnancy-induced hypertension. Toxemia of pregnancy is the general term that includes all these problems of late pregnancy.

Preeclampsia occurs most frequently in women who, prior to pregnancy, have been completely normal. Patients who are pregnant for the first time, who are carrying twins, or who have hydatidiform moles are especially prone to preeclampsia.

Observations of the course of preeclampsia led to the conclusion that the danger to the mother was materially reduced if she was delivered before convulsions ensued. Unfortunately, the fetus was then liable to succumb to the perils of prematurity. If delivery did not occur and coma or convulsions appeared, the fetus suffered from the mother's metabolic and respiratory difficulties. Attention had to be turned to treatment with drugs. In recent years several effective medicines which prevent convulsions have been widely used, and a number of drugs which safely lower blood pressure have become available. This has reduced the need for premature delivery.

Another factor has been the steady improvement in the care of prematures. The loss of mothers and babies has thus been significantly reduced. Unfortunately, we still see an occasional neglected woman who has suffered eclampsia and a fetal death.

The disease itself also appears to have been changing over the last several decades. In the 1950's in large city hospitals, it was not unusual to have several patients at once with eclampsia. Everyone who trained in obstetrics thirty years ago was likely to have had a number of experiences with eclamptic convulsions. However, eclampsia is now a rarity. Even large services giving care to the poor, among whom the condition continues to be more common, go long periods without actually seeing eclampsia. The milder forms of preeclampsia have become less common as well. We suspect that this is due to improved nutrition but there must be other factors in addition, since eclampsia can occur in very well-nourished women.

Acute toxemia, sometimes referred to as acute preeclampsia, does not tend to reappear in subsequent pregnancies and, indeed, even eclampsia rarely repeats itself. However, when toxemia occurs in a woman with chronic hypertension, the hypertension persists and the problem recurs in future pregnancies. There are unusual women, otherwise normal, in whom blood pressure elevation and protein in the urine reappear in each pregnancy, without becoming worse with the repetition and without resulting in hypertension in the nonpregnant state.

Lack of prenatal care is related to severity of the toxemia. This may reflect the lifestyle of the patients or it may simply mean that, not having appeared for prenatal care, they have missed the opportunity to detect the early mild forms of the disease and head it off with appropriate therapy. We do still, in the middle 1980's, sometimes see a patient who is admitted to the hospital having already had several convulsions and in a precarious state.

One group of pregnant women thought to be at risk for toxemia is adolescents. These young people notoriously tend not to appear for prenatal visits and the resulting incidence of neglected toxemia has led some observers to conclude that teenage pregnancy is per se high-risk pregnancy. This is probably an oversimplification. Studies show that age itself is not the most significant factor, but rather the young mother's diet is. Part of the problem is that, as I have indicated, the disease can be present without producing noticeable symptoms. Pregnant adolescents often neglect themselves.

Early Detection of Toxemia

Several clinical tests have been devised to detect the tendency to preeclampsia before it actually has made its appearance. None of them offers reliable enough prediction to make it actually useful among low-risk women. When the accumulation of body water goes to the point where there is obvious puffiness of hands and face (edema), it must be considered that acute toxemia has made its appearance. I have a vivid recollection of a patient who called on the telephone a number of years ago, at twenty-two weeks of pregnancy, to say that she had just been on a visit to one of America's smoggiest cities and had developed irritation of her eyes, which had then puffed shut. When, at my firm insistence, she came in for examination, she already had elevated blood pressure and some protein in her urine. This was followed shortly by fetal death. Fortunately the patient had no difficulty in conceiving again and subsequently proceeded to go through two completely uneventful pregnancies during which there was no evidence of toxemia.

A major element in the disease appears to be the development of a spasm of the small blood vessels throughout the body. The vascular system adjusts to this by increasing blood pressure in order to maintain blood flow to vital organs. There is then leakage of water into the tissues and leakage of protein into the urine. This by definition is preeclampsia. However, the elevated blood pressure at first does not produce symptoms. An ominous symptom is a severe, persistent headache. This symptom may be followed by the convulsions of eclampsia. When the blood pressure goes to markedly high levels, there may be injury to the blood vessels of the brain and leakage of blood. This produces symptoms like those of a stroke. This may complicate the convulsions of eclampsia; it has a high death rate when it occurs. If the blood vessels of the placenta are also involved it can cause premature separation of the placenta, as described above.

There does not seem to be much we can do to prevent preeclampsia from occurring. Improving the diet reduces the incidence of preeclampsia, but we have not learned very much more than that about prevention.

When the earliest signs of preeclampsia appear, it is advisable for the patient to reduce her activity considerably and to take a mild sedative, which functions as an anticonvulsant as well. The woman should be seen again in a few days to determine whether this is a rapidly accumulating severe toxemia or a transitory phenomenon that will correct itself with a reduction in activity. Some patients find it difficult to accept inactivity and sedation when they have no symptoms and do not feel sick. Nevertheless, this type of care may reverse the trend to more serious complications.

Care for Severe Toxemia

If it does not, then the patient should be admitted to the hospital, where she will be kept at bed rest, lying on her left side as much as possible. This is intended to take the weight of the pregnant uterus off the major blood vessels on the back wall of the abdominal cavity, with the immediate effect of improving blood flow to the kidneys and resultant loss of excess body water in the form of urine. At this time sedation may be increased to minimize the risk of convulsions. Repeated examination of the urine can be carried out in the hospital to measure the amount of protein loss. Sometimes these measures are all that is needed.

In some patients the disease is relentlessly progressive. The blood pressure steadily rises, with increasing loss of protein in the urine. The likelihood of convulsions then increases, as does the risk of fetal distress. In a hospitalized patient daily observations of the fetal heart rate pattern are made, to look for subtle evidences of placental injury. If the process worsens, the next step is intensification of anticonvulsant medication. The most commonly employed means for this is the intravenous or intramuscular administration of magnesium sulfate, a drug that minimizes electrical activity over the surface of the brain. It is the spread of such activity which is related to the convulsions. Magnesium crosses the placenta slowly and has effects on the fetus, but this does no harm *in utero* and the effects clear up promptly in the newborn. There is not complete agreement at present on magnesium sulfate therapy. For their anticonvulsant properties other drugs such as phenobarbital may be used.

When, despite treatment, the disease becomes more severe, it is necessary to consider delivery. The danger to the fetus in the uterus may outweigh the risks of prematurity in the nursery. This estimation calls for a judgment of the skills and facilities available for pediatric care.

In some cases it will be possible to induce labor by artificial rupture of the membranes and administration of oxytocin, and in this way to achieve safe vaginal delivery. During labor the fetus should be continuously monitored and the mother given substantial sedation. Where it is safely available, epidural anesthesia is ideal for late labor and delivery.

When induction is not feasible or when it is tried and fails, delivery by cesarean is the next step. These patients are not medically normal and skilled anesthesia is called for.

Toxemia sometimes becomes worse after delivery. Indeed, there are rare circumstances in which a patient who has appeared to be perfectly normal all through pregnancy and labor may without warning have convulsions after delivery. This phenomenon, known as postpartum eclampsia, is now possibly an even greater threat to the mother since it tends to occur so unexpectedly.

Toxemia of pregnancy is still a major complication of obstetrics, whose detection quite properly justify all the efforts we make in prenatal care. Fortunately, the women who experience toxemia rarely suffer long-term injury. The newborns, once they are delivered in good condition, do not exhibit any aftereffects. The fact that a woman had toxemia in pregnancy does not increase the likelihood that a daughter born to her in that pregnancy will herself have the disease.

Excessive Weight Gain

As mentioned previously, for a long time it was thought that excessive weight gain and excessive intake of salt had a causal relationship to toxemia of pregnancy. Weight gain is actually not a cause but a consequence of the disease, reflecting the fact that women with severe toxemia have abnormal accumulations of water in their tissues. So far as salt is concerned, even in the presence of acute toxemia the kidneys function normally to excrete the salt present in excess of the body's needs. Salt plays no causative role in toxemia. Thus, there is no merit in limiting salt intake while pregnant. It is certain that the administration of so called water pills, the diuretics that result in imposed loss of water and salt, do not have a place in the treatment of acute toxemia. They neither prevent it nor treat it.

Fetal Death *in Utero*

Once in a rare while a fetus dies, prior to birth, after the twentieth week of gestation, often without warning. There are many possible causes, most of them out of control of the mother and none of them common. The list includes congenital anomalies incompatible with life; severe maternal blood vessel disease resulting in marked delay of fetal development; severe long-standing high blood pressure; eclampsia; and premature separation of the placenta, all discussed earlier in this chapter.

Another condition that may result in fetal death is nonimmune hydrops fetalis. "Hydrops" is a term derived from the Greek word for water, and refers to the fact that in it the fetus becomes severely waterlogged. There is an excess of amniotic fluid, and the mother may become waterlogged as well. Hydrops was formerly observed most commonly when Rh-negative women who had been sensitized to Rh were carrying an Rh-positive fetus. This fetus was severely affected by the anti-Rh antibodies crossing the placenta from the mother to the fetus. This complication has become rare since the introduction of the Rhogam—the anti-Rh antibody—which is now administered to pregnant women to protect them and their babies against the development of Rh sensitization.

Mothers with severe unregulated diabetes may experience fetal death in the latter half of pregnancy as a result of the biochemical abnormality that results from an effort of the body to use sources of energy other than glucose. An accumulation of acids occurs, which seriously affects the ability of the fetus to excrete the waste products from its system.

Finally, fetal death may occur when pregnancy has gone well past term. This condition is called postmaturity. A postmature fetus ordinarily dies only if the mother is pregnant for the first time, is over twenty-five years of age, and is more than ten days beyond her carefully estimated date of confinement. In the presence of pregnancy complications there is a greater risk.

Clearly, all high-risk pregnancies require vigilance for signs of fetal distress. The mother should observe the activity of her fetus by recording its movements for one-hour periods several times a day at the same hour each day. In addition, non-stress tests (NST) are used to assess the condition of the fetus. An NST is done by having the patient lie down, tilted toward her left side, and placing a gauge on the skin of the abdomen, over the pregnant uterus. This gauge registers fetal movements and uterine contractions. Another sensor registers the fetal heart rate. These observations make it possible to assess the condition of the fetus. In addition, sonographic examination is done to determine whether there is a normal amount of amniotic fluid present, since fetal death is often associated with marked reductions in fluid.

In some circumstances, fetal death is silent. The mother simply notices the absence of fetal activity. Within a few days she may also note a loss of weight and a decrease in the size of her breasts, a sign of fetal death observed by Hippocrates twenty-four hundred years ago. The diagnosis can be suspected if the uterus is found to be markedly smaller than it ought to be for the known duration of pregnancy and if there is a significant loss of maternal weight in the absence of anything else to account for it. It can be confirmed by sonography to observe the absence of fetal heart activity. Although the uterus stops growing the mother is not likely to notice any change in contractions unless and until the placenta stops functioning.

When a condition that is associated with or aggravated by pregnancy is the cause of the fetal death, the mother is likely to improve thereafter. This is often the case with toxemia of pregnancy and with the maternal effects of hydrops fetalis. Otherwise women are neither benefited nor harmed medically by fetal death.

Labor after Fetal Death

The interval between the death of the fetus and the onset of labor will depend how early in pregnancy the death has occurred. The earlier the pregnancy the longer the interval is likely to be. Most labors ensue within two weeks. If labor does not commence spontaneously it is sometimes possible to use oxytocin or one of the prostaglandins to stimulate the uterus. Chances for success for this technique are greater if there have already been some changes such as softening, shortening, and opening of the cervix. As the stimulant drugs are very potent, however, they must be used with great care. There have been instances of uterine rupture (tears in the body of the uterus) from excessive stimulation: This is a surgical emergency on top of a medical tragedy.

There has been concern, when labor is delayed for several weeks following fetal death, that the patient may experience an abnormality of the ability of her blood to clot, known as disseminated intravascular coagulation (DIC). In this condition, the platelets, the tiny blood cells which assist in forming clots, clump together inside blood vessels, a location where ordinarily they remain free of one another. These clumps then use up some of the proteins in the blood which also take part in blood clotting. All this withdraws from the woman's blood many of the essential elements necessary for normal clotting. This of course sets the stage for serious hemorrhage. If DIC is suspected it can be identified by measurements of the number of platelets and the amount of the protein clotting factors in the blood. DIC tends to occur more frequently when the fetal death results from Rh incompatibility than when other factors are responsible.

If DIC is present at the time of delivery there may be serious hemorrhage from the site of the placental separation. DIC is also a major complication should cesarean section be required. It therefore has to be recognized promptly. Treatment consists of administering fresh whole blood or thawed-out frozen plasma, to replace the clotting factors lost in the disease process. Since the blood platelets which play a role in blood clotting are markedly reduced with DIC, platelet transfusion will on occasion also be used in its treatment.

On rare occasions evidence of the clotting abnormality appears without any sign of labor. It may then be proper to treat the condition medically, without undertaking to empty the uterus until the condition is reversed.

Sometimes, when all the facts are taken into consideration, it seems best to induce labor before full-blown DIC makes its appearance. As the situation is complicated and one patient is not exactly like another, it is not wise to state a rule for when one treatment rather than another should be chosen.

The greatest problem with fetal death is its psychological effect upon the mother, particularly if the onset of labor is

delayed. Her physical appearance late in pregnancy is unchanged but she is painfully conscious that she is carrying a
dead baby. She finds it hard to avoid the conviction that there
are adverse effects upon herself, a conviction not at all based
on fact. It is inevitable that the patient will go through the
same process of bereavement and grief that is experienced by
patients with stillbirth or the death of a newborn baby. But the
unfortunate women with a fetal death may have the additional
problem of working through the experience while still pregnant.

Patients in this predicament often feel a strong desire for
intervention to empty the uterus. It calls for sensitive insight
and tact on the part of the medical attendant to deal with this
psychological pressure, as well as necessary skill and judgment
to select the right time to induce labor with minimal physical
trauma to the mother. Awaiting the spontaneous termination of
the pregnancy is unquestionably the safest route to follow.

Danger Signals—When to Notify the Doctor

The pregnant woman is a competent adult able to participate
in her own care and to make many decisions about her own
health. She seeks professional help in order to have appropriate
advice from someone she knows and trusts readily at hand.
The patient herself can certainly make decisions about the
importance of minor injuries, transitory upper respiratory infections, minor stomach upsets, and the like. These are things
that she would ordinarily decide about if she were not pregnant,
and the existence of the pregnancy really does not impair her
judgment.

There are, however, some specific matters concerning which
you should consult your obstetrician, your family doctor, or
your nurse midwife, to use their experience in deciding what
steps to take and whether you ought to be receiving formal
treatment. A list of significant danger signals follows:

1. Vaginal bleeding at any time during pregnancy. If the
bleeding is simply staining, perhaps less than you would normally observe during menses, and if this occurs in the first
half of pregnancy, you can wait until a convenient time to get

in touch with your care provider. However, if you are well into the second or third trimester, bleeding calls for prompt consultation and may call for examination. A small amount of pink discharge accompanied by mucus can occur late in pregnancy as the cervix begins to shorten and open; this may be associated with some uterine cramps and is entirely normal. At the other end of the spectrum, there may be painless hemorrhage associated with placenta previa or premature separation of the placenta. In such an event it might even be wise for you to report promptly to your hospital without spending time in an effort to reach your care provider.

2. Puffiness of the face and eyes, particularly if this occurs suddenly. Swelling of the legs and ankles without involvement of the face and hands usually only signifies an effect of gravity on the extra water in the body. If swelling of your ankles is still prominent when you wake up in the morning, this is worth a telephone call and an inquiry.

3. Severe headache late in pregnancy may be a sign of severe toxemia. Then it is usually felt in the forehead and behind the eyes and does not respond to ordinary headache medications.

4. Dimness or blurring of vision in the second half of pregnancy may also signify toxemia, particularly if this is associated with marked puffiness of the eyelids that interferes with opening them all the way.

5. Severe abdominal pain, especially if it is constant, no matter where it occurs in the abdomen and no matter what the duration of pregnancy. It is more serious if it is associated with nausea and vomiting but less so if the latter are accompanied by repeated bouts of diarrhea.

6. Temperature over 100 degrees Fahrenheit, especially if this is associated with chills or if it persists.

7. Burning on urination and discomfort on finishing voiding.

8. Rupture of the membranes, which results in uncontrollable leak of the fluid from the vagina, if this occurs without signs of labor. The closer you are to the expected date of confinement, the shorter the delay between rupture of the membranes and the onset of the labor. Rupture of the membranes with a known abnormal lie of the fetus is a medical emergency, but the rupture of the membranes at the onset of normal labor is not. Membranes rarely if ever reseal once they have ruptured.

9. Beyond the twenty-sixth week of pregnancy, the unexplained absence of fetal movements for eight to ten hours, especially at the times when the fetus is ordinarily active, is occasion for investigation.

10

Spontaneous Abortion, Induced Abortion, and Premature Labor

Spontaneous Abortion (Miscarriage)

More than half of all fertilized ova are lost before the end of the first trimester. Many of these ova undergo a few cell divisions in the fallopian tube and develop no further. Some proceed to a many-celled stage but fail to implant in the uterus. Some implant too close to a blood vessel in the lining of the uterus and cause a hemorrhage which expels them. All these events take place before a woman can even miss a menstrual period and therefore they are not recognized as pregnancies. The hCG (see page 11) produced by an early embryo is detectable in the mother's blood somewhere about the fifth or sixth day after the fertile union (impregnation) has taken place. This is about the twentieth day of a normal cycle, before any other sign of pregnancy is present. It is now referred to as a chemical pregnancy. The evidence that has thus recently become available from this test confirms that about 45 percent of such chemical pregnancies are lost, quite unbeknownst to anyone.

Of the eggs that implant more successfully and therefore cause a delay in menses and symptoms that are recognized by the mother as pregnancy, approximately 15 percent are subsequently lost. These are what are ordinarily known as spontaneous abortions. The earliest of them may be taken for a heavier-than-usual menstrual period, as no material recognized as products of conception is passed.

Three-quarters of all known abortions occur prior to the twelfth week, and the greatest majority of these take place somewhere between the ninth and the eleventh week. Most abortions and miscarriages occur long before the twenty-fourth week. Only one in four pregnancy losses occurs between the twelfth and twenty-sixth week.

Factors Influencing Incidence

Three conditions are associated with a low frequency of abortion: youth, ability to conceive easily, and the absence of previous spontaneous abortions. A woman under twenty-five years of age who conceives within three months of her initial efforts to become pregnant and who has never aborted before is most likely to deliver a term baby without event. In this group of women the likelihood of abortion is less than 4 in 100 pregnancies. At the other extreme are women beyond the age of thirty-five who take six months or longer to conceive and who have a previous history of pregnancy loss. In this group the chance of abortion is approximately 40 in 100. But note that this means that 60 times out of 100 the patients will go on to term and have a normal baby.

Among women studied by ultrasound when they are between seven and twelve weeks pregnant and found to have an embryo with a beating heart, about 1.5 percent of those under thirty years of age subsequently lose the pregnancy. Between thirty and thirty-four the loss is about 2.5 percent, and above thirty-four years of age it is 4.5 percent.

These are of course generalizations. The process of formation of an embryo, its implantation in the uterus, and its growth thereafter is so complex that it amazes me that it works at all. When it fails repeatedly in a particular patient, it is certainly worth investigation, to determine whether the cause of these abortions is one that can be identified and corrected.

Repeated induced early abortion does not seem to have an adverse effect on the likelihood of subsequently completing a normal pregnancy. Whether or not this is true of second-trimester abortions is not as yet clearly established.

Specific Causes of Abortion

1. Abnormalities of chromosome number and, less commonly, chromosome form account for about 60 percent of spontaneous abortions. For example, a defect of the combination of sperm and egg may occur and result in tripling or quadrupling the number of chromosomes. This virtually always results in failure to develop a normal embryo and therefore the abortion of the pregnancy. In rare instances the embryo develops from chromosomes entirely of paternal origin; this results in the formation of a hydatidiform mole, a placenta without a fetus and therefore severely waterlogged. The placental villi become translucent vesicles, resembling seedless grapes. On occasion the mole may be malignant, acting like a very aggressive cancer. This is designated choriocarcinoma (Greek: *khorion*, "outer layer of an embryo"; *carcinoma*, "malignant growth of surface cells").

2. Endocrine disorders, the commonest of which is unregulated diabetes. This can be responsible for congenital anomalies in early pregnancy and may be related to early abortion. This does not occur in patients with well-regulated diabetes.

3. Uterine defects such as the inability of the cervix to remain closed until term. This results in the loss of an immature fetus. This is generally called the incompetent cervix syndrome. It may be a result of cervical injury but can occur quite without any known cause. It is a frequent cause of fetal loss in women whose mothers received diethylstilbestrol (DES) in pregnancy.

There are abnormalities of the uterus that result from the fact that it arises in the embryo from a pair of tubes, the Müllerian ducts, which later fuse together. They may fail to combine properly, or one duct may fail to develop. This results in a uterus with an inadequate cavity, which may reject the fetus long before it has become large enough to survive. Incomplete fusion of the two ducts produces an abnormal uterine cavity or even complete doubling of the uterine body and cervix.

4. Uterine infections may be responsible for abortion. This

may be true with herpes genitalis. A microorganism named Mycoplasma has been associated by some investigators with an increased rate of first trimester loss. All the data are not yet in on this however, and the results of treating patients with antibiotics for Mycoplasma have not been clear enough to prove the case.

5. Maternal disease is a rare cause of abortion. Severe chronic disorders in women of the childbearing age may be sufficient to halt ovulation and even menstruation; such women rarely become pregnant.

6. There is a small group of congenital defects in the infant that may not be dependent on genetic events or chromosomal anomalies and that result in fetal death. Examples of this are severe neural tube defects and an abnormality of blood vessel formation known as cystic hygroma. These are ordinarily associated with second-trimester fetal death and subsequent abortion.

7. Immunologic and environmental phenomena. There is some reason to believe that an occasional patient will have antibodies circulating in her blood that have an adverse effect on the fetus. The proof in this area has been difficult to obtain, possibly because of limitation on the precision of some of our laboratory tests. Curiously, Rh sensitization does not cause abortion. It is clear that environmental impacts can have an effect on abortion. This may be a result of excessive stress; an example of this occurrence is abortion following a severe life crisis.

8. By far the commonest general cause of abortion is a failure of either the embryo or the placenta to form normally. These are known as germ plasm defects. Approximately 60 percent of these have abnormal chromosomes. Approximately half of these are trisomies (see page 436). A quarter of them have only a single sex chromosome and some 20 percent have a total tripling or quadrupling of chromosome number.

Trisomy is more frequent among older women for reasons that will be discussed in greater detail later. Abortion, therefore, has a higher rate past the age of thirty-five. It also has a slightly increased incidence on genetic grounds prior to the age of sixteen.

The commonest form of abnormality of the sex chromosomes is the presence of only one X chromosome, with no other sex chromosome to match it. It appears that when there is a single Y chromosome without an X no embryo forms. With the single X chromosome, approximately 99 percent of the embryos abort. The cystic hygroma referred to above can be a manifestation of a single X chromosome.

An abnormality of shape in an individual chromosome is present in fewer than 5 percent of the 60 percent of abortuses with chromosomal abnormality.

How Do Abortions Take Place?

There are two forms of pregnancy loss that are called abortion or miscarriage. One is the form associated with defects of the uterus. In this instance the fetus is ordinarily normal and there may be restriction on the expansion of the uterus. The patient tends to go into premature labor or to experience painless dilation of the cervix. In either event an otherwise normal fetus is delivered substantially before it is viable.

The other form of abortion takes place because of defects in the embryo or the placenta. The level of hCG, estrogen, and progesterone in the mother drops. The general symptoms of pregnancy recede, and the uterus then begins to recognize the products of conception as a foreign body. The defective germ plasm conceptus often ceases development somewhere about six to eight menstrual weeks. The products of conception may remain in the uterus for another three or four weeks. Labor eventually ensues. It is marked by severe uterine cramps and bleeding. The process is uncomfortable but is ordinarily completed rapidly and with minimal blood loss. Occasionally the placenta does not come away intact. It may be necessary to use a suction device to empty the uterus of all the fragments of the products of conception. This is done to stop bleeding and to reduce the chance of infection.

Examination of the tissue of an abortion is crucial in learning something of its cause. If you abort unexpectedly at home it is essential that you save all the material that you pass and take it in for subsequent pathological examination.

These early losses are usually quite without complication, although they are certainly disturbing to the mother who has known that she was pregnant. Furthermore, the bleeding with such abortions can be somewhat more than with a normal period, and this is also rather frightening.

Since most spontaneous abortions are a consequence of untreatable defects in the embryo or the placenta, the patient can do no more, even with the best help that medical science can provide, than delay the completion of the event. For this reason I ordinarily do not recommend to women that they leave work or that they confine themselves to bed when early indications of abortion appear.

Many years ago this advice was studied carefully in a very large sample of patients who had previously had one spontaneous abortion. In a random manner they were advised either to continue being active in the ordinary course of events or to go to bed and stay there until all bleeding had ceased. There was no meaningful difference in the eventual outcome of the pregnancies between the two groups. This may be because, in a normal pregnancy, the embryo is very solidly implanted. It is not possible to shake a good fertilized human ovum loose from the uterus any more than you can shake a good unripe apple loose from the apple tree. If strenuous activity, hot baths, and the like were able to dislodge a normal embryo, generation upon generation of people would not have exerted themselves for the past several millennia to develop violent concoctions and surgical interventions for the purpose of inducing abortion. Nature sometimes makes mistakes, but normal seed and its fruits are jealously protected.

Since the great majority of spontaneous early abortions involve embryos that never could have become babies, it hardly makes sense to go to extreme measures to postpone the completion of the process. This principle does not apply to those abortions in the second trimester which may be associated with the loss of a normal fetus too immature to survive. The woman who is faced with the inevitability of a germ-plasma-defect abortion is probably well served by completing the event and returning to a physiological state of fertility as soon as possible. This, in any event, is the advice I give to my patients. However, do not become concerned if your personal attendant recommends another course of action for you, since there is room for individualization in this situation.

It probably can be safely said that the enthusiasm for hormone therapy to prevent spontaneous abortion has pretty much waned. To some extent this has been influenced by the realization that DES (diethylstilbesterol) therapy, from which so much was expected in the early 1950's, was actually harmful and, as a matter of fact, not effective for any of its intended purposes. Now, by measurement of hCG in the blood in very early pregnancy, combined with ultrasound examination, we can diagnose inevitable abortion due to embryonic failure. We can then prepare the mother for the loss and avoid the futile use of hormones. It is undoubtedly wiser to complete diagnostic studies than to undertake shotgun remedies. Contrariwise, when we are able to identify a fetal heartbeat by a Doppler device or by sonography, subsequent pregnancy loss is a rare event and there is no indication for hormone treatment.

When spontaneous abortion threatens well into the second trimester, management is entirely different. This subject is discussed on page 197.

Interval Between Abortion and Another Pregnancy

Many women having abortion inquire as to how long they should wait before initiating another pregnancy. There is no consensus on this subject. My own opinion is that if the previous pregnancy has aborted completely and the uterus is empty, the mother's ovaries will promptly return to normal function. While the lining of the uterus remains unhealed, it will be inhospitable to the implantation of any ovum that might be fertilized in the next period and pregnancy simply will not take place. On the other hand, if the uterine healing is complete, then a newly fertilized egg can implant without any difficulty and proceed quite normally through pregnancy. In fact, one of my own children is the product of such a sequence of events.

Some women go through a period of psychological stress after a pregnancy loss and, on these grounds rather than on physiological ones, they may wish to postpone a new pregnancy. I am sure that under no circumstances should a new pregnancy be undertaken as treatment for a bad psychological reaction to a pregnancy loss.

This advice is also dependent on a careful examination of

the abortus and an evaluation of the presence or absence of any repetitive factors of the sort mentioned below.

The Repetition of Abortion

What then are your chances of your having a successful pregnancy if you have previously aborted? As I have already said, if you have aborted on just one occasion your chances are as good and in some studies it seems even a little better than if you have never been pregnant before. This statement is true in the absence of any efforts at treatment. If you have aborted twice consecutively it may indicate that there is something going on, however unusual, that is worthy of investigation and possible correction before you become pregnant again. This is particularly true if you have never had a successful pregnancy. However, if you should become pregnant before a study can be completed the chance for a successful pregnancy following two prior spontaneous abortions is only slightly decreased as compared with that for a patient who has never miscarried. After three consecutive prior abortions the odds in favor of success go down a little further.

In other words, if you have aborted once, there is not much to worry about. If you have aborted twice, there may be a problem but even this is unlikely. If you abort three times it is well to seek consultation with specialized medical care.

We still do not know all the factors that influence abortion and cannot identify them even with the best technologies available at the moment. I have a sharp recollection of a woman who came in for prenatal care with the history that she had had six previous spontaneous abortions and no living children. On the very first pelvic examination, it was clear that this patient had multiple uterine fibroids and of course I came to the obvious conclusion that these had been the cause of the previous pregnancy losses. This woman sailed serenely through a completely unremarkable pregnancy. The fibroids grew with great enthusiasm but the baby, lost somewhere among them, grew even better. The patient went to term, fell into labor, and had a rapid, uneventful delivery. I was much impressed and, I must confess, quite puzzled by this. When the baby was a few days old I sought out the patient and asked her whether

she knew of anything that would account for this happy outcome. She smiled sagely and informed me that this new baby
was the product of a recent second marriage, her first husband,
the father of the six abortuses, having died in an industrial
accident.

All sorts of therapy have been employed with women who
have repeatedly aborted and never brought a baby to full term.
The full range of vitamins has been employed and a considerable spectrum of hormone therapies. The only one for which
there is any evidence, and even this is shaky, is treatment with
progestogens begun in the second half of the potentially fertile
cycle, and continued into the first trimester. It has been extraordinarily difficult to get satisfactory scientific proof of the
benefits of this therapy.

The surgical correction of uterine anomalies and submucus
uterine fibroids may make a tremendous difference in the prognosis for women with these rare problems.

The Story of a Typical Spontaneous Abortion

There are some dangers in enumerating signs and symptoms
for the benefit of lay readers. Jerome K. Jerome, an English
author, wrote an amusing story about this many years ago. It
concerned a hypochondriac who went to the British Museum
to read through an index of diseases by symptoms and concluded that he had virtually every disease in the book. He went
to his doctor who examined him, wrote out a prescription, and
suggested that he have it filled immediately. The patient took
this prescription to the drug store. The pharmacist read it,
laughed, and handed it back, with the statement that he couldn't
possibly fill it. It turned out that the physician had prescribed
a week's vacation. In describing a typical spontaneous abortion, therefore, I must caution you against making your own
diagnosis if any of this resembles your own problems.

In a typical abortion the couple have required several months
more than the usual two or three necessary for fertile people
to conceive. The patient has missed a menstrual period but has
otherwise minimal symptoms of pregnancy. She is not sure
about breast enlargement and there is a striking absence of

nausea. The woman reports in for care saying, "I feel great; if it were not that I missed a period I wouldn't even know I was pregnant." On pelvic examination, the uterus feels firmer and smaller than it should be. No fetal heart can be detected upon Doppler examination, although it should be present by the tenth week. A week or so later, approximately the tenth or eleventh week following the last menstrual period, the woman notices a small amount of brownish stain on toilet tissue after voiding. There is no pain or at worst a slight sensation deep in the pelvis, which is reminiscent to the patient of the sensations just prior to menstrual flow. This minimal brownish-red discoloration from the vagina may reappear with each voiding and a small amount of it may leak out with ordinary activity. Overnight nothing is noted but first thing in the morning some more of this discolored blood comes out of the vagina. This bloody discharge from the uterus does not cease overnight, but when the woman lies down, the blood pools in the vagina. When she gets up in the morning it comes out from the effect of gravity.

This early staining may then be followed by an increase in the sensation of impending menses. This is succeeded by cramps, which gradually increase in intensity, with the same kind of crescendo that occurs in normal labor. At the same time bleeding tends to increase and the color of the blood becomes brighter red. The bleeding may be so rapid that clots form. Eventually, when the cramps reached their peak, the woman may experience an urge to void or move her bowels. On attempting to do so, she may pass a mass of organized tissue, ranging in size anywhere from that of a plum to a moderate size peach. The outside appearance of this mass is clearly firmer and shaggier than that of a blood clot. At about this time the cramps stop, and bleeding slows down and diminishes to a volume typical of a menstrual period.

When the aborted tissue is examined it turns out to be a compact mass of placenta within which there may be a small sac containing a degenerated fetus or, in some instances, no fetus at all. If the bleeding uneventfully reverts to the average for the ordinary menstrual period, there is no need for curettage of the uterine cavity.

An Incomplete Abortion

In about a third of all patients, the process of abortion is not completely efficient. The uterus fails to push out the products of conception and cramping and bleeding continue without successful completion. Under these circumstances it may be appropriate to admit the patient to the hospital and stimulate the uterus with intravenous administration of oxytocin. This increases the contractions of the uterus and makes it possible for the abortion to be completed without any surgical manipulation.

Sometimes fragments of the placenta come out, but pieces remain behind in the uterus. The mechanism for aborting these is not completely efficient. If such fragments of placenta remain attached, the uterus has great difficulty in shutting off the blood to these areas, and the bleeding will continue. Under these circumstances nature has ordinarily dilated the cervix so that dilation by the physician is unnecessary. Indeed, if the cervix is not dilated there is some reason to wonder whether the diagnosis is correct.

It is possible to assist nature in emptying the uterus by introducing a hollow, semirigid plastic tube (catheter) into the uterine cavity. Once this catheter is in place, it is connected with a vacuum device that creates negative pressure. Since the placenta is relatively loosely attached to the uterine wall, creating this vacuum pressure sucks the loose fragments of the products of conception into the tubing. This then completes the abortion. This can be accomplished on an ambulatory basis, but since there may be considerable bleeding, it is often done within the walls of a hospital.

There has been a body of opinion to the effect that every spontaneous abortion should be followed by curettage to be certain that the uterus is empty and to make an early diagnosis in the rare event of an abnormality of the placenta. My conclusion is that if the process has completed itself spontaneously and the cervix has clamped down, dilation and curettage are unnecessary. If it is possible to examine the products of conception and be certain that they are complete and that no placental abnormality is present, curettage is not necessary either.

The Danger from Abortion

Today women only very rarely die from spontaneous abortion, and when they do it is almost always under circumstances of great neglect. Blood loss from this condition can be severe, but it is readily treated with transfusions. Uterine infection, an uncommon occurrence, is readily treated by antibiotics and by completely emptying the uterine cavity.

There are two forms of abnormal placental development that may have the appearance and produce symptoms that can be taken for those of spontaneous abortion. One of these is hydatidiform mole, a condition in which a placenta forms without an embryo. Curiously, it is usually derived from a sperm alone without an ovum, and it contains only genetic material from the father. The hormone-secreting cells of this placenta are usually hyperactive and so the patient's symptoms are those of a superpregnancy. The second condition is chorionepithelioma or choriocarcinoma, a true cancer of the placenta. This is discussed in more detail on page 000. Suffice it to say here that early diagnosis of these conditions, when they simulate spontaneous abortions, depends upon uterine curettage, and examination of the tissue from the uterus.

Induced Abortion

Induced abortions are terminations of pregnancy by artificial means, prior to viability. Spontaneous abortions, in contrast, are those which initiate themselves for the reasons described in detail above.

Induced abortions may be legal or illegal. A legal abortion is one carried out by or under the supervision of a licensed physician under circumstances prescribed by statute in the jurisdiction in which the abortion is performed. All other induced abortions are illegal.

Early History

Induced abortion is an ancient procedure and its first performance long antedates recorded history. It was practiced by
primitive people on every continent. Its universality is testimony to the antiquity of the procedure. The earliest medical
manuscript extant, a Chinese herbal five thousand years old,
recommends mercury as an abortifacient. The priest-physicians
of the Pharaohs, in papyri written four thousand years ago,
evidenced knowledge of induced abortion. Plato advocated
abortion on eugenic grounds for women less than twenty years
of age and over forty, believing that they created inferior infants. He advocated the same fate for pregnancies implanted
by men over fifty-five. Aristotle recommended abortion for
women who already had many children to help control the
population of the overcrowded city-state Athens. Soranus, the
greatest gynecologist of antiquity, in a famous book written
about A.D. 130, discusses which is preferable, abortion or contraception. With a modern tone to his words he argues for the
latter, since it is safer, he wrote, to prevent conception than to
eliminate it.

Religious Attitudes

The history of religious and ethical attitudes toward abortion
is interesting. The ancient Babylonian Code of Hammurabi
vigorously penalized induced abortion, specifying crucifixion
for the perpetrators. As abortion is only mentioned once in the
Bible, it can be assumed that it was little practiced by Jews
(Exodus xxi-22) in the Biblical period and that it presented no
problem to Christ's disciples. Judaism through the centuries
has prohibited abortion unless a recognized rabbinical authority
agrees in the individual instance that there is medical or social
need. One of the most interesting cases arose during the Hol-
ocaust, when any Jew who became pregnant was summarily
killed with special indignities. The chief rabbi of Kovno, Poland, ruled that under such conditions abortion was permissi-
ble, since if it was not done two lives would be lost, and if
done, only one life. Orthodox Judaism is still extraordinarily

restrictive about abortion, but the Conservative and Reform wings of the Jewish faith have become as liberal about abortion as most of the Protestant groups.

Christianity took early cognizance of abortion, and the first teachings of the Church forbade it under all conditions from the moment of conception. This decision was strongly reinforced by the fourth-century writings of Saint Augustine. Later the Church became concerned with the exact time of ensoulment, theorizing that before ensoulment there was no life and hence abortion would be no sin. The great thirteenth-century Church Father, Thomas Aquinas, promulgated the view that there was neither life nor ensoulment until the fetus moved and therefore abortion was not sinful in the first sixteen weeks of pregnancy. This view lasted for three centuries, and then the Church fixed ensoulment at forty days after conception. Abortion during the first forty days of pregnancy was considered no sin until 1869, when the Church ruled that life begins at the moment of conception and therefore abortion at any time is a grave sin. This is the position the Catholic Church holds today; it never sanctions abortion per se, even to save the life of the pregnant woman. For well over one hundred years the major Protestant sects have sanctioned abortion, at first only for saving the mother's life, and later for health and eugenic purposes. This permissive attitude toward abortion has now evolved even further, resulting in support by several of the major Protestant denominations of abortion on request, the decision being a personal one between doctor and patient.

Nineteenth-Century Abortion Laws

Before 1803 England had no specific abortion law, and the English Common Law had jurisdiction over abortion, holding that abortion was legal until the fetus moved. The 1803 English statute made all abortions a crime, but abortion before fetal movements was a lesser crime than abortion after fetal movements. The American Colonies, and subsequently the United States early in its history, were bound in many areas by English Common Law. Connecticut, the first state to pass an abortion statute, in 1820 made all abortions illegal, the penalty not being affected by duration of pregnancy. New York, in 1828, was the first political jurisdiction in the world to introduce an exception, abortion being permitted "to preserve the life of the mother."

Professor Cyril Means, a legal scholar, has researched the genesis of the New York law. The statute was passed by a Protestant legislature, not on ethical grounds but specifically to promote maternal health. This was in the days before anesthesia, asepsis, antibiotics, or transfusions, and death was common from the operative procedure of abortion, even within a first-class hospital. At the New York Hospital between 1803 and 1830, eight legal abortions had been performed with five women surviving, a death rate of 37.5 per cent. During the same period, childbirth at the New York Hospital was associated with a 2.8 per cent mortality. Therefore, to protect women against the inherent dangers of the operation, in 1828 the legislators insisted that its risk be permitted only when the physician involved believed there was no other means to preserve the life of the pregnant woman. Within several years all of the states either copied the exact wording of the New York statute or approximated it. In some it was phrased to promote "the safety of the mother," and a few stated that an illegal abortion was a criminal offense but did not define "legal abortion."

Present Legal Status of Abortion

By the late 1960's there was widespread dissatisfaction with the antiquated state of our laws on abortion. Legislatures began to approve laws authorizing abortion for reasons other than the few medical pretexts that had previously been accepted. Then, in 1970, New York terminated all restrictions on abortions done by physicians, except for requiring supervision by the State Board of Health. In January 1973, the U.S. Supreme Court recognized abortion as a privacy right to be exercised by the woman with the aid of her doctor, under no special supervision by local law until the second trimester of pregnancy. Once the fetus is viable, the state may assert an interest in its welfare.

Present Incidence of Legal Abortion

The Centers for Disease Control of the U.S. Public Health Service (CDC) reported 1,297,606 legal abortions in 1980 in the fifty states and the District of Columbia. These statistics are incomplete; the Alan Guttmacher Institute (AGI) collects more complete figures, since it includes the abortions done in the offices of private physicians, which are not necessarily reported to the CDC. The AGI statistics indicate that in 1982 the number of legal abortions in the United States exceeded 1.5 million. The national abortion ratio was 426 abortions per 1,000 live births for the period from July 1982 through June 1983, ranging from a low of 100 in Utah to over 1,517 in the District of Columbia. The national abortion rate was 25 abortions per 1,000 women aged fifteen to forty-four in 1980.

Twenty-nine percent of the women aborted in 1980 were nineteen years of age or younger, and another 35 percent were from twenty to twenty-four. Seventy-seven percent of the women were unmarried, the abortion ratio being very much higher for them than for married women. Racial distribution is also unbalanced. The abortion ratio for black women was 543 per 1,000 live births and for white women, 332.

More than half of all the abortions were performed at under eight weeks of gestation and 89 percent at less than thirteen weeks. A remarkable 95 percent was done by dilation and suction or dilation and evacuation. These are the safest techniques at the present time; a detailed description of each is to be found below.

It is noteworthy that the younger the woman the later in pregnancy the abortion tends to be done. Young women with no living children continued to account for an increasing proportion of abortions, while women with four or more children have experienced a steadily declining abortion ratio.

Most meaningful are the statistics that demonstrate the effect of legalization on maternal deaths. In 1972, when a few states had already enacted laws permitting abortion in certain specified circumstances, abortion mortality had begun to change for the better; abortion-related deaths still amounted to 90 among 586,760 reported abortions, or 15 per 100,000. In 1980 there were 16 deaths among 1,297,606 abortions, or 1.1 per 100,000. Six of these deaths were complications of spontaneous abortions and one was of unknown cause. The one illegal abortion that resulted in death was actually performed outside the United States, although the patient returned and died here. There were

8 deaths associated with legal abortion, a rate of 6 deaths per 1,000,000 among legal procedures. The most significant change for those of us who work in large public hospitals is that we are no longer repeatedly confronted with the need to try to rescue desperately ill women from death due to infection from illegal abortions.

For the years 1972–1981, surgical evacuation procedures, except dilation and evacuation (D & E), had a mortality rate for the mother of 0.9 per 100,000 procedures as compared to 9.6 for intra-amniotic instillations (amnioinfusion) of material to induce abortion and 60 per 100,000 for abdominal operations for the purpose. The rates for each of these have declined steadily during this eight-year period and continue to decline at the present time, but the relative rates are unchanged. The present maternal mortality for evacuation of the uterus prior to the eighth week of pregnancy has to be considered to be in the vicinity of 3 per 1,000,000 abortions. As the thirteenth week is approached the death rate climbs even for suction evacuation, and beyond this point, where dilation and evacuation is required, the death rate is probably in the vicinity of 5 per 100,000. This is still approximately half the mortality encountered for intra-amniotic instillations.

In 1982 in New York City there were 162,000 abortions completed. Well over 90 percent of these were done by suction evacuation. In 1981 there was only one death from legal abortion, and none in 1982. In the small percentage of abortions late in the second trimester, done by amnioinfusion or by abdominal operation, there were eighteen births of live fetuses. This deplorable accident can be appropriately avoided by more careful estimation of the duration of pregnancy and the size of the fetus by ultrasound examination.

Effects on Future Childbearing

What are the effects of abortion on future childbearing? It is quite solidly established now that abortion prior to the tenth week of pregnancy has no impact on the safety of subsequent pregnancies, even with repeated procedures. We do not even now have sufficiently good follow-up information on abortions in the second trimester by any appropriate procedure. There is some suggestion that the dilation of the cervix in these late procedures may increase the incidence of subsequent premature labors. Intra-amniotic instillation to induce abortion in the second trimester may result in a particularly violent labor. This has been observed to produce rupture of the uterus or rupture of the cervix, each of which may produce serious hemorrhage. Both require surgical repair.

Opposition to Abortion

Even though legal abortion appears to function well and to meet a great need, as witnessed by the fact that more than one and a half million abortions are done in the United States each year, this has not silenced the opposition. It is politically significant that the approximately 1.5 million women who request abortion tend to be young, disproportionately poor, disproportionately black, and not politically potent. The most effective segment of the women in favor of legal abortion are those who identify reproductive freedom as essential to their personal and professional lives. On the other side, the women who oppose abortion tend to be those who see motherhood as their most important role in life and who feel that ready access to abortion denigrates that role. The opposition to abortion is predominantly found among men. With few exceptions those individuals who have been involved in bombings and arson against abortion facilities have been males.

There are surely earnest individuals who equate abortion with homicide and on such grounds find it unjustifiable. Others feel that abortion is immoral unless it is necessitated by serious medical conditions in the mother; these people believe that abortion on socioeconomic grounds cannot be justified. There are those who have argued against abortion on the ground that it has serious psychiatric consequences for the mother. Careful follow-up studies have demonstrated that this is not the case, although in many instances the interruption of a pregnancy may be followed by a period of guilt and grief. No unbiased study has yet demonstrated any long-term unfavorable psychiatric reactions to abortions except for abortions carried out under duress.

In early 1985 it appeared that the organized and well-financed opposition to abortion had made some headway in its campaign, particularly since they had the outspoken support of the President of the United States. It is, however, still the case that a substantial majority of the population supports the availability of abortion and this even includes people who would not themselves be willing to be aborted. There are many who support the position that a pregnant woman should have the right to decide what happens to her body. As I have indicated, the mortality rate from term pregnancy is substantially higher than that from early abortion. It has been argued for this reason that a woman's request that pregnancy be terminated could be considered a form of self-defense against what she perceives to be a threat to her life. The recent court decisions (and with the efforts that are being made to obstruct the provision of abortion, these are fairly numerous) have steadfastly declined to turn back the clock in this area of women's rights. Those of us who in the past witnessed the damage due to illegal abortion and on occasion struggled to save a woman's life at such a time find it dreadful to contemplate that we might ever return to such circumstances.

Abortion Techniques in the First Trimester

At present, the basic technique for early abortion is suction evacuation of the products of conception from the uterus. When the abortion is done up to about the ninth or tenth week, it can occasionally be accomplished with minimal dilation of the cervix, especially in patients who have previously had term deliveries. Dilation and curettage, the procedure known as D & C, is outmoded under almost all circumstances.

The important first step is an accurate determination of the duration of the pregnancy. This is readily accomplished if the woman is known to be normal, has kept careful records of her menstrual periods and her contraceptive practices, and can provide a reliable description of her symptoms. The next step after taking the history is to do an abdominal and pelvic examination. The uterus may prove to be larger than would be expected for her menstrual dates—if for example, she has a uterine fibroid—or substantially smaller. It is then necessary to resort to sonography for an objective determination of the duration of pregnancy. The sonogram may on occasion disclose an empty uterus, in which case the diagnosis may be ectopic pregnancy.

The safest time to carry out abortion in the first trimester is at about seven or eight weeks of pregnancy. When abortions are done earlier than this, occasionally the cervix has not yet been softened by the hormonal effects of the pregnancy. Gaining access to the uterine cavity then involves use of considerable force to open the cervix, particularly in women who have not had previous pregnancies. When the cervix is unusually firm and the patient is seven or more weeks pregnant, it is appropriate to employ local anesthetics, injected into and around the cervix. This not only obliterates most of the discomfort of the procedure but induces relaxation of the cervix, making manipulation easier. Many patients are benefited by sedation and analgesia with a combination of drugs like Valium and Demerol. General anesthesia ordinarily should not be used, as it markedly increases the risk and lengthens the immediate recovery time, though it does enable the procedure to be done more quickly. The abortion can be done on an ambulatory basis.

Since the body of the uterus is itself not anesthetized, the patient is able to feel the contractions with which the uterus responds to the evacuation of its contents. These cramps are essentially the same as those of the menstrual period. The patient should be warned in advance that this cramping may occur. Some of the discomfort may be due to negative pressure involved in the procedure; it is always possible to turn off the suction machine temporarily if the discomfort becomes severe.

The operation is carried out with the patient lying on her back and her thighs spread apart. An antiseptic solution is used to wash the external genitalia. A sterile speculum is placed in the vagina and the cervix brought into view. The antiseptic solution may then be applied to the cervix and upper vagina. The local anesthetic, if it is to be used, is instilled into and around the cervix. Next, the cervix is held by a surgical instrument and a probe inserted through its canal to verify the size of the uterine cavity.

Now a catheter is passed into the uterus. This tube has an

opening at the side of its internal end. Its outer end is attached to the vacuum device. For pregnancies at about seven weeks the catheters are about the same diameter as an ordinary lead pencil. For more advanced pregnancies they have to be larger and may be as much as two-thirds again larger in diameter. When the plastic tube is in the proper place and the suction has been established, the catheter is rotated. The negative pressure within it draws the products of conception into the tube and thence into the receptacle in the suction device. Since the tube is translucent it is possible for the operator to see the products as they are passed and thus be sure that the procedure is successful. All this takes a few minutes. Very little bleeding occurs, since the uterus responds promptly with contractions, which reduce the blood loss. With somewhat more advanced pregnancies it may be necessary to use an increasingly large series of metal dilators to open the cervix. These dilators are tapered probes that gradually stretch the cervical canal open to allow room for the larger catheters.

At the conclusion of the procedure the catheter and the speculum are withdrawn and the patient is allowed to rest for a brief while to recover from whatever discomfort she may have had. The operator is obligated to inspect the tissues that have been removed to be certain that there are products of conception among them. Inadequacy in the amount of tissue suggests an ectopic pregnancy.

Postoperative care is minimal; it generally requires no more effort than the patient would ordinarily undertake for a menstrual period. There is no reason why the patient cannot return promptly to her normal activities. The administration of antibiotics for a few days after the procedure may reduce the occurrence of fever and infection.

Abortion Techniques from the Twelfth to the Sixteenth Week

The technique most commonly used at this duration is dilation and evacuation (D & E). It is essential to know the size of the fetus because this will determine the selection of instruments to be used for the evacuation. An accurate estimate of the duration of pregnancy is obtained by sonography. At less than sixteen weeks it is difficult to place a needle into the amniotic sac and therefore amnioinfusion, which will be described in some detail below, cannot be employed.

The patients are prepared for D & E by methods to soften and open the cervix, at least several hours and sometimes a day or two before the procedure itself is undertaken. The method most commonly employed and the one that has the fewest side effects is the insertion of osmotic dilators into the cervical canal. These swell in the presence of water. One or more is introduced into the cervix. There they absorb water from the cervical canal and gradually enlarge, sometimes sufficiently so that further dilation of the cervix is not necessary at the time of abortion. The cervix also softens so that it can be readily dilated further if necessary. The commonly used osmotic dilator is laminaria, a seaweed that can be gas-sterilized prior to use. Individual laminaria are approximately the diameter of a lead pencil and about three inches long. It is possible to put several side by side into the cervix of a pregnant woman who has previously had children. The laminaria are removed before the initiation of the evacuation of uterine contents.

As is the case with suction abortion, the patient lies on her back with thighs apart, and a speculum is put into the vagina to visualize the cervix. Some sedation is generally given before this, with the same drugs used in first-trimester abortion. A local anesthetic of the cervix is then established and the cervix grasped. After the cervical canal has been adequately dilated, a catheter of a diameter appropriate for the duration of pregnancy is introduced through the cervix up to the membranes and negative pressure applied. This empties the amniotic fluid from the sac and brings the fetus down to the tip of the suction device.

Using forceps, the fetus can then be grasped and drawn through the dilated cervix. Once the fetus is completely evacuated, the suction device can be put back in and the placenta removed by suction.

This technique has several advantages at this duration of pregnancy, not the least of which is its safety compared with other techniques. Although it is several times more hazardous than an abortion early in the first trimester it is also materially less risky than abortion by any other technique beyond the sixteenth week.

The procedure can also be done on an ambulatory basis. It is important that women who are Rh-negative, unless they know with certainty that the father of the pregnancy is also Rh-negative, should be given a prophylactic dose of hyper-immune anti-D globulin (Rhogam).

Abortion Techniques at the Sixteenth Week or Beyond

At the present time these abortions are done in less than 5 percent of all women coming for abortion. Some are women found to have fetuses with congenital abnormalities. Since genetic amniocentesis is ordinarily done at about the sixteenth week and it takes three to four weeks to establish a diagnosis, many of these women are as far as the twentieth week before procedures to interrupt pregnancy can be decided upon.

Abortion can be done by dilation and evacuation at this duration of pregnancy, and reports have appeared of D & E done as late as the twenty-second week of pregnancy. In some jurisdictions this is contrary to law, but even where it is legal, fewer and fewer such procedures are being done this late. D & E is a more formidable undertaking this late in pregnancy, since the fetus is substantially larger and much more difficult to extract. It is necessary to achieve a much greater degree of cervical dilation, in some cases up to as much as two inches in diameter. Special instruments are required to achieve this. It is also necessary to put in laminaria on at least two occasions, so that the procedure takes an additional day. The abortion can be done under local anesthesia with general sedation and is therefore feasible on an ambulatory basis, but some of the physicians doing this have preferred to use general anesthesia.

Warren Hern, who has done as many of these late second-trimester abortions as anyone else in the United States, reports that, with the proper preparation with laminaria and careful selection with sonography, his actual time to do the abortion is less than ten minutes. He also reports a major complication rate of 3 per 1,000 procedures. However, the risk of this procedure in the hands of someone less experienced will be substantially larger than that.

The other technique available at this duration of pregnancy is amnioinfusion. This involves placing a needle through the abdominal wall and the uterine wall into a pocket of amniotic fluid inside the uterus. A few hundred milliliters of fluid are withdrawn and drugs intended to bring about fetal death and uterine contractions are injected into the amniotic sac. The original material used for this purpose was a strong salt solution but this has now been replaced with other medications, the commonest of which is prostaglandin F_2, used by itself or in combination with urea, a nitrogen-containing chemical that is a normal component of the blood. The prostaglandin causes intense spasm of the umbilical cord, in addition to stimulating uterine contractions. The use of urea increases the safety of the mother, because urea is a normal body constituent and a healthy person can tolerate considerable concentrations of this chemical. At some time not entirely predictable after the injection of the abortifacient materials, the fetus dies and uterine contractions begin. These eventually become quite forceful and are more painful than the normal term labor since the uterus has not had an opportunity to prepare itself for labor. The total time from injection to abortion can be shortened by the application of laminaria prior to the infusion.

Women undergoing late abortions are best cared for in a hospital. The majority of patients require drugs to alleviate pain. They are frequently unable to eat during this period and benefit from the administration of intravenous fluids. There are occasionally transitory adverse reactions to prostaglandin. Fortunately, prostaglandin is destroyed quite rapidly in the lungs as the blood containing it passes through, and these toxic responses are of brief duration.

Once the cervix has been opened by the uterine contractions, the products of conception are passed quite easily in about 50 percent of the instances. The placenta often does not come out readily and it may be necessary for the physician to undertake an instrumental removal. This is ordinarily accomplished through the opened cervix with little difficulty.

It is quite clear that prostaglandin and prostaglandin/urea

combinations are safer than the administration of concentrated sodium chloride for amnioinfusion. With all these methods a very rapid labor can result in injury to the unprepared cervix.

We have inadequate information at the present time of the later effects of these late abortions on future childbearing. It is difficult to suppress the suspicion that there may be increased risk of subsequent pregnancy loss, but it is not yet possible to show that this actually is the case.

The Rh-negative women should also receive Rhogam.

Once the abortion is complete and the bleeding minimal the women can be discharged from the hospital to their own care. Little more is required than they would do for a heavy menstrual period. Those patients who have more than the usual amount of bleeding are advised to take iron by mouth for two or three months after the completion of the abortion.

Since with amnioinfusion it is desirable to hospitalize the patients, ambulatory abortion by D & E is considerably less expensive.

Postabortional care for all should include counseling on preventive health maintenance with specific reference to contraception. There have been some studies of the insertion of intrauterine devices after the completion of abortion. It is not clear whether this is ideal for every woman. Although it certainly can be readily done at the conclusion of early abortions, with abortions in the second trimester, the dilation of the cervix and the size of the uterus are such that an intrauterine device tends to fall out. However, IUDs may not be available in the United States in the future (see IUDs, p. 480). In some situations it may be wise for the patient to start using oral contraceptives immediately after the completion of the abortion.

Sterilization either by laparoscopy or abdominal operation at the time of first-trimester abortion does not increase the complications of either procedure.

There have been studies of the outcome of term pregnancy among the patients who are refused abortion because they have gone too far in pregnancy. These studies suggest that there is really no difference in subsequent maternal or neonatal complications among them as compared with women who have never considered abortion. There is no evidence of serious psychiatric disorder among women who have had abortions, although there are periods of grief and bereavement over the loss of the pregnancy.

Induced Abortion after Cesarean

Previous cesarean does not complicate first-trimester abortion done with a suction catheter. The same probably applies to D & E. However, since amnioinfusion aborts by inducing uterine contractions, there have been uterine ruptures at the site of a previous cesarean with this method.

Abortion by Hysterotomy and Hysterectomy

Hysterotomy (emptying the uterus by opening it through an abdominal incision) and hysterectomy (removal of the intact uterus) are major operations and present an unacceptable degree of risk when used for abortion. An intent to facilitate sterilization does not justify doing unnecessary major surgery. Hysterotomy, by producing a defect in the uterine wall, has the potential of imperiling future pregnancies.

Abortion by Medical Means

Abortion by using a drug that will stimulate the uterus to contract and thus empty itself of the products of conception has long been considered to be the ideal method because it eliminates the risks associated with surgical approaches. Medical abortion is an ancient idea and the pharmacology of every century has included such methods. Thus far, however, no drug has been found that is both safe and effective; none that we know of works with certainty unless it makes the woman so ill that her life may be endangered.

In the past, quinine and ergot powders were tried as abortifacients but were rarely successful. More recently, attention was directed to intravenous oxytocin: a very potent hormone that induces uterine contractions. It is impressively effective in the last trimester and increasingly so as the pregnancy approaches term. However, it is useless in inducing abortion during the first and second trimesters, when the amounts needed to cause abortion are prodigious, and have undesirable side effects.

In the past fifteen years investigators of medical abortifacients have turned to the use of one of the prostaglandins. The trail to this class of drugs was broken by a gynecologist who observed, when he was carrying out artificial insemination by injecting semen into the uterine cavity, that the uterus reacted with violent contractions. He concluded that there was some component of semen that was powerfully stimulating the uterine muscle. Subsequently, Dr. Ulf von Euler in Sweden studied this effect and isolated the active material. Since he concluded that it was produced in the prostate gland, he named it prostaglandin. A long series of related chemical compounds has now been synthesized and tested for human use. The search has been for a prostaglandin that will induce uterine contraction without affecting the muscle of the gastrointestinal tract at the same time. Prostaglandins have been administered by dilute intravenous drip and or as suppositories in the upper vagina. There is little question that they stimulate sufficient uterine activity to result in abortion. However, these abortions tend to be protracted and to be accompanied by considerable blood loss. Since the uterine contractions themselves are quite forceful, an exaggeration of the contractions of menses and labor, the women require large doses of pain-relieving drugs. But a more serious obstacle to their use in practice is that many women experience severe nausea and vomiting, and even a greater number have repeated bouts of diarrhea during the peak of effectiveness of the drug. Experimentation with various routes of adminstration, various doses, and various prostaglandins has not yet identified a method that separates the abortifacient action from these formidable side effects.

Making Decisions about Abortion

The Supreme Court in 1973 in the case of *Roe* v. *Wade* established the right of a pregnant woman to request an abortion, in consultation with her physician. The physician's role is largely to give advice on medical issues that might for one reason or another indicate that abortion is not appropriate. Some doctors are not willing to do abortions but may be prepared and able to refer a woman to another doctor or clinic. If this is not possible, the woman may have to conduct her own search for the help she needs. A good resource is the nearest Planned Parenthood clinic.

There have been a number of efforts all over the country to require that the parents of adolescents be notified of their daughters' request for abortion. Because a woman's right to make her own reproductive choices is a constitutional right under the Supreme Court, parents cannot veto the decision of their teenage daughter either to have or not to have an abortion. There exists, in many jurisdictions, but varying from state to state, a rule known as the "mature minor rule." This protects the young woman's autonomy, provided she is found to be sufficiently mature to make up her mind in a rational way. If she has been able to confide in her parents, has consulted with them, and has secured their agreement to her having an abortion, the problem of whether she has mature enough judgment does not arise. However, difficulties may arise if she is alienated from her parents, has no parents effectively functioning, or she and her parents disagree.

A requirement of parental consent would probably do nothing to remedy bad family relationships in cases of this sort. Some jurisdictions require that the young woman secure permission from a court, in lieu of parental consent; the court may decide in terms of the best interests of the minor, or may determine that the young woman is capable of making her own decision and allow her to do so.

In any case, ideally one would want pregnant young women in their teens to have a strong support system upon which they can rely rather than have the delicate question of abortion decided in the daunting atmosphere of a courtroom.

Ambulatory or In-Hospital Abortion?

The question arises whether abortion should be provided in what is generally called an outpatient clinic or whether it should be done in a hospital. Most health departments have made rules governing facilities providing services on an ambulatory basis, whether inside the walls of the hospital or freestanding, that is, physically separate from a hospital. There is not very much to choose between the two types of facility, provided they meet health department guidelines. Since ambulatory services do not have to include the cost of a hospital bed, they are materially less expensive than being admitted to a hospital. Many hospitals provide an ambulatory abortion service that is essentially equivalent to that provided by a freestanding clinic.

If you need local information about abortion facilities it will probably be best for you to get in touch with the nearest Planned Parenthood facility, whether or not that facility itself provides abortion. Advertisements in the Yellow Pages of the telephone book are not a reliable indicator of the quality of the service provided.

For some patients the decision to seek abortion is simple and the experience not materially different from that of making a visit to the physician for any other minor surgical procedure. Such patients as this are able to take off a morning or an afternoon from work, have the abortion, and resume their daily lives.

Other patients may suffer major psychological trauma, which leads them to delay making the abortion decision; this in turn results in their having to undergo a second-trimester procedure rather than the brief and simple early abortion. Furthermore, the fact that abortion may be available on request may not be helpful in dealing with a woman's moral qualms arising from her personality, upbringing, and education. The legality of the procedure simply emphasizes that the patient herself has the responsibility for the choice, which may be easy or difficult. It would be wrong to underemphasize the importance of these psychological factors. My impression, for example, is that patients who have had several elective abortions tend to have a rocky emotional time during the first pregnancy that they decide to carry to term. Fortunately, there is no evidence that early abortions properly performed have any effect on future fertility.

Premature Labor

There is no exact physical or physiological point at which a fetus ceases to be a premature and becomes mature, no matter how precisely the pregnancy is dated. All the changes that occur are gradual, especially in the latter two-thirds of the third trimester. There are no great leaps forward in baby behavior from one day to the next.

Some sixty years ago a perceptive Finnish pediatrician, who dedicated his entire life work to the care of small newborns, proposed that for purposes of classification a weight of 2.5 kilos be considered the dividing line between prematurity and maturity. This has the convenience for users of the British and American systems of weights and measures of being almost precisely five and a half pounds. His suggestion was universally adopted and has remained the basic definition ever since.

Prior to delivery, the date of the last menstrual period is the best single piece of information as to the duration of the pregnancy. For this reason, birth certificates in most of the States now call for entry of both that date and of the weight of the newborn. However, as many women do not have an exact recollection of the date, this information is probably less reliable than the objectively verifiable weight of the newborn in deciding whether or not it is premature.

On the average, maturity of the fetus, by the weight criterion, is reached at about thirty-five weeks. This does not mean that smaller babies cannot be saved. Newborns have survived whose birth weights were less than 400 grams, a gestational age of about twenty-five weeks, but this is quite rare. If we accept the weight criterion, for all births in the United States the overall rate of prematurity in 1982 was 6.8 percent.

However, there is a significant difference between the rate for white women (5.6 percent) and for black women (12.4 percent), which runs consistently through almost all statistics on the newborn, and which suggests that the standard of the weight of the newborn in determining prematurity may have to be modified for ethnic factors. Socioeconomic background (poverty, inadequate nutrition, and other such matters) may account for some, or even most, of the statistical differences in birth weight between American black and American white newborns. It is also true that some ethnic groups tend to have smaller babies and some to have larger ones.

I recall noticing while traveling in the western part of Guatemala how small the adults were; their newborns are correspondingly diminutive. On the other hand, as an obstetrician in Minnesota, I became quite familiar with the nine- and ten-pound infants regularly produced by patients of Swedish extraction.

Shortly after World War II a very careful study was done in Aberdeen, Scotland, on the incidence of prematurity among the various social classes. Because of the stability of the population and a clear identification of not only the employment and social status of the baby's mother and father but also of its grandparents, it was possible to identify the long-term social background of the mothers. It became quite clear that the incidence of prematurity doubled as one proceeded from the financially best-off group of patients to those least advantaged. It was also clear that the social status of the mother's parents affected the rate of prematurity in the same way, even if the mother herself had moved up in social class. Although we do not have the exquisite detail that was provided to us by the Scots, it is fair to conclude that the broad differences in the United States between the outcomes of pregnancies among white women and those among black reflect the same mix of inheritance and socioeconomic status.

There are other factors that bear on the size and maturity of the newborn. In the United States the rate of premature birth is distinctly increased among adolescent mothers and among those over forty years of age. This probably reflects dietary inadequacies among the teenagers and an increased incidence in pregnancy complications among the older women, for example, placenta previa and hypertension. As I have mentioned, placenta previa often makes it necessary to deliver the baby prematurely. High blood pressure similarly may force the doctor's hand to bring the pregnancy to an early termination.

One factor is the occurrence of multiple births, which are more common among black women. Twins and triplets deliver substantially before term, the average among twins being approximately twenty-two days early. This results in a distinctly increased proportion of prematures among multiple births. Furthermore, multiples increase in frequency as women become older and have more pregnancies.

There is no question that dietary improvement will add weight to the newborn, although it has not been conclusively demonstrated that this weight difference alone makes a significant difference in the outcome for these babies.

Cause of Premature Labor

Unfortunately we know very little about the cause of most of the instances of the premature labor. Occasionally it is obviously due to some abnormality of the uterus. The two such causes that have been clearly identified are malformations of the body of the uterus and abnormalities of the cervix.

The uterus forms from two tubes, one on each side of the body, which come together early in embryonic life to fuse to form a single structure. On occasion one tube or another develops insufficiently, resulting in a distorted uterine cavity or in one that derives from only one of the two tubes. These defects tend to result in a uterus that fails to expand normally in the course of pregnancy and for that reason ejects the fetus prior to term. This is apparently the explanation for the premature onset of labor in DES daughters, the women who were exposed when they themselves were fetuses to diethylstilbestrol given to their mothers.

The defects of the cervix manifest themselves by a dilation of the cervix, commonly rather painless, in the middle of the second trimester. On rare occasions this occurs in the first pregnancy. It may also occur with increased frequency in patients who have had late second-trimester abortions.

Even more uncommonly, premature labor can be associated with the presence of uterine fibroids that restrict the ability of the uterine body to expand to accommodate the pregnancy. Causes of premature labor of this sort generally are repetitive unless some measures are undertaken to correct the abnormality.

Another cause of premature labor, one that remains an enigma despite much study, is premature rupture of membranes. When the membranes rupture at or close to term, labor is likely to ensue shortly thereafter. The earlier the rupture, however, the longer the interval before labor. If membranes rupture far enough before term, a premature birth will be inevitable.

Treatment of Premature Labor

The initial step is to establish the diagnosis. In many cases this is easier said than done. The pregnant uterus normally contracts, and a woman may well become aware of this by the twenty-fourth week. On occasion these contractions are rather severe. Furthermore, the cervix shortens and occasionally dilates during the early part of the third trimester. If these two events combine in a single patient it may be extraordinarily difficult to decide whether or not the patient is in early labor. If in fact she is not, any therapy or none at all will be equally successful. Evaluating the treatment thus is very difficult, as the measure of success is that nothing has happened, and one cannot be sure that there even was a condition that required treatment.

Assuming, however, that the woman actually is in premature labor, we still do not have a completely safe drug that will predictably and reliably turn it off. The usual treatment starts with bed rest and a period of observation, sometimes combined with narcotics to dull the patient's awareness of her discomfort and assuage her anxiety and drugs to help her sleep. We must suppose that those patients salvaged from what appeared to be premature labor by this therapy have not been in labor at all.

We now have a series of medications that do have provable effects on uterine contraction. One of these is alcohol, which may be taken by mouth as beer, wine, or whiskey, or intravenously as the pure drug. The latter route is more readily controlled. In adequate doses, alcohol blocks some of the hormonal mechanisms responsible for uterine contraction and thereby markedly diminishes the frequency and force of contractions. This effect is not quite as potent as one would wish. It has been difficult to demonstrate whether its use in women who appear to be in premature labor does more than delay delivery for a few days. A difficulty is that, when adequate doses of alcohol are used, the patients become serious nursing problems. Many of them are quite drunk. The procedure must be done in a hospital for that reason and cannot be continued for long periods.

Another effective medication is magnesium sulfate, given

either intramuscularly or intravenously. The latter route has come to be preferred because of its greater predictability. Magnesium given in this way must be administered in a hospital. In doses close to those which eliminate uterine contraction, it can also depress maternal respiration, so that the patient must have continuous observation while the drug is being given. Magnesium eventually crosses the placenta and may affect newborn respirations as well; babies with elevated magnesium levels at birth require special attention.

The final group of drugs effective in stopping the uterine contractions are the beta-mimetics. They mimic the action of adrenalin, the secretion of the adrenal gland which is part of the emergency system by which the body reacts to danger or fright. It is known that fright can delay or halt labor, and that adrenalin given intravenously in labor will temporarily halt contractions and relax the uterus. This property is shared by betamimetics such as ritodrine and terbutaline, which can have a more prolonged effect. All these drugs speed up the pulse rate, increase blood pressure and blood sugar, and cause tremors and a sense of anxiety. Since they cross the placenta, they have similar effects on the fetus.

They are at first administered intravenously in low concentrations. These are steadily and cautiously increased until the desired effect in stopping uterine contractions is achieved. The women unfortunately often become aware of the fact that their hearts are speeded up and that they are anxious. These side effects may limit the amount of drug that can be employed to less than needed to stop the uterus. Other serious side effects such as chest pain and formation of fluid in the lungs make it necessary that these patients be under observation while the drug is being used. When labor has been brought to a halt, it is possible to switch to oral administration and then to begin to ambulate the patient.

It must be clear from what I have said that we do not have an ideal drug to stop premature labor. The search for safer and more predictable drugs continues. As is the case with uterine stimulants such as the prostaglandins, it is difficult to slow down or speed up the uterus without affecting other body systems.

Corticoid drugs have been employed in recent years in an

effort to hasten the development of the lungs of the fetus in hazard of premature birth within the next few days. This has also turned out to be something very difficult to study. It appears that by about the thirty-third week of pregnancy the fetus has developed the ability to respond to stress by producing enough of its own adrenal cortical steroids to mature its lungs. For babies scheduled to be delivered before the thirty-third week in the absence of fetal stress, for example because of maternal disease, it is presently thought helpful to give the mother substantial doses of steroids to encourage lung maturation in the fetus. There is some question whether this therapy might have long term effects on the fetus; this possibility must be weighed against what appears to be an improvement in the respiratory performance of these small newborns.

Premature Rupture of the Membranes

This is by definition an uncontrollable leakage of fluid, occurring more than twelve hours before the onset of labor, resulting from tears in the membranes. It seems to make a difference in the outcome whether the tear in the membranes is in the region close to the cervical os, in the low uterus, or whether the tear is up high in the fundus. The risk of infection is substantially greater when the tear is low and the likelihood of the prompt onset of labor is less when the tear is high.

We would all be delighted to have some kind of blowout patch with which to reseal the membranes, but nothing of this sort exists. The consensus is that when labor ensues following premature rupture of the membranes, efforts should not be made to restrain it.

Surgical Approaches to Premature Labor

When the premature onset of labor is clearly due to abnormalities of the uterine fundus, surgical approaches may be considered for subsequent pregnancies. Where the problem is uterine duplication, there is a group of operations designed to unite the two halves into a single adequate uterine cavity. There have been some elegant successes with this undertaking. This can also be said for those women in whom fibroids have clearly been a causative factor in premature labor. The treatment is removal of the fibroid or fibroids, not always an easy operation. In the event of either of these procedures, subsequent deliveries are probably better done by cesarean.

Where the defect is in the cervix, it may come to attention because the patient notices a pinkish watery discharge in the early second trimester. On speculum examination the cervix is found to be softened, its canal shortened and anywhere from two to five centimeters dilated, with membranes protruding through the canal. Occasionally the membranes fall through the cervix into the vagina in an hourglass fashion. Most of these pregnancies are doomed because of damage to the membranes, which shortly results in their rupture. However, even this late it may be possible to sew the cervix closed with one of several operations that fall under the general title of cerclage. Heavy suture material is placed in the cervix in a purse-string or similar fashion. When this is successful, it holds the cervix closed until term. Some doctors prefer to cut the suture out at that time and allow the patient to go into labor, while others leave a successful cerclage in place and deliver by cesarean.

It is now accepted that a patient who has a history of previous pregnancy losses due to such to a defective cervix is probably best served by a prophylactic cerclage, done toward the end of the first trimester as soon as it is possible to demonstrate by sonography that the fetus is normal.

Route of Delivery for Premature Infants

There has been debate as to whether elimination of the stresses of labor by delivering all significantly premature babies by cesarean section would increase the newborn survival rate. The best evidence now is that this is not the case, although there are times when cesarean is clearly indicated for other reasons. Examples of this are situations where the fetus is presenting abnormally, where placenta previs is present, where there is infection, or when the cervix is rigid and fails to dilate. Of course, these are reasons for doing cesareans to deliver mature babies as well.

11

Diseases and Operations during Pregnancy

Having a baby today is a very safe undertaking. With competent care, serious illness and mortality from childbirth are rare events. My own estimate of the inevitable maternal death rate from unavoidable accidents of pregnancy and labor is about 3 deaths per 100,000 births. The discomforts of labor are relatively brief, and have yielded to effective pain relief by medical and psychological means, all of which tend to increase speed and safety of birth. The trend to educated, family-centered care in which the patient's support system is encouraged to participate at times of crisis has been of immense help to pregnant women.

Concerns about the fetus and newborn are real, but the risks continue to decrease. Once you have safely reached the twenty-eighth week, you have a 98 percent chance of having a surviving child and better than 99 percent chance that it will be without serious abnormality.

There is no illness to which a pregnant woman is immune unless it be some menstrual disorder. There is no complaint that a pregnant woman may not experience—with the exception of infertility. It would take an encyclopedia to consider in detail all the major deviations from normal health, their effects on the course of pregnancy and, in turn, the influence of pregnancy on the ordinary life cycle of every disease. This book is not an encyclopedia, but within its confines we can discuss some of the commoner major medical and surgical problems as they occur in a pregnant woman.

Diabetes

Prior to the introduction of insulin in 1922, diabetic women rarely became pregnant and when they did, the outcome was ordinarily catastrophic for both mother and baby. The death rate for each was alarmingly high. With the use of insulin, diabetic women have become normally fertile and the threat to the mother's life has virtually vanished. Until very recently however, this could not be said for the welfare of the fetus.

For one thing, uncontrolled diabetes appears to lead to a small but significant increase in the rate of congenital anomalies. If the embryo escapes this damage, it is by no means in for smooth sailing unless the diabetes is very carefully regulated. The excess sugar present in the mother's blood crosses through the placenta so that as the mother's blood sugar rises, the blood sugar of the fetus goes up, too. Under these circumstances, the cells in the fetus's pancreas that are responsible for regulating blood sugar produce excess insulin, which then functions as a growth hormone in the fetus. Consequently, when the mother's blood sugar is constantly elevated, the fetuses tend to become very large. Their appearance is so typical that it has earned an acronym among pediatricians, who call such newborns "IDM," meaning Infant of a Diabetic Mother. The size of such a fetus may hinder normal birth and result in serious complications of labor. Furthermore, efforts of the mother and baby to regulate their blood sugar create a metabolic stress that alters a number of the baby's other chemical systems, sometimes so severely that the baby dies before birth. To complicate the matter, some women with apparently normal sugar metabolism when not pregnant become diabetic in pregnancy.

In modern obstetrics, all these problems can be managed successfully through careful regulation of the diet and the use of insulin to keep blood sugar within normal limits.

Screening for Diabetes

Any pregnant woman who has had a baby over nine pounds at birth or an unexplained stillbirth or has a strong family history of diabetes has to be considered diabetic until proven otherwise. The proof is obtained by first determining the blood-sugar level under fasting conditions and then giving a standard oral dose of glucose. This is the screening test. If the blood-sugar level one or two hours later is increased above normal, then a glucose tolerance test (GTT) is done. After the oral glucose load, blood sugar levels are measured half an hour, one, two, and three hours later. In diabetics the blood sugar rises higher than normal and the rise is sustained.

If during the prenatal course sugar is found in the urine, a blood-sugar test is done. In some pregnant women, the increased flow of blood through the kidneys results in leakage of sugar even though the blood sugar is normal. These women do not have diabetes. If the measurement of blood sugar does not rule out diabetes, then the screening test is done and this may be followed by a GTT.

The trend now is to do screening tests on all pregnant women at the start of the third trimester in order to identify those who have become abnormal through the stress of pregnancy but who do not as yet have sugar in the urine. The expectation is to head off trouble by early diagnosis.

Care of the Diabetic Mother

Once either true diabetes or gestational diabetes is established, it is important to maintain the maternal blood sugar within normal limits. This is monitored by taking frequent tests of sugar in the blood. The mother can even take small samples of her own blood from her fingertip and test them at home to find out the range of her blood sugar. If the mother is unable to do this she can be admitted to the hospital and these tests done on an inpatient basis. The goal is to maintain the mother's blood sugar at completely normal values by diet and the administration of insulin. There is clearly a need for meticulous individual attention to the mother.

For a long time, it was felt that the threat of stillbirth was so serious that babies of diabetic mothers should be delivered just as soon as they were mature enough to survive without serious respiratory problems. At present, however, the trend is to begin fetal monitoring by the non-stress test (NST) as the patient nears full term, and to continue frequent determinations of blood sugar. If these tests are completely normal, there seems to be no reason to deliver the baby early.

In the past few decades, a great majority of diabetic women were delivered by cesarean section. With the improvements in testing and treatment, very large infants are encountered less and less often. The section delivery rate among diabetics is, however, still substantially higher than that in normal patients.

Management of the diabetic mother in the first few days after delivery can be difficult if there are rapid, wide, or unpredictable changes in the mother's sugar metabolism. The infant of the diabetic mother also requires meticulous care by experienced pediatricians. This is described in Chapter 23.

Hypertension

Maternal hypertension or high blood pressure is another condition of major concern. Since hypertension is, for the most part, of unknown cause, its impact on pregnancy is difficult to predict in an individual case. Some hypertensive women go through pregnancy without any change whatever in their condition and without any sign of hypertension affecting the pregnancy, while others become materially worse. Their blood pressure rises farther and protein appears in the urine. This is called superimposed toxemia, and it may require prompt delivery if medical management fails to achieve control of the blood pressure. In general the hypertensive woman will experience a lowering of blood pressure in the second trimester of pregnancy exactly as does her normal sister. As the pregnancy approaches term the patient's blood pressure tends to return to its prepregnant level. Hypertensives usually produce small babies with small placentas. These babies are ordinarily more mature than their weights would indicate, a common observation in the fetuses exposed to chronic stress. There is a small incidence of fetal death.

The hypertensive woman who is on long-term medications designed to lower blood pressure must continue these medicines during pregnancy and, if the blood pressure seems to be eluding control, the dose of medicine must be increased. Contrary to the impressions of some, starting the medication during pregnancy does not in any way improve the outlook for the fetus. Such late complications of hypertensive disease as stroke and heart enlargement are no more common during pregnancy than they would be otherwise, nor are they in any way accelerated over the long run. Antihypertensive medication has no adverse effect on the fetus. Diuretics (water pills) must be used with great care in pregnancy, however.

Sexually Transmitted Diseases (STD)

When this book was first written, and until very recently, these were called venereal diseases (VD). The one of principal concern at that time was syphilis. In the effort to prevent its effects on the baby *in utero*, testing for syphilis was required by law and all pregnant patients had to have a "Wassermann," the then current screening blood test. The picture has changed dramatically in fifty years. Untreated maternal syphilis is now so rare that in many areas the cost of testing every pregnant woman for it is no longer felt to be economically justifiable.

Fortunately, treatment of syphilis with antibiotics is relatively cheap and simple and provides complete cure of the infant.

Herpes

Meanwhile, herpes genitalis has emerged as a common threat of fetal injury. It is true that death from a generalized virus infection can occur in infants who become infected with the herpes virus either late in pregnancy or in the course of childbirth, as they come through a birth canal that harbors the virus. Many women carry the herpes virus without having any obvious evidence of disease.

The situation is further complicated by the fact that among patients known to have had herpes in the past, it is extremely unlikely for the newborn to develop the disease. The reason for this is not clearly understood, although it seems to have some relationship to the formation of antibodies to the herpes by the mother. The antibodies cross the placenta into the baby's circulation and give it some immunity to the disease.

Fortunately, laboratory tests for the detection of anti–herpes genitalis antibodies are now being developed. The confusion with herpes labialis (fever blisters), which affects the lips and may be only remotely connected with herpes genitalis, may then be cleared up. Caution at present dictates that the mother or any nursing personnel or physicians with open lesions of herpes labialis ought to take precautions against transmitting this virus to an infant.

A mother who is actively shedding virus from the vagina or the labia should have an abdominal delivery, to avoid having the fetus go through an area with active virus particles. It is not presently known whether intact membranes act as a barrier against infection to eliminate or significantly reduce the fetal risk in vaginal delivery. In any case, if you have had in the past, or now have, the painful ulcers associated with herpes or if you have had a diagnosis of herpes genitalis proven, it would be wise to have herpes cultures done from your vagina as you approach the time of delivery. If these cultures are consistently negative and there are no lesions present, there is probably no problem. On the other hand, if the cultures have been positive, your doctor may wish to deliver your baby by cesarean section, unless it is possible to get at least two consecutive negative cultures from the birth canal just before delivery. A word to the wise is timely here: The highest incidence of herpes infection in newborns occurs among those born to mothers who do not know they have herpes.

Of the infants who develop herpes in the newborn state, 20 percent of the mothers have had a first genital infection, while 25 percent have recurrences of previous involvement. Another 10 percent have ulcers around the mouth—the oral form of herpes. One third of the mothers have herpes antibodies but no clear history of the disease.

There may be a glimmer of hope in the care of this problem. A few patients with persistently positive cultures for herpes have been treated with acyclovir (Zovirax) by injection in late pregnancy. The cultures have reverted to negative and mother and baby did well. But these cases are as yet too small in number to make us certain that the treatment is safe as well as effective.

To protect the infants from infection after birth, careful handwashing by the mother is adequate. Breastfeeding is not precluded by herpes.

Gonorrhea

Gonorrhea also is a threat, because it is an infection that the baby can acquire from its mother as it comes through the birth canal. The baby's eyes are particularly susceptible to infection. Infection under the eyelids and in the cornea can result in serious visual loss. The preventive treatment, consisting of instillation of antibiotics under the eyelids, is simple. The diagnosis of infection is not difficult, because there is a profuse discharge of pus from the eye. In those jurisdictions where silver nitrate instillation to prevent such gonorrheal infection is still practiced there may be a temporary discharge due to silver nitrate itself. You should call any such discharge to the attention of your pediatrician.

It is not yet clear how much impact chlamydia infection (another STD) has on the pregnancy or the newborn. The onset of chlamydia conjunctivitis in the baby does not occur until the second week of life, as compared with the rapidly occurring conjunctivitis that results from gonorrhea. At present, we do not believe that there is any long-term injury attributable to chlamydia conjunctivitis, particularly if it is treated properly by antibiotics.

Rubella

The virus of rubella (German measles) formerly caused a great deal of fetal injury but the development of an effective and safe vaccine, Meruvax II, has almost eradicated the problem.

Rubella in adults is a relatively mild disease associated with low fever and discomfort, a light rash that tends to be slightly itchy, and enlarged lymph nodes, particularly those at the back of the head and behind the ears. It is unusual for the discomfort to last more than eighteen to thirty-six hours.

For the fetus, who can become infected because the virus readily crosses the placenta, the impact is much more severe. If the rubella occurs early in pregnancy the infant may have eye cataracts, deafness, heart defects, and hernias. The likelihood that one or more defects will occur has been variously estimated but is probably greater than 50 percent in a woman who has had rubella in the first eight to ten weeks of pregnancy.

For this reason rubella is widely accepted as a reasonable indication for abortion. The decision whether to abort has to be made in light of the fact that most of the congenital anomalies induced in the first trimester are amenable to corrective surgery after the child is born.

The diagnosis can be proven by blood tests for antibodies to the virus, even if the illness in the mother has been so mild as to leave doubt as to the diagnosis.

When rubella occurs in the second trimester, congenital anomalies do not ensue, because the fetus already is fully formed, but the fetus can acquire the virus disease itself. These active infections in the second trimester are not treatable. Under these circumstances, the baby may be born with congenital rubella. Many such babies are small for gestational age and at least half of them become seriously ill sometime in the first year of life. In addition to everything else, they can transmit rubella to those with whom they come in contact. About 20 percent of the fetuses infected with the German measles virus develop diabetes later in life.

The conscientious public health effort to vaccinate all female children and young women so that they are immune to rubella prior to pregnancy has markedly reduced the public health importance of the disease. We have not had any serious epidemics for several decades.

AIDS

Acquired immune deficiency syndrome (AIDS) due to HTLV III virus is rarely encountered in pregnant women. However, it is of obstetrical importance since it can be transmitted to the fetus and the newborn.

Most infected women have been intravenous drug users, but the disease can also be spread by sexual contact, blood transfusion, and artificial insemination. The mothers who have transmitted the disease to their children all have either had AIDS or have had antibodies to the virus. Delivery by cesarean may not prevent infant infection since the fetus may already be infected.

Once a mother has had an infant with AIDS there is a greater than 50 percent likelihood that subsequent children also will be infected.

It is not established whether AIDS can be transmitted by breast-feeding. It appears wise to test the newborn of infected or antibody-positive mothers for antibodies. If none are present, the voice of caution says to bottle-feed.

Other Viral Diseases

The other relatively common viral diseases, such as influenza, measles, and mumps, ordinarily do not have any impact on the fetus and have no more effect on a pregnant than on a nonpregnant adult. The chicken pox virus (Varicella) is capable of crossing the placenta and infecting the fetus in utero. If the baby remains in the uterus until the pock marks have healed, it ordinarily will not have any scars. The timing of the infection may of course be such that the baby is born with chicken pox. Such newborns are not very sick.

The commonest viral disease affecting the fetus is cyto-megalic virus, which can cause death in the newborn period. The likelihood of this is thought to be somewhere between 2,500 and 7,500 cases among our three million annual births. It is not now considered feasible to screen all pregnant women for this virus, partly because we do not have any effective preventive or curative treatment.

Hepatitis B virus can cause hepatitis and liver failure in the newborn. If the mother has chronic hepatitis B she can transmit it to the fetus across the placenta or by contact with the infant in the newborn period. There appears to be an increase in prematurity among babies born to mothers with hepatitis B. The mothers can be screened for hepatitis B disease by testing for an antibody which is presently designated HB_2Ag. If the result is positive, newborns should be protected by giving them human immune antibodies against hepatitis B virus. It is at present not settled whether breast-feeding plays a role in the transmission of the virus to the newborn.

Hepatitis A, which is a brief, relatively acute infection, is apparently not a problem either to the pregnant woman or the newborn infant.

Parasites

Diseases due to parasites such as malaria and the intestinal worms endemic in certain parts of the United States are not risks to pregnancy except for the illness that they cause in the mother. Parasites do not ordinarily cross the placenta. An exception is toxoplasmosis, a condition caused by a microscopical protozoon, Toxoplasma gondii. The disease is spread in two ways. One is eating raw meat from an animal that has had the disease, or handling such meat prior to cooking. The more common source is a household cat, which sheds a form of the parasite in its feces. These then dry out and the toxoplasma ovocysts can be inhaled by people handling cat litter. The ovocysts ordinarily are shed by the cat only during the initial phases of infection and are generally acquired by the cats themselves when they eat infected small animals while out foraging on their own. The disease does not occur in cats who have always lived indoors, were not born to mothers with the disease, and who have not been exposed in close quarters to other cats who have the infection.

The acute disease in an adult is marked by flulike symptoms of fatigue and aching muscles. It has no particular characteristics that would make the diagnosis easy without laboratory tests. The diagnosis cannot be confirmed unless the mother had a blood test for toxoplasmosis early in the pregnancy and was found not to have toxoplasma antibodies. A subsequent test with a high antibody value then is presumed to be evidence of the disease. Toxoplasmosis normally is treated with Pyrimethamine combined with an appropriate sulfa drug. However, since Pyrimethamine may cause congenital anomalies if the patient is in the first trimester of pregnancy, treatment at that stage must be with sulfa drugs only. If the mother is diagnosed as having toxoplasmosis during pregnancy, it is best to treat the infant preventively at birth, rather than wait to see whether the newborn has not been infested with the toxoplasma.

In a study done on 180 pregnancies in which the mother acquired toxoplasmosis during gestation, 110 of the newborns were not infected at all.

Of the 64 babies found to be infected by laboratory tests, 46 were otherwise entirely normal. Eleven babies had some mild involvement. Seven had severe toxoplasmosis and six of these infants died of the disease. The problem in the babies is that the toxoplasma organisms infect the brain and produce a rather serious illness in the newborn. In a slightly less severe form, these organisms may involve the eyes and later result in partial loss of vision.

Heart Disease

The tremendous reduction in heart disease due to rheumatic fever in the last generation has changed the entire picture of heart disease in pregnancy. Most young women are now successfully treated for this disease in its early phases and are given preventive treatment for a number of years after an initial episode, so that defects of the heart valves, which were distressingly common when I was an intern, have virtually vanished. Where medical treatment alone has not sufficed, heart surgery has done much to make these patients close to normal.

Heart diseases have no impact on the fetus. Those mothers who are in good health, without evidence of heart failure, ordinarily will handle pregnancy well. In some instances it may be necessary to reduce their activities as they approach full term. There is an unavoidable expansion of blood volume in pregnancy and, therefore, an added load on the heart. A patient whose heart status is unstable may need an increase in cardiac drugs and increased rest. But in general, the future for the mother is not affected by a pregnancy.

Cystic Fibrosis

Cystic fibrosis, a genetic disorder, is being encountered in pregnancy more often than formerly. Women with cystic fibrosis are increasingly reaching reproductive age in a state of relatively good health, thanks to antibiotic treatment, which has prevented the severe pneumonia to which they would otherwise be prey. The chances for a pregnant woman with cystic fibrosis, therefore, depend entirely on her state of health when she became pregnant. Those women whose disease is well controlled apparently tolerate pregnancy without event. Those who are severely affected, particularly with pulmonary complications from repeated bouts of pneumonia, have increased respiratory difficulty as pregnancy proceeds.

Cystic fibrosis is a hereditary disorder that can now be diagnosed in the fetus by amniocentesis. Early warning is of value, since cystic fibrosis can cause obstruction of the large intestine in the fetus prior to birth.

Blood Diseases

Various abnormalities of the blood system present some problems for pregnancy. Perhaps commonest are defects of the red blood cells. The most familiar one of these is sickle-cell disease. In this condition the molecules of hemoglobin, the chemical that transports oxygen in red cells, acquire an abnormal shape when their oxygen is given up to the tissues. This shape disrupts the red blood cells to the point where their plasticlike envelopes break and the hemoglobin is dumped into the fluid portion of the blood. The consequence of this, when it is severe, can be an acute illness associated with a great deal of chest and abdominal pain. These patients are commonly also severely anemic. It appears that the health and welfare of the mother with sickle-cell disease during pregnancy is helped by multiple blood transfusions, to keep her red blood cell count fairly close to normal. This treatment is not totally without risk but seems to result in an improved outcome for the pregnancy. Fortunately, virtually every adult woman who has sickle-cell disease is aware of it and therefore can participate in making careful plans for her care during the pregnancy. Mothers with sickle-cell disease or one of its variants have an increased rate of miscarriage and premature delivery. Parents with sickle-cell trait, a condition in which the individual carries the hereditary gene in a mixed form and therefore is not ill, may have normal children, or children with either the trait or the disease itself.

The disease can be diagnosed in the fetus by amniocentesis early in the second trimester of pregnancy.

Leukemia is now much more efficiently treated than in the years prior to the availability of chemotherapeutic agents. The health of pregnant women with leukemia is thus much better than it used to be. However, the disease is still a major complication and each case must be dealt with on an individual basis. Transmission of leukemia to the fetus is virtually unheard of. Chemotherapeutic agents that do not affect the welfare of the fetus are employed in the treatment of the pregnant woman.

A disease with the lengthy name of thrombocytopenic purpura occasionally occurs in pregnancy. This name derives from a series of Latin and Greek terms that mean that the patient develops hemorrhages under the skin (*purpura*, from which we derive the adjective purple), due to a shortage of blood platelets in the circulating blood (thrombocytopenia: *thrombocyte*, the blood cell which assists in clotting and *penia*, meaning a shortage). The disease is in many instances due to a circulating antibody, which the mother unfortunately forms against her own platelets. This substance may cross the placenta; thus the fetus of the mother with thrombocytopenia may itself be thrombocytopenic. It is not as yet fully settled whether these babies need to be delivered by cesarean section to protect them from bleeding during vaginal birth. Precisely how to deal with the management of delivery in a patient with thrombocytopenia probably has to be left to individual decision by the obstetrician, assisted by a skilled hematologist.

Surgical Complications

In general, the management of acute surgical emergencies, such as an automobile accident, involves caring for the injuries caused by the accident and ignoring the pregnancy, except to prove by ultrasound whether the fetus has survived the accident. In rare instances, violent trauma such as can be incurred in automobile accidents may cause serious damage to the fetus without injury to the same degree in the mother. I saw one such woman in Salt Lake City. She was returning from a visit to her obstetrician late in pregnancy when her car was struck amidships by an automobile driven by another pregnant woman. The other driver was not injured. My patient developed abdominal pain and she thought her membranes had been ruptured by the crash. She was therefore brought to the hospital for observation. Unfortunately, by the time she arrived, the fetus was already dead. After an uneventful labor, it turned out that the baby had sustained a fatal skull fracture without any corresponding damage to the mother.

Other instances of this sort have also been observed. In general, the policy of treating the acute maternal injury and ignoring the pregnancy is appropriate. A leg broken in a skiing accident or a fall downstairs is no threat to the fetus. I have seen a seriously inebriated woman who fell from a second-story window, incurring extensive bruises but no damage to her fetus. There is the occasional gunshot or knife wound of the uterus; these must be dealt with on an individual basis.

As far as surgical diseases are concerned, the ones of real concern in pregnancy are those involving abdominal conditions, the overwhelmingly most common one being acute appendicitis. Here again, the important lesson is that the appendicitis is cared for as if the mother were not pregnant. The diagnosis is much more difficult in the third trimester of pregnancy than in a nonpregnant individual because the appendix is behind the growing uterus and some of the commonly observed signs of appendicitis do not appear. My own principle is that the patient should have an appendectomy if there is any doubt at all about the diagnosis of appendicitis in pregnancy. When an infected appendix ruptures late in pregnancy, at the time of operation the surgeon should first deliver the fetus and then correct the surgical problems.

Occasionally, diseases such as ulcerative colitis, or terminal ileitis, also known as Crohn's disease, are encountered in pregnancy. Their treatment, too, is that which would be appropriate in the nonpregnant state.

Occasional gynecological emergencies occur during pregnancy. Fibroids, the common muscle tumors of the uterus, can become twisted and quite painful. Ovarian cysts may occur during pregnancy. They may twist on their stalks, or rupture, and cause acute pain. The treatment of these conditions is exactly the same as it would be in a nonpregnant patient.

Incarcerated hernias, in which a portion of intestine is trapped in the hernia sac, causing an acute intestinal obstruction, clotting in a hemorrhoid, a kidney or ureteral stone, and acute gall bladder problems, all should be given appropriate emergency treatment.

Elective surgical treatment for other conditions such as hemorrhoids, varicose veins, and cosmetic purposes is better postponed until the pregnancy is completed; there is no need to subject the patient to an extra operative risk. However, even major operations during pregnancy are unlikely to result in abortion or a premature labor, or indeed to have any other effect on the fetus. Fetuses tolerate maternal anesthesia without any evidence of congenital anomaly or circulatory difficulty.

This principle extends to open-heart procedures in which the mother is put on a cardiopulmonary bypass while external machines oxygenate and pump her blood. Some patients have undergone such operations as late as the thirty-first week of pregnancy and given birth to normal infants at term. Since there is cooling of the mother's body during bypass, the fetal heart slows down. It recovers well at the conclusion of the cooling. Bypass operations except for those that are essential for the survival of the mother are best postponed until after delivery.

Dental Care

Dental care can certainly be given at any time during pregnancy with complete safety. The local anesthetic agents presently used by dentists are safe. If the dentist considers that general anesthesia is necessary, the pregnant woman should be hospitalized.

Psychiatric Illness

Pregnancy is a time of considerable stress for most women. Rightly or wrongly, a pregnant woman often suspects or is made to feel that whatever she may do or think will adversely affect the outcome. In a first pregnancy, she may uneasily anticipate the trivial but numerous discomforts she is about to suffer, or feel anxiety about the normality of the labor and of the newborn. Or she may be concerned about her adequacy as a mother, extending from breast-feeding to diapering to bathing (all simple tasks but threatening to one who has never done them before); or worry that the arrival of another person in the family will disrupt established emotional ties. The catalog is familiar and lengthy. It is not surprising that the first trimester may be a mixture of depression and euphoria. In the first trimester, the depression may be aggravated by nausea, which is actually a sign of a well-functioning placenta and a good pregnancy.

Formal psychiatric illnesses such as schizophrenia and organic depression are not materially changed in pregnancy. I have seen psychotic women go through pregnancy and labor without any notable awareness that their bodies were changing. One such woman seriously explained to me that a vastly increased appetite obviously accounted for her great weight gain and expanded waistline. She totally ignored the movements of her fetus.

The treatment of these major illnesses in pregnancy is, again, the same as it would be in the nonpregnant state. Shock treatment can be used, but with precautions against long periods of interference with breathing. Lithium is under suspicion of causing fetal abnormalities and should not be used in the first trimester of pregnancy.

Bereavement, Suicide

A serious and only recently acknowledged psychiatric illness commonly follows the birth of a dead infant or the early loss of a newborn. It was once the practice to isolate the mothers from the event, by using general anesthesia for a stillbirth and by rushing the mother out of the obstetrics area and even prematurely out of the hospital. We have since learned a great deal about the proper care in this situation, a matter discussed elsewhere in this volume in more detail.

Suicide appears to be infrequent in pregnancy. United States statistics are limited, but they seem to indicate that an unmarried adolescent having her first pregnancy is most likely among all pregnant women to take her own life.

First Resources

The pregnant woman can and should turn to her support systems for help when and how she needs it. The most obvious resource is her partner. The second can be the women in her family, mother, sisters, mother-in-law, and sisters-in-law. Her care provider, whether doctor or midwife, comes next on the list. A book such as this (and there are now many in the field) can be reassuring. Education for childbirth has been a major assistance in this area.

12

The Mechanics of Labor

A Labor Pain

The neophyte always wonders how she will know when labor actually begins. Can she distinguish the pains of childbirth from intestinal cramps or an ordinary backache? The throes of labor are unique for several reasons. In the first place, unlike other pains, they rise in *slow crescendo*, remain *fortissimo* for a brief period, and close in moderate *diminuendo*; or they are like a scale that makes a leisurely ascent to its high tone and is held aloft for a few beats before the several descending notes are sung. The transcription of a labor pain into music would be:

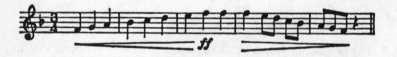

It has been suggested by Mrs. Susan Peterson, a reader of a previous edition of this book, that a major scale does not convey the "grinding and twisting" sensation of a labor pain. For musically literate readers she offers this transcription as "a probably more accurate and certainly more contemporary idiom":

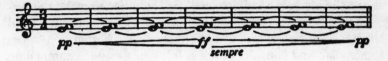

Labor Pain for Two Oboes

Another distinctive feature is that a labor pain is always associated with a contraction of the uterus. If a woman feels her
abdomen during the acme of such a pain, she notices a large,
board-firm mass, which becomes a softish, indentable mass
once again when the pain is over. The chief characteristic of
these pains is their rhythmic nature, their recurrence at fixed
intervals. As labor progresses, the interval from the beginning
of one pain to the beginning of the next is gradually shortened
from fifteen or twenty minutes at the onset to three or four
minutes when labor is well under way. In addition, the total
length of an individual pain increases from less than half a
minute at the start to more than a minute toward the end. Unlike
most pains, labor pains have a complete remission between
them, a happy respite in which the patient is comfortable.
Usually labor pains occur first in the small of the back and
after a few hours migrate down the flanks to center in the whole
lower abdomen. Many compare them to exaggerated menstrual
cramps, which are grinding and twisting in type. The pinkish
vaginal discharge that ordinarily accompanies the pains of true
labor is termed "show." It is blood-tinged mucus dislodged
from the cervix as the latter begins to dilate. Sometimes this
normal show, which is to be distinguished from abnormal
bleeding (frank, undiluted blood), anticipates the onset of labor
by a day or more.

False Labor

As I mentioned in Chapter 9, true labor may be preceded by
one or more discouraging bouts of false labor. A woman who

has already borne children will find it easier to make the distinction between the two. If she has previously had a very rapid labor, caution dictates that she report what is going on to her attendant and consider the possibility of a pelvic examination to be certain of the true state of affairs. In false labor dilation of the cervix does not change and the presenting part of the baby does not descend. However annoying or painful contractions may be, in the absence of these signs of progress the diagnosis of false labor is quite secure. There is no need to keep the patient under immediate observation. Nor is it necessary to keep a record of the frequency of contractions. The patient should not alter her eating or sleeping habits.

Cause Not Known

What causes labor to begin? Why does it start approximately 280 days after the first day of the last menstrual period? These are simple and definite questions which no one as yet can answer. From the appearance and disappearance of the hard abdominal mass, we know that contractions of the uterus occur irregularly throughout pregnancy (Braxton Hicks contractions), but suddenly, for no explicable reason, these painless contractions become regular and painful; then labor has begun. Quite commonly, particularly in early labor, the entrance of the obstetrician is followed by a temporary lull in the intensity and frequency of pains.

Time of Day

Everyone knows that there are more babies born at night than during daylight hours. There is no question that a hurried dash to the hospital after midnight is a more memorable event than a leisurely trip in the late morning. But actually the common consensus is borne out by objective facts and is not to be relegated to the domain of popular superstition. If deliveries were scattered at random in the twenty-four-hour period, simple arithmetic shows that 4.17 percent of deliveries would occur during any given hour. As a matter of fact, by studying more than six hundred thousand spontaneous births, Franz Halberg and I were able to demonstrate that the highest rate of delivery really did occur between four and five in the morning and constituted 4.77 percent of all births. The low point was spread out between four and seven o'clock in the late afternoon and accounted for only 3.63 percent of the births per hour.

The onset of labor follows a similar curve, which swings smoothly between the high and low points in the twenty-four-hour period. It does not make much difference whether labor begins with spontaneous rupture of the membranes or with contractions, or whether it is a first labor or a later one. The length of later labors is shorter but the times of onset are essentially the same. When delivery is accomplished by elective cesarean section and by induction of labor for convenience it is not surprising that there is a marked increase in the number of births during the day. The same is true to a lesser extent of deliveries by forceps, which tend to cluster in the early morning and late afternoon. These are the artifacts of human intervention.

Day of the Week

In recent years the incidence of births in the United States has not been equally distributed among the days of the week. Deliveries are increasingly concentrated on Monday through Friday with a deficit of weekend births. Within this pattern, the frequency of births is highest on Tuesday and lowest on Sunday. There is undoubtedly a result of the increased rate of cesarean deliveries, particularly of elective repeat sections, which are usually done on weekday mornings.

Time of Year

For many years the monthly incidence of births has consistently peaked in August and September and has been significantly lower in December and January. Figures issued by the National Center for Health Statistics for 1982 showed an overall difference of about 12 percent between the two periods, reflecting a difference of about 110,000 births between the summer high and the winter low. On the other hand, the fertility rates for the same year appeared to be highest during the spring months of April, May, and June. The birth rates, based on the total population for 1982, month by month were as follows:

Month	Percentage
January	15.2
February	15.6
March	15.6
April	15.3
May	15.6
June	16.2
July	16.7
August	16.7
September	17.1
October	15.9
November	15.5
December	15.2

This kind of distribution makes clear that the greatest number of conceptions occur in the fall.

Rupture of the Membranes

About 10 percent of all labors begin with rupture of the membranes. This event may be preceded by contractions of which the patient is aware, but often it occurs quite without advance notice. There can be a trickle of fluid, and the patient who has been leaking a little urine when coughing in the last few months will have difficulty being certain just what is happening. When the fluid is tested is it found to be considerably more alkaline than urine. It also contains more sodium chloride, so that when it dries it exhibits a phenomenon called ferning, a picturesque term describing the appearance of the salt crystals that form in the drying process. Additionally, amniotic fluid near term may contain flecks of vernix caseosa, which is unmistakably of fetal origin.

The term dry labor has occasionally been used to refer to a labor initiated by rupture of the membranes, with the loss of a great deal of fluid. There is in actuality no such phenomenon. The cells which line the amniotic sac constantly filter water and the fetus continues to void urine, at a total rate of a quart every two hours. The uterus does not wring itself dry although it may diminish in volume. These labors are not materially different from those in which membranes remain intact.

Amniotic fluid does act as a cushion on the baby's head. When membranes are ruptured, patterns of fetal heart rate slowing (decelerations), which have been referred to as head-compression patterns, tend to be more frequent. They are well within the baby's ability to adapt and have no long-term or short-term consequences.

Rupture of the membranes is called premature when the bag of waters breaks twelve or more hours prior to the onset of labor. When this occurs near term, labor usually ensues within twenty-four hours. The earlier in pregnancy membranes rupture, the longer the interval. Membranes form a barrier to the movement of bacteria from their usual location in the vagina up into the uterine cavity. We assume that the baby has been colonized with its mother's bacteria by the time membranes have been ruptured for twenty-four hours.

When this takes place, it may result in bacterial infection of the membranes, the placenta, and the fetus. The initial fetal response to this infection is an increase in its heart rate. The evidence of maternal infection is an increase in the pulse rate, an elevation of temperature, and an increase in white-blood-cell count. The mother may feel vaguely ill—like the flu. The early stages of infection of the membranes (chorioamnionitis) may produce very little by way of symptoms and it may be necessary to do laboratory tests such as a white-blood-cell count to detect it.

The proper treatment of these infections is intensive antibiotic therapy, and prompt delivery. If there is not rapid response with the expectation of birth within a few hours, labor should be stimulated with oxytocin, or the baby should be delivered by cesarean section. With vigilance and prompt treatment, the outcome for mother and baby in these cases is usually excellent.

The colonization of the uterine contents and the infection that may follow become increasingly likely the longer the membranes are ruptured. A number of studies have been made to determine whether the outcomes can be improved by inducing delivery within twelve hours or by giving antibiotics prophylactically. Such intervention seems to make no particular difference. If the membranes rupture when a woman is close to term and about to go into labor, labor ordinarily ensues promptly.

In this group it does not really matter whether we await the spontaneous onset of labor or undertake measures to bring it about a few hours earlier.

The serious problem occurs with premature rupture of the membranes when the baby itself is premature. This accident may happen at any time in the latter half of a pregnancy. It is not, however, common enough to allow us to make a meaningful comparative study of various possible modes of treatment. One suggestive study surveyed fifty-three patients who ruptured membranes before the fetus was viable. The policy at the institution where the study was made was not to induce labor; as a consequence, eighteen of the fetuses went past the twenty-sixth week, and thirteen of these produced surviving infants. This is a significantly greater salvage than would have been possible if labor had been induced directly following the rupture of the membranes.

When membranes rupture after the twenty-sixth and before the thirty-fifth week, for example at thirty or thirty-two weeks of pregnancy, the decision whether to intervene turns on individual factors, particularly other complications of pregnancy which may be present. Where premature rupture of the membranes occurs with an abnormal presentation such as a high footling breech or a transverse lie, the decision will be to do cesarean section promptly.

When the membranes rupture two months or so prior to the expected day of confinement (EDC) and a policy of nonintervention is decided upon, the patient should remain at home or in the hospital until the onset of labor. Maximizing rest seems to delay labor, although this has been very difficult to prove. When premature rupture has occurred, there is agreement that the use of drugs to halt labor is contraindicated.

Artificial Rupture of the Membranes

Artificial rupture of the membranes (AROM) has recently had a bad press, mostly because a few investigators have published the view that the fetuses are endangered by an increased incidence of fetal heart rate decelerations after membranes are ruptured. Unless there are complications, however, the increased incidence of decelerations of itself does not create a risk for the fetus. AROM remains our chief reliance for induction of labor. In such cases it is usual to rupture the membranes with the patient in the hospital and then to await the spontaneous onset of labor. If labor does not ensue in twelve to sixteen hours, then stimulation with oxytocin is initiated.

Artificial rupture of the membranes has no effect on the course of normal labor once it has started. When there is a delay in progress, however, AROM may help the patient get back into good labor. AROM is of course a necessary result of the attachment of an electrode directly to the skin of the fetus for internal monitoring, unless the membranes have already ruptured.

How Many Labor Pains Are Required?

"How many pains make a baby?" is the facetious form in which the layman phrases a serious scientific query. As can be surmised, there is extraordinary variation, just like the number of strokes in a tennis match. According to one Swiss study, first labors required an average of 135 contractions and multiparous labors, 68.

The Forces Involved in Birth

Before discussing delivery, we must first consider the forces involved in birth.

Imagine the baby confined in a large, gourd-shaped, elastic bottle, the muscular uterus. This lies upside down within the mother's abdomen, the bottom of the bottle under her ribs, and the mouth deep in her pelvis. The cervix is about a half-inch long when labor begins, and it is almost closed. Before a full-term baby can be expelled from the uterus, the round neck must be stretched to a diameter of four inches (ten centimeters), the minimum necessary to allow the baby to pass from the uterus into the narrow, stiff-walled, five-inch corridor (pelvis and birth canal) that leads to the outside world.

The motive power that dilates the mouth of the uterus and propels the child through the resistant birth corridor is mainly the force generated by the contractions of this large muscular

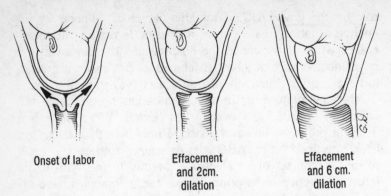

Onset of labor   Effacement   Effacement
and 2cm.   and 6 cm.
dilation   dilation

From left to right, the changes in the mother's cervix late in pregnancy. The fetus is head down, and only half of the upper end of the vagina appears. In the illustration on the right the cervix is open, and the membranes are pushing down into the opening.

In some women these changes do not take place until labor has begun. In others they may have occurred even before the first noteworthy contraction.

organ. This largest muscle of the body, far heavier and greater than the powerful biceps of a heavyweight weight lifter, forms a complete elastic casing about the child except for the small opening at its neck—the relatively weak point in the wall. When the muscle fibers contract, the pressure within the uterus is greatly increased—the process is like compressing a water-filled rubber bulb—and this increased pressure is transmitted to the constraining walls.

Many computations have been made of the force of a single labor pain, and figures varying from four to one hundred pounds have been obtained by separate investigators. From their data, an average of between twenty-five and thirty pounds seems likely. This force is directed against the cervix in two ways. The uterus has a completely separate inner lining, the membranes which contain the child and the amniotic fluid. During a pain both the baby and the fluid surrounding it are put under thirty pounds of pressure in all directions. When the membranes are intact, this force drives the fluid against the cervix; when they are ruptured, the baby is driven against it. Through pressure exerted by either the fluid or the baby, the cervix is forced open, stretched from within. In addition to this pressure from within (dilation), the neck of the bottle is shortened and pulled open by the contraction of the muscle fibers of the lower portion of the uterus, to which the muscle fibers of the cervix are attached (retraction). About six or seven of the hours of a primiparous labor and three and a half of the hour of a multiparous labor are occupied in stretching the opening in the cervix to its maximum four-inch diameter. This phase of labor is called the first stage, the stage of cervical dilation. When the cervix is fully dilated, the baby no longer meets resistance in the upper birth canal, and the whole force of the uterine contractions is spent in driving it through the lower birth canal. In this stage of labor (the second stage) the force of the uterine contractions is greatly augmented by involuntary contractions of the woman's abdominal muscles, to which are added her own bearing-down efforts. Instinctively she fills her lung with air, fixes her diaphragm by closing her epiglottis, and increases her intra-abdominal pressure by straining as though at stool. These activities increase the uterine pressure to about sixty pounds.

The woman having her first baby ordinarily delivers her infant in about seventy-five minutes of the second stage of labor. This is the expulsive stage, timed from the complete disappearance of the cervix as a separate structure in the birth canal and the actual birth of the baby. When contractions are somewhat decreased or the baby is unusually large the process will take longer but may still be well within the normal limits of the health and welfare of both the fetus and the mother. For women having second and later babies the second stage of labor varies from fifteen minutes to forty minutes, once again depending upon the force of contractions and size and presentation of the infant. Prolongation of the second stage of labor in the absence of any other evidence of difficulty is not a necessary indication for a surgical intervention.

The third, or placental, stage of labor is the time elapsed from the birth of the baby to the delivery of the placenta. This may last as little as two minutes. In the absence of bleeding, there is no particular hurry about the delivery of the placenta. If there is any unusual delay in the spontaneous delivery of the placenta, or if partial separation of the placenta initiates hemorrhage, it is proper for the medical attendant to carry out a manual removal. The operator introduces a hand through the open cervix into the uterine cavity, feels for the plane of separation between the placenta and the uterus, and sweeps a hand through this plane. When the separation of the placenta from the uterine wall is complete, the placenta is then drawn out by the hand. It is ordinarily wise to administer oxytocin or methergine to a patient under these circumstances to assure a forceful uterine contraction and thereby limit further bleeding.

Normal Length of Labor

There have been a number of careful studies on the ordinary length of labor, and, as in most such studies of large groups, many individual cases fall far outside the average. Further, if the calculation is based on the patients' own reports, there is a great variation in perception from one woman to another as to when she believes that labor has begun. There are women who come to the hospital asking to be told whether they really are in labor, only to be found far advanced in the first stage and within an hour of delivery. These women may be matched with those who are certain they are in labor because they have been conscientiously timing what they feel as hard contractions for a number of hours. When the latter come to the hospital they may show no objective evidence of labor and may not deliver until a number of days later, after an interval without uterine activity. For this reason the best information as to the start of labor would be based entirely on patients who have been carefully studied by pelvic examination before and after they believe they began labor. This is particularly true because of the large variation in the length of the latent period, during which uterine contractions may occur without any change in physical findings.

At one extreme I have observed several patients whose entire labors lasted less than half an hour. One such woman repeatedly delivered either at home or on the way to the hospital despite her serious efforts to get to the hospital in time. Another patient I remember only sensed that she was in labor and steadfastly denied having any pain. She was however aware enough of her own body to drive the forty minutes to the hospital in sufficient time to deliver there. At the other end of the time spectrum, during my internship I saw two patients who had labors lasting several days. One was having her first baby and had experienced serious obstruction of labor in a small hospital in rural Maryland. Shortly thereafter we saw a patient having her fourth baby who made steady progress in the dilation of her cervix over a period of six days. The labor was so gradual that it did not disturb her eating or her sleep. Eventually, when she got into the second stage of labor, she had a normal delivery. Events such as these are, of course, extraordinarily rare.

Anticipation of a very rapid labor need not be a source of apprehension. The patients who deliver shortly after arrival at the hospital and the even less common patients who deliver while en route or in the lobby rarely experience serious difficulty. The women with difficulty in labor remain pregnant until they get to the delivery area.

A number of years ago some ten thousand deliveries at the Johns Hopkins Hospital were summarized in regard to the length of labor. They were divided into two groups: patients having a first baby and those having later babies. The interval was measured from the onset of the first pain the patient was aware of until the delivery of the placenta. Three values were reported, the mean, the median, and the mode. The mean is what is commonly called the average. It tends to give a misleadingly high value since the very long labors seriously outbalance the brief ones. One thirty-hour labor counts as much as five six-hour labors. The median is the value at the center of the group, which is to say that half as many women have longer and half as many have shorter labors than the median figure. The modal value is probably the most informative since it is the duration of labor most commonly observed. The results were as follows.

	Mean (Hours)	Median (Hours)	Mode (Hours)
Primipara	13.04	10.59	7.0
Multipara	8.15	6.21	4.0

What this means is that from the onset of labor until the time you deliver if you are having your first baby you can reasonably expect that the labor will probably last about six to ten hours and for a later labor, three and a half to six hours.

Several investigators have reported on the incidence of very rapid labors—labors lasting less than three hours—and relatively long labors—those requiring more than twenty-four hours. One woman in a hundred may anticipate that her first child will be born in less than three hours, and seven in a hundred may expect such good fortune in subsequent births. Approximately every ninth woman requires more than twenty-four hours to deliver a first child.

"Back Labor"

The concept of back labor, which describes the situation in which the discomfort of uterine contractions is felt over the low back, has gained some currency recently. In fact the discomfort of false and true labor may both be felt in this area.

There are two possible causes for the sensation of back labor when the patient is in true labor, and they may be present simultaneously. One is the rapid opening of the cervix. This pain results from the stretching as the cervix shortens up and dilates. In this event there may be more than the ordinary amount of bloody show, since the small blood vessels in the cervix are torn before the pressure of the presenting part has given the blood within them enough time to clot.

The other cause of back pain may be that the head of the fetus is positioned in the pelvis so that it faces the front of the mother rather than her back (occiput posterior position, or OP). This position of the head has a mechanical disadvantage that may result in a delay in the progress of the labor. With first labors an OP presentation often requires a longer period of bearing down to bring about delivery. The baby has to rotate 180 degrees to be born in the usual position, facing the mother's back (occiput anterior, OA).

Back labor does not exist as a separate condition but rather as a symptom of something in the labor process that may not be in the least bit abnormal.

Effect of Maternal Age on Labor

The effect of maternal age on labor is a matter of interest at both extremes of woman's fertile span.

In many cultures, sexual activity for women begins before the start of fertility. Fortunately, in almost all instances ovulation and consequent pregnancy do not occur before hormonal maturity. The maternal bony pelvis thus reaches its adult shape and size and the deposition of the body fat and breast development are also at "grown-up" levels by that time. That a pregnant woman is an early adolescent can be told by her facial expressions and behavior more readily than by physical examination.

Not too long ago, it was thought that difficult labors, toxemia of pregnancy, and premature delivery were frequent problems among these teenagers. It has now become clear that these conclusions were influenced by societal disapproval of the patients' life-style and not on the basis of careful statistics, which do not confirm the suppositions. The serious issues of adolescent pregnancy are social and not biological. Given proper nutrition and prenatal care, early adolescents do quite well in pregnancy and labor.

Women having first pregnancies past the age of thirty-five were also considered to experience increased risks in labor. This was attributed in some vague way to stiffening of the soft tissues of the cervix, vagina, and perineum. Whether this is true becomes increasingly important as the birth rate among women over thirty comes to rise. I know of no unbiased evidence for it. My deduction is that society has tended to consider the pinnacle of woman's achievement to be motherhood and that postponing this merits some sort of penalty. We have learned, however, that given good prenatal care, much like the adolescent, the woman over forty can be certain that she will have a safe first pregnancy and labor.

Ironically, she is now expected to be much concerned about fetal trisomies (the condition in which an excess number of chromosomes in the fetus may result in serious congenital abnormalities), the likelihood of which is still only one in a hundred at thirty-nine years of age.

When one compares women over thirty-five in labor with first children with women in general, the selected older group experiences labor about one and one half hours longer. If the comparison is made with women under twenty, the increase is nearer to four hours. But remember, these are still mostly relatively brief labors.

In all studies of women over thirty-five years of age, the maternal and fetal risks are slightly higher than for younger pregnant women. For the mothers this probably is a result of age-dependent increases in the occurrence of such complications as hypertension and diabetes. In a large series studied in the 1960's as part of a nationwide collaborative study of pregnancy outcome, the perinatal mortality (loss of fetuses and newborns) observed among mothers seventeen to nineteen years of age was 25 per 1,000, whereas after the age of thirty-nine it was 69 per 1,000.

Stillbirths accounted for 92 percent of the difference at that time and 14 percent were due to congenital anomalies. At present, twenty years later, there has been a significant improvement in perinatal mortality, so that the rates are much less, although the relative position is the same. With early diagnosis of abnormal fetuses in women in the older age group the difference due to congenital anomalies is considerably smaller. Genetic diagnosis by chorionic villus sampling and amniocentesis allows abortion of defective embryos. Fetal monitoring reduces loss due to stillbirth.

What this boils down to is that women aged thirty-five or over undertaking their first pregnancy with appropriate obstetrical care can confidently anticipate a happy outcome more than 96 percent of the time.

Youth and Childbearing

Despite the fact that the forty-year-old woman does well, there is no gainsaying that the best ally of successful childbirth is youth. It is a message that the medical profession must constantly reiterate to the women of America. This in no sense should be interpreted as a clarion call for teenage motherhood.

Ideally, young couples should have their families at a time when they are emotionally and economically prepared to plan for the future of their children, how many they want, and how far apart to space them. Such plans are always subject to change and adaptation to unforeseen events, but on the whole it seems better to me not to let one's family occur by accident.

No couple need feel that they have a debt to mankind to replace themselves. All children should be born with the invaluable heritage of being keenly wanted by parents who are capable of caring for them and anxious to do so.

Apart from all socioeconomic considerations (of course in actual practice they can never be ignored), the ideal age for a woman to start a family, from the purely obstetrical viewpoint, is between the ages of eighteen and twenty.

Despite the obstetrician's preference for youth, in the United States at present the great majority of babies are born to women in their twenties who are part of the baby boom of the 1960's.

In recent years we have also experienced a steady increase in the average age of women having their first baby. Figures from the National Center for Health Statistics (NCHS) demonstrate the trend in data from 1979 to 1982. The table below shows the number of women per 1,000 in each age group who had live-born first children.

Age Group	1979	1982
15–19	39.7	41.0
20–24	52.6	54.7
25–29	34.5	38.4
30–34	10.1	14.6
35–39	2.1	3.3
40–44	0.3	0.4

All rates have increased, but note that in the age group from twenty-five to twenty-nine, the rise was 11 percent, whereas for ages thirty to thirty-four it rose 45 percent and for thirty-five to thirty-nine an astonishing 57 percent. Preliminary data for 1983 from NCHS makes clear that the trend to later motherhood continues.

Similar figures appear when total births, irrespective of whether they are first or tenth births, per 1,000 women in each age group are reported.

Age Group	1979	1982
15–19	52.3	52.9
20–24	112.8	111.3
25–29	111.4	111.0
30–34	60.3	64.2
35–39	19.5	21.1
40–44	3.9	3.9

In the lower age brackets the numbers have become smaller and in the upper, larger.

Despite these changes, the total fertility rate for the U.S. in 1984 was calculated by the NCHS as 1,819 per 1,000 women in the reproductive age group. The total fertility rate is the number of children anticipated over the reproductive lifetime if present birth rates continue. This rate predicts less than two children per couple.

13

Spontaneous Labor and Delivery

The Start of Labor

Labor usually begins with the onset of contractions that are sufficiently forceful to draw themselves to the mother's attention. At first she may not be able to distinguish them from the Braxton Hicks contractions of the third trimester of pregnancy except by the fact that they persist and steadily become closer together. The contractions of normal labor are not ordinarily carbon copies of one another, in either duration or spacing, early in the game. When contractions are not occurring frequently the interval between them tends to be somewhat irregular.

Certain specific signs occur that will help to identify true labor. In pregnancy the cervical canal is closed by a plug that consists of mucus deposited in the canal by the glands on the cervix. This may come out from the vagina prior to labor, but if it appears at a time when contractions are increasingly forceful, labor has probably begun. When the cervix begins to open fast enough to tear its blood vessels, you may notice a bloody discharge. When this is mixed with the cervical mucus it is referred to as "bloody show" and is also a characteristic of true labor.

About one time out of ten labor actually heralds its appearance by spontaneous rupture of the membranes. This is painless. The membranes are actually fetal tissues and have no nerves in them. Rupture of the membranes can occur independent of events that do cause pain such as forceful uterine contractions and rapid changes in the cervix. Some patients do actually feel the membranes "pop." When rupture of the membranes is followed in short order by forceful and uncomfortable uterine contractions the diagnosis of the onset of labor is quite certain.

Some labors take a slow and majestic start that allows ample time for personal business such as arranging care for older children. Other labors begin like a violent storm sweeping across the landscape, the contractions resembling the rolling thunder of the approaching clouds. One cannot predict with any certainty which labors will be slow and which rapid, but in most cases the patient having her first baby will have enough time to identify what is happening to her and take the necessary steps.

Among the things I do not recommend, when the patient suspects that labor has begun, is timing the contractions. Few things are more futile and frustrating than sitting for several hours with a clock, a pencil, and paper writing down the intervals between "labor pains" that turn out to be false labor, or to be part of what is known as the latent phase. It is much better to seek some sort of diverting activity that will occupy your mind until labor becomes unmistakable, or until you feel you should consult someone to find out what is really happening.

That someone may be the person who is going to help you with the birth, or it may be convenient for you to proceed directly to the hospital. Signs that suggest the need for a phone call include noticeable discomfort, or an inability to sleep or to distract yourself from what is going on in your body. If you feel this way you should make the call, no matter what time of day or night it is. Your doctor or midwife will tell you how they want you to call them, and they are accustomed to having these crucial events happen at odd hours. It is better to resolve doubts by calling when you feel the need than to wait until too late. A definite decision whether labor is present, however, may depend on vaginal exams done several hours apart. It is also wise to consider the time of year and the weather. When

I practiced in Minnesota and knew that a severe snowstorm was on the way I took care to advise patients to go to the hospital earlier rather than later. In an urban area you may have to allow for traffic conditions, which may cause delays in getting to your hospital. Babysitting arrangements for your older children can create last-minute problems. I advise my patients, in such an event, simply to take the children along to the hospital. There is sure to be someone resourceful enough to take care of unexpected young visitors.

Women are advised not to eat or drink after labor starts because of the danger that they might aspirate stomach contents if they have to have a general anesthetic later in labor. The odds are that nothing of the sort will happen. Although there is evidence active labor delays emptying of the stomach, nature seems to provide protection in the form of loss of appetite and even vomiting later in labor. Nevertheless, no matter how adequate your preparation, no matter how smooth your pregnancy, no matter how many easy and safe deliveries you have had, there is no way to guarantee that you will not need a general anesthetic on an emergency basis during labor. Even so, I am not aware of any evidence of harm from eating early in labor or early in its latent phase or during false labor. You may wish to be cautious and limit your intake to fruit juice or clear soup. Probably the message is that if you are in doubt you ought to avoid solid food, but it is also not wise for you to go for many hours without fluid intake.

Sexual intercourse at the onset of labor is a custom in a number of primitive cultures. In some it is explained as an aid to lubricating the vagina and in others it is thought to accelerate the labor. There may be physiological basis for these explanations, since we now know that orgasm releases oxytocin and stimulates uterine activity. However, the practice can increase the incidence of infection during and after delivery. For precisely the same reason, I advise against douching at the onset of labor.

Why the Hospital for Delivery

We use hospitals and their facilities for labor and delivery for the same reason that we have fire departments in our communities. We would all much prefer to have the fire trucks and the firefighters stay in their station year-round without ever having to come out. But on the other hand, safety in the community calls for their being available in the event of calamity.

Every now and then, in labor, an accident occurs that calls for the immediate application of experienced judgment and anesthetic and surgical skills. For example, the umbilical cord may fall through the cervix ahead of the leading part of the baby. This accident inevitably creates a mechanical obstruction of flow through the cord as labor advances. The fetus is literally choked off from the placenta and death can ensue in moments. Another accident, which is almost impossible to predict, is separation of the placenta from the uterine wall, shutting off the fetus from access to the maternal blood supply and thereby from proper exchange of oxygen and carbon dioxide, water and nutrients.

Sometimes a newborn unexpectedly has difficulty in establishing breathing patterns, even when it is born at full term following a completely normal labor. I still vividly remember the birth of such a baby following a completely uneventful and rapid labor in a young woman in glowing good health. The baby gasped just once and then lost all signs of life. We had appropriate resuscitation equipment at hand and went to work promptly, administering oxygen under positive pressure. It took this newborn almost ten minutes before she managed to come around and breathe on her own. In reviewing the mother's labor, the placenta, and the baby herself we never found any explanation for this event. I have since had the pleasure of seeing pictures of her when she received a master's degree from a major university and others taken shortly thereafter at the time of her marriage. Had this birth occurred in the absence of suitable equipment for resuscitation I am quite certain that even had this young woman survived she would not have done so undamaged.

At present, approximately 99 percent of all births in the United States takes place in hospitals. The most recent statistics that we have relate to the deliveries in the United States in 1981. In that year the highest ratio of out-of-hospital births was 4.4 percent, in Oregon. Washington was next with 3.5 percent, then Texas with 3.1 percent and Idaho with 2.6 percent. All the other states had rates lower than 2 percent. In Texas, 60 percent of the out-of-hospital births occur in four counties along the Rio Grande where there are large numbers of low-income Hispanic women. The population of Oregon includes a sizable religious cult that avoids medical care. There has recently been a study of a similar religious cult in Indiana. Although the members of the cult have not permitted the public health authorities to inspect their privately held birth records, there is substantial evidence that the perinatal loss rate is three times greater than the statewide rate. The maternal death rate is probably a hundredfold higher than for other Indiana women.

About 50 percent of the babies born outside the hospitals are delivered by physicians and all but a tiny fraction of the remainder by midwives. About half of the latter are lay midwives, a term that describes people who have not completed any formal training and are not registered by a health department as qualified to provide care. In the countries of Europe, which earlier organized their health services to encourage delivery at home, the practice has changed materially in recent years. In 1965, Holland had the highest rate of home births in Europe, but today the majority of Dutch babies are born in hospitals under the care of trained midwives.

This is not to say that we should not make changes in the traditional forms of hospital care. We can provide facilities equal to those of the hospital in a birthing center, located outside the walls of the hospital but sufficiently close to it so that the transfer of problem patients can be accomplished in a matter of minutes. With the proper selection of patients during pregnancy and in early labor, I am sure we can achieve a degree of safety equal to that of the hospital.

But what seems to me more promising is to revise the facilities that we provide for patients within the hospital in such a way to make them more supportive, more homelike, less institutional. This includes not only the physical facilities but also the way in which the women and the members of their support system are dealt with by the hospital personnel. There is simply no incompatibility between the highest quality of obstetrical care and the provision of all that natural childbirth means. Sympathetic support can also be provided to the patients in labor with such complications as prolongation of labor, hypertension, postmaturity, and the like. These call for increased monitoring but do not in every case necessitate barring family members, restricting activity, confinement to bed, or the need to give birth in a delivery room.

I counsel pregnant women strongly against placing themselves in the care of lay midwives. I know that some patients feel that because childbirth is a natural process, they do not wish it to become cluttered and complicated by artificial maneuvers and the application of technology. For this reason some of them place themselves in the hands of untrained and even unskilled persons. But while I fully agree that childbirth is natural, and do not believe in the use of technology for its own sake, I do believe in being prepared—with skill and the necessary equipment—to recognize and handle the emergencies when they occur. I would no more want a patient in the hands of an untrained practitioner, armed only with good intentions, than I would want my local fire department staffed only with terrified amateurs. For those patients who prefer the care of midwives, certified nurse midwives in the United States have the skill and ability to meet the needs of normal patients who want family-centered care. And there is now no place in the United States where care of this sort is not available.

In addition in all urban areas in the United States there are obstetricians who are also willing to meet patients' expectations for simplified, compassionate care with a minimum of interference with normality.

Preparations for the Hospital

The first step is to arrange for a visit to the hospital where you expect to deliver. If you expect to drive to the hospital, learn the route and where to park the car. Some hospitals have excellent parking facilities available twenty-four hours a day, whereas others may rely on on-street parking in crowded areas. Find out whether the security personnel at the entrance to the hospital will be able to help you if you arrive at an inconvenient hour. You should find out where the nighttime, weekend, and emergency entrances are located and get some idea of the relationship of these places to the portion of the hospital set aside for labor and delivery. No one ever plans it, but it is possible to arrive at a hospital in the middle of the night and at first find no one who can help you.

If you have the leisure to do so, you should probably set aside a small suitcase or a backpack into which you have placed the comfort items that you will want to have in the hospital after you deliver. This includes such things as books to read, playing cards, toilet goods, and one or two nursing brassieres. In most hospitals you will be encouraged to shower and take a shampoo as soon as you are comfortable after delivery. You may therefore want to take a hair dryer and other items you are accustomed to using.

Some women are more comfortable with their own bed-clothes. Most hospitals will not make any objection to your bringing pillows, pillow slips, and sheets, which you can use while you are in labor and in your hospital room after delivery. Remember that these things may become soiled and therefore should be items that are readily washable.

There probably is no need whatever to bring baby clothes to the hospital when you go into labor except perhaps for the minimal items that are essential for the baby when you take it home. This minimum includes a cotton shirt, a simple washable cotton gown, and a small washable wrapping blanket. In the winter you will want to have additional covers, but in the summer the baby will hardly need to be wrapped at all for its first trip out into the cruel world. Now, to be sure, these items are minimal and it is possible to dress the baby up considerably more than this, but additional clothing is not necessary from a health standpoint. It is wise, however, not to overdress the baby in hot weather.

When You Arrive at the Hospital

Each hospital has its own system of admitting patients, including finding the documents to indicate the status of your reservation. Each hospital has its own set of forms that have to be filled out and signed. Some hospitals attach an identification bracelet to the mother and prepare a plastic card to be used for printing her name and other vital statistics on the various pages of her records.

In many labor and delivery areas the staff is aware of the

fact that some women come in simply to be observed and not necessarily to stay. A certain amount of the bookkeeping and paperwork is then deferred until it becomes clear that the patient is in labor and will remain in the hospital. In that case the paperwork is completed later by clerks who come to the patient's bedside or who interview the patient's partner to secure the necessary information.

In most hospitals it is routine to escort any patient who is in active labor directly to the labor area. But, for example, when a woman enters the hospital for regulation of diabetes there is no hurry, and she may make a leisurely trip through the admitting office paperwork.

Many hospitals routinely require that women in labor be taken to the labor area in a wheelchair despite the fact that, moments earlier, they rode to the hospital in a car or a bus and walked in through the door. It is probably wise not to object too much to this. Allow the staff to give you a ride, however brief and however unnecessary, from the entrance to the labor area. Take along with you those personal items you have brought to the hospital, particularly the valuables you may have brought (although those might better be left at home). If you arrive at the hospital in very active labor, be sure to say so immediately, emphatically, and directly to the people who greet you as you come in. I have known patients, too diffident to do this, who have spent most of a short labor sitting in an admitting office or an emergency room, waiting for a busy clerk or nurse to take them in turn. Do not be shy. Make clear what your needs are.

Admission to the Labor Area

The staff on duty in the labor area will greet you when you arrive there. These are people who are fully accustomed to providing emergency care and doing it with maximum efficiency.

Your hospital will probably have a copy of your prenatal record immediately available to the staff of the labor area. If you have called in before coming, and things are not too busy, they will already have looked at the record to get some idea of who you are and whether you have any complications. When you arrive they will talk to you, ask you what is going on, and why you decided to come to the hospital. They will need to know, for example, if you have already consulted your doctor or midwife, and whether anything of note has happened to you since your last prenatal visit.

When the staff has interviewed you, they will take you to the labor room and give you a hospital gown to put on, unless it is apparent that you are in very early labor or not in labor at all.

A word about hospital gowns. They are unprepossessing in appearance, made of materials tough enough to withstand the rigors of a hospital laundry, and not designed for style or warmth. They have short sleeves and come to about mid-thigh in length; they close with tapes, which may be worn either in front or in back. The purpose of this design has nothing to do with appearance. It is to allow access to your body for purposes of examination and treatment.

If you are obviously in advanced labor when you come in, someone will see you promptly: either your personal attendant, if he or she is present, or a resident or staff nurse-midwife if they are on regular duty in the labor and delivery area. Should you become ready to deliver before your personal attendant can get to the hospital, a resident or nurse-midwife will be ready and able to give you the necessary assistance. That is what they are there for, and every professional on an obstetrics service knows from experience that a baby will not wait to be born once it is ready.

When I was an intern there were still hospitals in which the staff made efforts to restrain patients from delivering until their own physicians could be present. However, this is recognized as unsafe for the baby and the practice has fortunately been abandoned.

Assuming you are not on the point of having the baby at the moment of your arrival, whoever examines you will begin by feeling your abdomen, to make sure that the size of the fetus corresponds with what you and the hospital record say is the expected date of confinement. If the fetus appears to be premature, preparations will have to be made for the special care the baby will need after birth. The examiner will then listen to the fetal heart rate. In some hospitals, if the patient is in labor a fetal monitor will be attached to make a written record of the force and frequency of uterine contractions and the response of the baby's heart rate. It takes only fifteen or twenty minutes to identify indications of abnormalities of labor. The examiner will also routinely take your pulse, temperature, and your blood pressure, and if you have recently had a respiratory infection or otherwise been ill, will examine your lungs to be sure they are clear.

The next step is pelvic examination, to check whether the membranes are ruptured, to find out what the presenting part is, and to gauge how deep it is in the pelvis. The examiner will also observe and write down the condition of the cervix, how long it is, and how far it has opened. These measurements are recorded in centimeters: 2.5 to the inch. Until the opening is 3 to 4 centimeters across, it is not possible to be certain that the patient is in labor. (Full dilation is 10 centimeters, or 4 inches.) Lastly, some hospitals take a bacterial culture of the lower vagina, chiefly to look for Group B beta-hemolytic streptococcus, a germ that can cause rapid and severe infection in the baby.

If time permits, the examination will also include taking a urine specimen to test for the presence of protein and sugar; and some blood for tests such as a repeat serologic test for syphilis, a red-blood-cell count, and a repeat identification of the patient's blood group, in case a transfusion should be necessary.

In all emergency admissions, at the time that the blood is drawn, the needle or catheter is kept in the vein and administration of intravenous fluids begun.

For patients with adequate prenatal care who are in normal labor, precautionary administration of intravenous fluids, which many patients find a nuisance, may be omitted.

If You're Not Surely in Labor

If status of your labor is unclear, you may be advised to wait around the hospital for another few hours. Some hospitals provide pleasant facilities for this sort of waiting; others may expect you to go out into a nearby lounge along with visitors and other patients. But in any event, the passage of a few hours will make clear whether or not you are actually in labor. Some patients note that when they get to the hospital contractions cease and then after a pause begin again.

—And If You Are

When the decision is made that you are actually in labor, further steps may be taken. When I first entered obstetrics it was routine to give an enema to every patient to whom it could possibly be given. It was thought that it was necessary to empty the large intestine and that the enema accelerated labor. This practice has happily largely vanished from obstetrics with the realization that the administration of enemas is of no medical value and, from the patient's standpoint, it simply adds one more form of discomfort.

Another source of unnecessary discomfort that has been commonly eliminated in the years since I was a young doctor is the shaving of the sexual hair. This used to be done to all patients in labor, who then underwent the doubly unpleasant experience of first being shaved with a dry razor and no lubrication on sensitive skin and then enduring the itching sensations during the period of regrowth. We all now generally agree, however, that this shaving carries no medical benefit to the patient that would justify the disagreeable nature of the experience, and I am glad to say that it is no longer in vogue. I have myself not had any of my patients shaved since 1950, and none has suffered any medical detriment from this policy.

Conversely, some hospitals encourage patients to have a shower on admission. This too is a medically insignificant procedure. Whether to shower or not at this stage is a matter of the patient's personal taste and comfort.

With the growing respect being paid to family-centered obstetrics, the woman's partner is now being encouraged to stay with her through most of her labor. The most distressing thing for many women in labor is to be left alone. The patient's partner is the appropriate person to be with her.

In Bed or Not
The patient can be in labor in bed or sitting in a chair or walking in the hall at least during the first stage of labor; it is probably

wise for her to be in the most comfortable position that she can find. If the woman prefers to lie down she ought to turn partly onto her left side. The fetal monitor equipment in use at present produces the best records with patients lying down in bed. However, there is some newly developed equipment that can be attached so that the patient can be up and around. The practicality of this equipment awaited the recent perfection of lightweight radio transmitters, which broadcast the signals created by the uterine contractions and the fetal heartbeat to nearby equipment that then prints the recording.

When labor is not normal, continuous fetal monitoring is of great value, and for this purpose, the patient should usually be in bed. There are, however, some patients who benefit from walking and at the same time need continuous monitoring. And it is in this group of women that we foresee the greatest benefit from the new technology, which frees the patients from the wires that have up to now attached them to the fetal monitor.

Let me emphasize that there is no absolutely necessary or ideal position for the first stage of labor. Some patients are more comfortable propped up in bed, others are more comfortable standing on the floor and kneeling over a bed, others prefer to walk. I think what is important is for you and the people working with you to find the position that is best for you. You can generally trust what your body has to say about this, in terms of the discomforts that you feel in labor.

As labor goes on, your medical attendant or members of the hospital staff will examine you from time to time to follow your progress. You may even ask them to do so, and unless there is some reason why you should not be examined at that time, they will ordinarily be glad to oblige, and tell you what they have found. The examiner will again feel your abdomen to locate the baby and find its presenting part and how far it has come through the birth canal. A vaginal examination may also be done at this time, to check how far the cervix has opened, but if you come in with prematurely ruptured membranes, it is not wise to do many vaginal examinations. If you are having your first baby, these examinations will be a considerable help to you in following your labor, though with later babies you may be able to estimate your own progress pretty well without repeated examinations.

Unless there is some medical reason why you should not do so you can expect to go to the toilet to empty your bladder. Urinating is much easier if you do it naturally than if you attempt to balance yourself on a bed pan. The staff may want you to urinate into a container so that the amount of urine can be measured and so that chemical tests for evidence of acidosis can be carried out. This is as easy to do sitting on a toilet seat as it is on a bed pan.

In the best of all possible worlds, a patient's labor is sufficiently tranquil so that she can maintain her fluid balance by taking fluids, such as ice chips, clear broth, fruit juice, or tea, by mouth. In strong, active labor, many patients are nauseated, and some vomit. Under these circumstances they should receive intravenous fluids, because if there is inadequate intake of water the patient can become dehydrated and shrink her blood volume. Her circulatory system is then unable to maintain adequate blood flow to the placenta. To prevent this from happening we have learned to maintain the patient's fluid intake at normal levels during labor.

The Criteria of Progress in Labor

There are two criteria for progress in labor, closely related to one another. One is the level or station of the presenting part (the head or the breech) of the fetus in relation to the mother's bony pelvis, the space through which the baby must pass to be born. The point of reference for level or station is an imaginary line drawn between a pair of pelvic bony structures, the ischial spines. They jut into the birth canal off its side walls about halfway down through the true pelvis and are usually its narrowest point. The muscles and ligaments that surround the vagina and anus attach to the bony pelvis at about the spines and, hanging below them like a hammock, form the support of the abdominal contents (the pelvic floor). The presenting part of the fetus stretches these tissues and passes through them to emerge from the vagina at the time of delivery. The hammock also serves to rotate the head to occiput anterior, the position of normal birth of the head, in which the face of the baby is toward the mother's back.

The level or station of the presenting part has no significance when the fetus is in transverse lie, with its spinal column not parallel to that of the mother. Vaginal birth is not safe for either mother or infant when labor ensues with such a lie. The proper treatment is cesarean section.

You will hear doctors using terms such as "minus one" or "plus three." Decoded, these terms mean, respectively, that the presenting part is one centimeter above the imaginary line joining the pelvic spines, or in the case of plus three, the presenting part is three centimeters below this level. When the baby comes down to about four centimeters below the level of the spines, the head or breech presses on the pelvic floor; this pressure creates an additional urge to push which results quite soon thereafter in the birth of the presenting part.

The other criterion, the state of the cervix, is described under two headings. One is the description of the size of its opening. Not all cervices are perfectly circular, but they are idealized as such for the statement of their diameter. For first labors the cervix is very much shortened and thinned out before it starts to dilate. The extent of this shortening can be expressed in two ways. Some of us describe the length of the cervical canal in centimeters, whereas others express this as a percentage of the expected length of approximately two centimeters. Labor may begin with later babies while the cervix still has some length to it. If it is one centimeter long, it may be described as being fifty percent effaced. Many times when a cervix has dilated beyond four or five centimeters it is completely effaced, which is another way of saying that it has no significant length.

These, then, are the items that the attendant checks in doing a vaginal examination. They are ordinarily recorded in the patient's chart at the time the exam is done.

If continuous fetal monitoring is being used, the electronic device will make a record of the fetus's heart rate and the frequency of contractions. In addition to this, in well-managed labor rooms the patient's blood pressure is recorded every half hour or every hour and the patient's pulse similarly jotted down at frequent intervals. The patient's temperature is taken every three or four hours in labor and more frequently if the patient has a fever. The fetal heart is listened to about every fifteen minutes during active labor if it is not being continuously recorded and its rate and the frequency of contractions are entered in the chart. All this monitoring can be accomplished with a minimum of annoyance to the patient by sympathetic and gentle personnel. It is even possible to administer intravenous fluids in such a way as not to limit the patient's mobility or increase her discomfort.

Pain Relief in Labor and Delivery

Labor, whether lengthy or brief, is hard work, as the word implies. The work itself is well within women's ability to handle it. The work of the first stage of labor is done by a very competent smooth muscle that does not need any specific exercise to prepare it for its task. The work of the second stage of labor is carried out by voluntary muscles of the abdominal wall, and they too do an excellent job. Patients who have had lengthy labors sometimes feel a great sense of frustration and sometimes even inadequacy to the task, but when the time comes to bear down and push the baby out they almost always find resources of energy that are quite equal to the needs.

For the great majority of women labor is also painful. Women who are by nature stoic and those who have been well prepared for labor deal with this discomfort quite competently. They do so vastly better in the presence of an active, warm, and sympathetic support system such as can be provided by their partner, by labor coaches, by labor room nurses, and by the attendants they have chosen to help them with the process. Medical science has stepped forward to provide both psychological and medicinal interventions in an effort to reduce this experience of pain.

The History of Pain Relief in Obstetrics

Early in the first book of the Old Testament it is said to women that "in sorrow thou shalt bring forth children." It was taken for granted that pain was an appropriate accompaniment of the labor process. One can search the authoritative obstetrical texts on the sixteenth, seventeenth, eighteenth, and the first half of the nineteenth centuries without encountering a single reference to the use of drugs for the relief of pain in labor, despite the fact that pain-relieving drugs were known and were employed commonly in medicine and surgery. The greatest obstetrician of Renaissance France, François Mauriceau, in his influential textbook of obstetrics, comments that he was asked to see a kinswoman who had injured her back when six months pregnant. Writing in 1668, he states that he prescribed "at two different times a small grain of laudanum (the available preparation of opium at the time) in the yolk of an egg, a little to ease her violent pains." However, in this same authoritative textbook there is no comment on the relief of pain in labor. Many pages are devoted in these early books to the proper management of very long, very painful labors, whose conclusion was achieved by crude surgery that must have been the source of extreme pain, without any reference to pain relief as part of the care.

In one of the fabled episodes in the late seventeenth century, the Dr. Chamberlen who had invented obstetrical forceps was invited to demonstrate them in the delivery of a woman with severe pelvic deformity due to rickets. He struggled unsuccessfully for three hours in a woman who had had nothing for pain relief, before having to admit failure to deliver the baby. It was taken for granted in that era that survival of the baby itself was not a consideration, and we are not told whether the mother survived.

The credit for bringing this dreary epoch to an end goes to Sir James Young Simpson of Edinburgh, the intrepid innovator who conducted the very first delivery under anesthesia as we know it today. Simpson himself actually searched medical literature fruitlessly in an effort to find any earlier reference to pain relief during childbirth. He administered the first obstetrical anesthetic for the delivery of a woman in the slums of Edinburgh. She was "etherized shortly after nine o'clock" on the evening of January 19, 1847. Simpson had personally experimented on himself with the use of the primitive anesthetic agents available at that time before using it on this patient. By coincidence on the very same day he was informed of his appointment as one of Queen Victoria's Scottish physicians. He considered this appointment the less important of the two events. He wrote to his brother that "flattery from the Queen is perhaps not common flattery, but I am far less interested in it than having delivered a woman this week without any pain while inhaling sulphuric ether. I can think of naught else." Simpson was vigorously attacked for having given pain relief in violation of the proscription in the Bible. His opponents underestimated him. His prompt reply to their criticism was that before Adam produced Eve from his rib, God caused him to fall into a deep sleep. Whatever the theology, in short order, and encouraged by Queen Victoria herself, anesthesia became established as a technique for use in delivery.

The use of medication to relieve pain during labor, prior to the discomforts of delivery itself, was introduced by Gauss of Freiburg, Germany. In 1907 he introduced the combination of two drugs, morphine and scopolamine, for this purpose. The morphine eliminated pain and the scopolamine impaired memory. Under the influence of these drugs the patient remained in a dream state somewhere between consciousness and unconsciousness. Gauss therefore called the technique "twilight sleep" (*Dämmerchlaf* in German). Interestingly enough, the most commonly used drug for pain relief in obstetrics in the United States is Demerol, a name derived from Gauss's name in German for twilight sleep.

The sole addition to the medical armamentarium since the contributions of Simpson and Gauss has been the development of regional block anesthesia for the relief of pain in labor and at delivery.

Methods of Pain Relief

The four decades following the end of World War II witnessed a great deal of experimentation with methods of pain relief both for the conduct of labor and for delivery. Some of these consist entirely of the use of drugs and others are directed mainly to psychological training.

A few of these techniques have emerged as both acceptable to patients and safe for use. This does not mean that we have a perfect solution, only that a period of intense investigation and broad experimentation has brought out several useful methods of pain relief that can be used, individually or in combination, with generally satisfactory results.

Pain relief in labor can be achieved in three principal ways. One is the administration of drugs to change the patients' threshold for pain. Second is the use of nerve-blocking agents that interrupt the transmission of pain from the abdomen and low back to the brain. The third relies on techniques for prepared childbirth which range from Lamaze through psychoprophylaxis to hypnosis.

No pain-relief method using drugs is entirely free from the potential of causing undesirable side effects on both mother and fetus. But the failure to use drugs where there is a clear medical indication may also have adverse effects. The woman who is in labor for a very long time needs some relief. If she fails to get this she may develop metabolic acidosis resulting from inadequate calories and hard work. The acidosis potentially has an adverse effect on the baby. Since patients in labor ordinarily are not able to take in calories in adequate amounts, in a prolonged labor the patient suffers the effects of acute starvation, often aggravated by a lack of sufficient rest. Women who are in severe discomfort in labor may nevertheless require oxytocin stimulation because of a delay in the normal process. It would be inhumane to stimulate labor in such cases without taking measures to assure pain relief. Moreover, there is good evidence that oxytocin stimulation, when given to treat delay in labor, is more effective in the presence of an epidural block.

General Considerations

There is still no perfect anesthetic for obstetrics. From the standpoint of safety, the ideal forms of pain relief for labor and delivery use the absolute minimum of medication that will achieve their purpose. The most-effective anesthetic methods have the highest incidence of serious complications. The least effective ones are safest but are not adequate for the major operative procedures which, however infrequent, are an essential part of obstetrical care.

It is unfortunate but true that throughout the United States a significant fraction of the deaths in childbirth are due to anesthesia. In some instances a formidable anesthetic has been used as a necessary part of the treatment of a major accident of pregnancy, with fatal but unavoidable results. Unfortunately, there are also instances in which the fatal outcome is the consequence of ineptitude or poor judgment. Nevertheless, there are no completely safe anesthetics. In a serious emergency, the greatest safety factor is a skilled and careful anesthesiologist.

Drugs for Labor

Chief among the drugs used to change the threshold for pain is Demerol (meperidine), which is carried by the bloodstream to the pain centers in the brain. Nisentil (alphaprodine) and Stadol (butorphanol) are closely related to Demerol but are in less common use. All of these are members of the general class of narcotics. They differ from such drugs as heroin and morphine in that they are more likely to encourage drowsiness rather than euphoria, the technical term for a "high." Since all of them can slow breathing in both the mother and the newborn infant, they are usually used in modest doses and combined with other drugs, principally tranquilizers such as Phenergan (promethazine) and Vistaril (hydroxyzine). The tranquilizers do what their name suggests with minimal side effects. Combined with the narcotic-related drugs, they tend to produce a reassured, less anxious patient who tolerates pain better than an unmedicated, unprepared woman.

On occasion a decision may be made to combine one or another of these drugs with barbiturates such as Seconal or Nembutal. The advantage of these is that they tend to induce sleep with almost no effect on respirations, and they are rapidly eliminated by the liver.

The goal of this form of pain relief is to relax the woman in labor and to assist her in tolerating the pain. It is surely not to "knock her out" and not to wipe out the memory of labor. When I was an intern, perfect analgesia in labor was expected to remove all recollection of having had a baby. We had to awaken patients hours later and to convince them that they had delivered. There are still a few patients who request this kind of care.

But the great majority of women today wish to be aware of the labor and delivery. We now concentrate on reducing the unpleasant aspects of the process without removing the woman's awareness and memory. This is not always easily done.

Individual women react quite differently to identical doses of narcotics and tranquilizers. With the customary dose some fall asleep for an hour or two and others have only a slight response. Most patients are alert during uterine contractions and doze off between them. They are awake enough to help with their care.

It fascinates me that patients who have been very subdued during labor come brightly awake with the birth of the baby and its first cry. By using emotional support, encouragement, and repeated small doses of drugs, most women are kept reasonably comfortable and fully able to participate.

There has always been concern about the effect of these drugs on the fetus. Prior to birth there are no adverse effects. When the birth has been easy it is not possible to show any evidence of drug effects except by delicate chemical tests on the baby's blood and urine. There is no difference in newborn behavior or ability to breathe unless there has been a difficult delivery. In that event the baby may be sluggish and delayed in crying and breathing.

If a woman given a narcotic drug inadvertently receives too large a dose or unexpectedly proves to be highly sensitive to the drug, its effect on breathing can be reversed by the administration of Narcan (naloxone). This drug has its principal use in the treatment of a baby whose breathing is diminished or delayed as the result of the administration of one of the narcotics to the mother.

All of these preparations are ideally given by injection; at the present time they are almost all used intravenously in doses somewhat less than would be used if they were given into the patient's muscle. If the patient is receiving intravenous fluids it is feasible to add small doses at frequent intervals.

None of these drugs has any significant effect on uterine contractions, although there is an impression that their use may prolong labor. No major study, however, has borne out this impression. What actually happens is that, if these drugs are given before labor is truly under way, the interval from the moment that the drug is given until the birth will be longer than if the drug is withheld until patients are in active labor. In treating the discomfort of prelabor it is usually better to use appropriate drugs by mouth rather than by injection.

Conduction Anesthesia in Labor

Epidural anesthesia is a form of pain relief that does not affect either the progress of labor or the alertness of the mother or the baby. For these reasons it might seem to be an almost perfect method, but it is accompanied by drawbacks that must be taken into account in any decision to employ it.

The epidural space is located within the bony ring that forms the spinal canal. The backbone is made up of twenty-four vertebrae, which rest on one another like a pile of poker chips. The bodies of the vertebrae have cartilage pads between them and are connected to one another by dense ligaments. Behind each vertebral body toward the back there is a bony ring; the spinal cord comes down from the brain through this series of rings, encased in a dense membrane named the dura mater. Nerves emerge from the dura and go out through the spaces between the rings of the several vertebrae to the arms, legs, head, neck, chest, and abdomen.

The spinal fluid in which the nerve tissue of the spinal cord floats is within the dura. This fluid communicates with the fluid of the brain itself inside the skull. There is a space between the spinal cord and dura and the spinal canal. The size of this epidural space is greatest at the level of the two vertebral bodies just below the rib cage in the lumbar region.

The technique for injecting blocking agents is to insert a fine catheter through a needle into this space, inside the spinal canal but outside the dura. The blocking agents flow through the catheter and bathe the nerves as they emerge from the dura. This stops the pain sensation from reaching the brain and removes the brain's control over the muscles served by the nerves. Anesthetic doses are given from time to time through the catheter as needed to produce an effective pain block. It is sometimes possible to do this and still maintain some muscle control, an asset in managing the second stage of labor so that the patient can cooperate in bearing down.

Although an epidural block does not affect the mother's awareness of what is going on, except for the relief from the pain of labor, it may cause the blood to pool in her legs and in the tissues below the level of the block, as the blood vessels in this area are widely open. The consequence of the pooling can be a drop in the mother's blood pressure, but this can be prevented by giving her at least a half liter (a little over a pint) of intravenous fluids shortly before administering the anesthetic agent.

Epidural must be given with precaution against accidentally introducing the anesthetic agent into the spinal fluid in the intradural space. The doses of drugs given in the epidural space are substantially larger than those given with a direct spinal. On occasion despite all precautions the drug given through a catheter can leak into the intradural space and engender a profound spinal anesthetic. The effect can extend up the spinal cord and, by paralyzing the muscles of the chest, interfere seriously with respirations. Epidurals therefore must be given slowly and deliberately, with several test doses, before the full dose to produce pain relief is administered. This means that it ordinarily takes twenty to thirty minutes to establish an effective epidural; the method cannot be used in a hurried situation.

Because of the weakness of the lower extremities that is produced by epidural, the patient will almost always have to remain in bed. In that event she should be lying with her right hip up to take the weight of the uterus off her major abdominal blood vessels, to prevent blood from pooling below this level, which might decrease the output of the woman's heart. This in turn can diminish the flow of blood to the uterus and thus bring about changes in the fetal heart rate.

The drugs used for epidural anesthesia do reach the mother's general circulation in small amounts. They thus cross the placenta and get into the fetus, and they can also get into the mother's milk. However, there is no evidence that the fetus or the newborn suffer any effects at all from the minute amounts to which they are exposed.

Because of the weakening of muscle response in the mother, the second stage of labor, particularly in first labors, tends to be somewhat longer with effective epidurals. This can be minimized by allowing the epidural to wear off once the second stage of labor is reached. This is not quite as lacking in compassion as it may sound. Most patients who labor with minimal medication testify that the discomfort of the second stage of labor is less than that of the latter part of the first stage of labor, and the second stage is likely to be much shorter than the first.

Caudal Anesthesia

Shortly after World War II a form of epidural under the name of caudal anesthesia enjoyed considerable popularity. Its effects in general are quite similar to that of epidural except that the catheter is put in at the tailbone. If the technique is used for pain relief in labor it produces its most profound effect in the area around the vagina, which, as I have explained, is not the area of maximum discomfort during the first stage of labor. Caudal entails the same dangers of unintended overdose due to injection into the dura as does epidural. Because of the difficulties in placing the needle for caudal anesthesia, this method has very largely been supplanted by either continuous epidural or terminal saddle block, which is a very low intradural spinal injection.

Paracervical Block for Labor

There used to be some enthusiasm for paracervical block for pain relief in labor. This block is produced by injecting a local anesthetic agent alongside the cervix, using a vaginal approach for the injection, with the intention of blocking the nerves near at the uterus. This technique is no longer widely used for two reasons. One is that its effectiveness is not entirely predictable. The other is that every once in a while there has been severe slowing of the fetal heart rate after the drug is given. This is probably due to passage of the drug into the placenta and thereby into fetal circulation, and also to spasm of the uterine arteries from its local effect.

Nerve-Blocking Drugs

The nerve-blocking drugs in present use are all synthetic progeny of cocaine, and their names all end in "-caine." Chemists have developed forms that are rapidly broken down in the body, thereby increasing their safety. Some have powerful local anesthetic effect when applied to body surfaces, notably the mouth, throat, vagina, and anus, whereas others must be injected into the area where a block is desired. When introduced into the tissues in excessive doses, they are absorbed into the blood and carried throughout the body. They cause agitation and then convulsions. An excess dose given as a spinal (intradural) injection can stop the patient's breathing. Yet these drugs are almost without harmful effects when swallowed or placed on body surfaces.

Recently there have been reports of effective spinal conduction anesthesia with small doses of morphine. We do not have enough experience with this method to allow a reasoned judgment of its usefulness in obstetrics.

Psychoprophylaxis

There are a number of such methods currently available. I have commented on them elsewhere in this volume. The education that goes along with them is of value in itself, and probably plays a large role in their effectiveness. For this reason I advise all patients to take such preparation whether or not they expect to rely on a particular technique for pain relief.

Hypnosis and acupuncture have been used with some success for pain relief in labor and delivery, but their effectiveness is, unfortunately, unpredictable. Although much publicity has been given to cesarean section done under acupuncture it has largely escaped notice that the women treated with acupuncture have also received substantial amounts of such drugs as Demerol.

Choice of Pain Relief in Labor

An essential final point to make is that you need not and probably should not make a firm commitment in advance of labor to using or not using any method of pain relief. Decisions as to how much to use, when to use it, or whether to use it at all can be made from moment to moment as labor goes on. I prefer to consult with my patients as to what will be helpful to them as labor progresses. You should discuss, with the people who are going to help you in labor, what their attitudes are on the use of these methods and in particular what will be available at the hospital where you expect to deliver. Epidural, for example, requires a high level of skill and experience in anesthesia. If your hospital does not have anesthesiologists on call at night or on weekends for labor patients, epidural may simply be unavailable.

Anesthesia for Cesarean Section

Abdominal delivery is ordinarily carried out with the patient lying on her back. With either general or regional anesthesia there may be pooling of blood in the lower half of the body, partly due to the anesthetic agent, and partly to the weight of the pregnant uterus resting as it does on the major blood vessels in the back wall of the abdomen. The woman's blood pressure falls and blood supply to the fetus is reduced. Therefore, it has become the usual practice to put a wedge, often a pillow or a folded blanket, under the patient's right hip to rotate the patient slightly to her left. This shifts the weight of the uterus off the blood vessels and restores normal circulatory and blood-volume conditions.

Cesareans can be done under either general anesthesia or one of the types of intradural or epidural. Local anesthesia, hypnosis, and acupuncture have also been used, but only seldom.

General Anesthesia for Cesarean

A general anesthetic for cesarean ordinarily is begun with a very short-acting drug, such as a barbiturate, given intravenously, to put the patient sound asleep. The patient is then given an intravenous dose of a drug related to curare, the effect of which is to paralyze the body's voluntary muscles. This stops breathing as well as all other body movement and brings about considerable relaxation. Taking advantage of this relaxed state, the anesthesiologist then passes an endotracheal (Greek: *endon*, "within," *trachea*, "windpipe") tube through the patient's mouth, through the vocal cords, and into the upper portion of the trachea. A small balloon wrapped around this tube is then inflated so as to fill the trachea, thus eliminating any possibility of breathing in food or gastric juice while the tube is in place. The anesthesiologist connects the tube to the anesthesia machine, which artificially breathes for the patient while she is paralyzed by drugs. From then on, the barbiturate is given intravenously to keep the patient soundly asleep and enough of the curarelike agent given to keep the patient fully relaxed. The anesthesiologist maintains continuous observation of the patient's heart rate and blood pressure. Since the curarelike drugs do not cross the placenta and only enough barbiturate is used to keep the mother asleep, this form of anesthesia has virtually no effect on the newborn.

This general anesthetic method is ideal whenever a cesarean needs to be done in a hurry or when it is done for hemorrhage. It can be established in a matter of a few minutes, in contrast to twenty to thirty minutes for an epidural. As mentioned above, epidural and intradural anesthesias tend to result in the pooling of blood in the lower half of the body which in turn aggravates the effect of blood loss by further reducing the amount of blood available for the heart, brain, and kidneys. General anesthesia has no such effect and is thus materially safer in the presence of hemorrhage.

The obvious disadvantage of general anesthesia is that the mother is asleep during the birth of her baby. She also tends to be in a somewhat detached dream state for varying periods of time after she has begun to awaken from the anesthesia at the conclusion of the operation. This interferes with early bonding with the newborn.

Spinal and Epidural for Cesarean

Spinal, which can be given in a matter of two to three minutes, is the anesthesia of choice in some institutions when cesarean has to be done in a hurry and there is no maternal hemorrhage. The mother loses all sensation below the rib cage for the duration of the spinal anesthetic, which may last for a matter of several hours. Since this is a so-called one-shot technique, it is necessary to give enough anesthetic drug on the initial injection to last the expected duration of the procedure.

The margin of safety with an intradural is not as great as it is with an epidural, since the drug is put directly into the spinal fluid and can spread farther in that fluid pool than is intended. The drug then weakens the muscles of the chest and produces a decrease in breathing activity. The patient, as she realizes her inability to breathe properly, may experience considerable anxiety. We are alert to the possibility of this complication: Its warning signs are a drop in blood pressure and a speeding up of the pulse rate. The treatment is to give early support to the woman's breathing, making use of oxygen and the anesthesia machine.

Epidural is now firmly established as the anesthetic of choice for cesarean section in hospitals that have the skilled anesthesiologists necessary for its safe performance. Epidural anesthesia for cesarean is more intense and rises to a higher sensory level in the abdomen than epidural for labor and vaginal delivery, but the technique of giving it is identical. For women in whom I anticipate that a cesarean section may be the eventual outcome, I am likely to recommend an epidural during labor so that the anesthetic will be in place should the need later arise to deliver the baby abdominally.

With these conduction anesthetics the patient remains awake and alert. She can see and hear and hold her baby. She may feel motion and pressure in her abdomen, but pain is eliminated. The loss of muscle control wears off in a matter of a few hours, and all functions return to normal.

Anesthesia for Vaginal Birth

From a strictly medical standpoint a fully normal birth does not require an anesthetic for the safety of either the mother or the fetus. The passage of the baby through the vagina, a structure that readily expands to accommodate it, does not ordinarily cause pain. As the presenting part descends through the pelvis, the tissues and muscles composing the pelvic floor are stretched, producing a tearing sensation and some actual tears. This is most striking in first deliveries, but may recur in later births if the mother has had an episiotomy or repair of a tear in the past.

The area at the entrance to the vagina can be readily anesthetized by nerve-blocking agents injected locally. These can either be placed in the tissues of the perineum or injected along the side of the pelvis at the point where the nerves that serve this area emerge. This latter technique is called a pudendal block because the anesthetic agent is placed in the vicinity of the pudendal nerve. When either a local or a pudendal block is put in place it causes a loss of local pain sensation but no loss of the normal bearing-down reflex. The mother can complete the vaginal birth without any impediment. These two anesthetic methods are ideal as well for operative deliveries done with a vacuum extractor since this technique is most efficient when the extraction is carefully timed to coincide with the mother's bearing-down efforts.

Forceps are used in the second stage of labor when the mother is unable to complete delivery by her own efforts or when the condition of the fetus requires its prompt birth. The obstetrician must be certain that the head of the baby has moved down in the pelvis and that its failure to be born naturally is not due to pelvic narrowing or excessive fetal size. It is also essential to be certain that the mother's cervix is fully out of the way. If the head of the baby can be seen in the vaginal opening, the forceps operation requires little pulling by the doctor and has no ill effects on baby or mother. Such a procedure is called a low or outlet forceps.

When the head has not yet come into contact with the pelvic floor, even though it has come low in the pelvic canal, the operation is likely to be more difficult and to require greater force, thus presenting greater risks than low forceps. It is called a mid-forceps operation; being more painful, it calls for more intense anesthesia than does low forceps or normal birth.

Epidural anesthesia is appropriate for forceps delivery. The anesthetic agent, which settles down in spinal fluid, is given with the patient sitting up so as to use gravity to intensify the block in the low pelvis and perineal floor. This is referred to as a perineal dose; it can be given as a single shot or through a catheter that has been used for pain relief during labor.

Another choice for forceps delivery is the saddle block: this is a very low intradural spinal, administered with the patient sitting up, for the same purpose and effect as with the perineal dose of an epidural. The most intense portion of the anesthetic is in the perineum and the lower part of the abdomen, while anesthesia in the legs is minimized. The patient usually continues to be aware of uterine contractions, although she will not feel any discomfort in her vagina or perineum. She can then bear down as requested by the obstetrician who is doing the forceps maneuver. The safety of the forceps operation is enhanced by the improved relaxation available with saddle block as compared with local anesthesia in the vagina.

There is no significant recovery period from any of these anesthetic techniques for vaginal delivery. The mothers are awake and can immediately receive the baby and start to nurse it if they so desire.

Complications of Anesthesia

It is a general practice for anesthesiologists to keep the patients in the operating room or delivery room until they have fully reacted from a general anesthetic. This makes certain that the patient's cough reflex has returned so that the danger of aspiration should the patient vomit is reduced to a minimum. Various methods, such as administering antacids, have also been used to reduce the acidity of the gastric juice that may be present in the otherwise empty stomach of a patient in labor.

There are occasional patients who are deficient in the enzyme necessary to break down the curarelike drugs to a harmless form. These women take substantially longer to reestablish their own breathing. There may therefore have to be a delay in removing their endotracheal tubes. As soon as the patient's own respirations have resumed the problem is resolved.

Because the endotracheal tube has been passed between the vocal cords, some patients have a hoarse voice for a day or two after a general anesthetic has been given. There are no late complications related to this and it clears up without difficulty.

The immediate problems related to spinal anesthesia have already been mentioned. An occasional patient experiences a severe headache following a spinal. This is believed to be due to a leak of spinal fluid out through the hole in the dura made by the spinal needle. The pressure inside the patient's head decreases as it does with a slow leak in an automobile tire. It is thought that the pain is due to pulling on the nerves that pass from the brain stem through spaces in the skull. The headache is ordinarily worst toward the back of the head. It is not present when the patient is lying down. The severity of the headache may impair the patient's ability to be up and around.

Two methods are effective in relieving the pain. In one, a clot of the patient's own blood is used as a patch over the hole in the dura. In the other, the patient is given two or more quarts of intravenous fluid for the purpose of restoring a normal amount of spinal fluid volume.

The Second Stage of Labor

Many descriptions of late first-stage labor make reference to "transition": the moment when the cervix is almost fully dilated and the baby's head is being released into the vagina. This is associated with severe pain, attributed to stretching of the cervix. Many patients do not experience transition, however. Instead, the pain of the uterine contractions undergoes a subtle change and the patient feels the urge to bear down. This feeling is identical with the sensation that all of us have when we are about to have a bowel movement. Toilet training taught us long ago to restrain this impulse for social acceptability, but we also know from experience that, when we have a severe bout of gastroenteritis and diarrhea, the urge may be irresistible. This is what happens in the second stage of labor.

The force of uterine contractions is sufficient to push the baby's head into the vagina but not enough to push it out through the connective tissue and muscle sling around the entrance to the vagina. The stretching of the upper vagina and the anterior wall of the rectum, which is loosely attached the vagina, seems to create the bearing-down reflex. This occurs simultaneously with the peak of uterine contractions. In bearing down, the woman holds her breath, contracts the muscles of her abdominal wall, and makes every effort to push the baby out through the vaginal opening. Even when a patient is under epidural anesthesia, unless it is intense, the patient can feel some of this urge and can organize her bearing-down efforts.

With a first baby the duration of bearing down is often between half an hour and one hour. If contractions occur approximately every three minutes, the whole process takes between ten and twenty effective contractions.

What is accomplished during the second stage? For one thing, the baby's head descends even deeper into the pelvis.

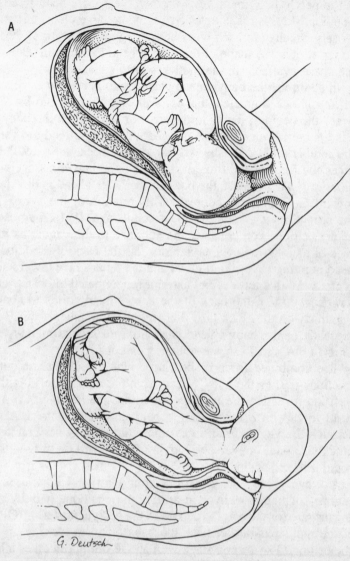

The second stage of labor. The mother is on her back, with her head to the left and her left leg in a raised position. The right half of the mother's body is transparent. The fetal head in A is well into the pelvis. The cervix is so thinned out and opened that it is continuous with the vagina, which is also opening. In B the largest part of the baby's head has been born, although its nose and mouth are not yet beyond the vagina.

If the pelvic bony passage is narrow, the baby's head molds. The fetal skull is made up of five separate large plates of bone loosely attached to each other at their edges. Shifting of these bones allows the shape of the baby's head to accommodate to the space available in the mother's birth canal.

In addition, the baby's head usually enters the lower pelvis in an oblique diameter, that is, with the back of the baby's head, the occiput, partly to the right or left. When the baby's head is born it emerges with the baby looking directly toward the mother's back. If she is lying on her back the baby then faces the floor at the time of birth. This is known as occiput anterior (OA), because the back of the baby's head is directed toward the mother's abdomen. This rotation of the vertex is the second major feature of the second stage. If, for purposes of orientation, you consider the entrance to the vagina as the face of a clock, an occiput anterior has the back of the fetus's head pointing to twelve o'clock and the fetus's face toward six o'clock. With a left occiput anterior (abbreviated in obstetrical jargon as LOA), the back of the baby's head points to about one thirty on the clock face. For right occiput anterior (ROA), the back of the baby's head is pointing to approximately ten thirty. LOA and ROA are oblique positions.

The combined force of bearing down and of uterine contractions pushes the baby's head from the oblique to OA, the position in which the baby presents the smallest width of its head to the birth canal. If the baby has started its descent through the vagina in an LOA, the rotation of OA is counterclockwise and, conversely, moving from an ROA to OA, the rotation is clockwise.

Not every baby delivers in occiput anterior. I have seen a number of babies deliver in an oblique position. It is by no means rare for the baby to deliver in the occiput posterior (OP). If the mother is on her back the baby emerges looking up at the ceiling. The second stage with an OP ordinarily takes a bit longer, particularly with first babies, because the OP presents less-favorable diameters of the baby's head to the sling of muscle and connective tissue that surrounds the vagina.

On occasion, because of inadequate uterine contraction, the head does not rotate well. In that event, the head usually fails to complete descent and delivery. There are two ways of dealing with this difficulty. One is to administer an anesthetic and assist the forces of labor with either a vacuum extractor or forceps. The other is to increase the force of uterine contraction by the administration of oxytocin. Whether and when to administer these therapies is a matter of obstetrical judgment.

In good labor, the head moves steadily down in the vagina until it encounters the perineum, the technical name for the muscles and connective tissue that I have referred to as the pelvic floor. The perineum is attached to the arch formed by the pubic bones and surrounds the opening of the vagina. The advancing fetal head stretches these maternal tissues until the baby's scalp begins to be visible. This may give the mother a burning sensation in the stretched area.

The Birth of the Head

The head, now in OA, flexed, with the chin on the baby's chest, begins to extend, as if the baby were trying to look up. As the head descends further and the vaginal opening enlarges with each bearing-down effort, more and more of the scalp is seen. Then the forehead comes over the perineum. The extension continues with each push—the eyebrows, then the eyes and nose, and finally the mouth and chin. The greatest vaginal stretching is now over and the mother can take a brief breather as the head, released from the vagina, turns back to its earlier oblique position.

If everything goes well and the perineum stretches adequately there is no need for a perineal incision. However, in many patients, particularly with first babies, it is quite obvious that a tear is likely to occur. At the patient's choice, this can be accepted as part of the process and whatever tear takes place subsequently repaired. It is equally reasonable to make an incision—an episiotomy—employing a scissors and a local anesthetic. This incision is generally straighter, with less tissue damage and therefore considerably easier to repair than a tear. It used to be thought that episiotomy helped to prevent vaginal relaxation later in life. However, since the episiotomy is made principally in the skin and connective tissue of the perineum it has little to do with subsequent relaxation of the supports of the rectum, of the bladder, or of the uterus itself.

The pressure in the vagina on the baby's chest at this time usually squeezes some amniotic fluid out through the nose. Babies are ordinarily quite alert at this point and if they are stimulated with small blasts of air from a syringe they blink. If meconium has been present in the amniotic fluid efforts are made promptly to suck the meconium-laden material out of the baby's nose and throat.

The remainder of the birth of the baby may very well proceed by itself with the next uterine contraction. The shoulder, which is in the anterior or twelve o'clock position, delivers under the bony arch. The other shoulder delivers at the six o'clock position, and it is just a matter of moments or one additional contraction until the mother pushes out the remainder of the baby, completing the second stage of labor.

In recent years I have been handing the baby directly to the mother, putting it down on her bare chest and throwing a towel over it. There are studies to indicate that if the baby is immediately placed in skin-to-skin contact with the mother that its loss of body temperature in the first half hour after birth is at a minimum. If the baby is wrapped in towels the heat loss is a bit greater. If the baby is placed in the air under an infrared warmer the loss of body temperature is even greater. A normal baby placed on the mother's chest, directly next to her heartbeat and in contact with her warm skin, remains quite tranquil. It will cry substantially less than babies who are tickled, rubbed, dried off, or otherwise stimulated. The baby will generally look around in the room and slowly but steadily start breathing. It will become pink more slowly than stimulated newborns. A mother who wants to do so can nurse the baby at this time. A fair proportion of the newborns will take to the breast and its colostrum with considerable vigor. This is more likely to be successful with the later babies of mothers who have nursed previous children and who therefore have some of the moves down pat.

There is no hurry to clamp the umbilical cord of a normal baby. The cord can be allowed to stop pulsating and then clamped about half an inch away from the skin edge that surrounds the cord. It is then cut. If the cord blood vessels have contracted and the flow of blood has come to an end, there is not actually any need to clamp it. If it is cut twelve inches or so away from the baby's abdominal wall, it will not bleed. The clamped stump dries up and falls off on about the fourth or fifth day of life.

Where to Deliver

In most hospitals patients move from the labor room to a delivery room for the actual birth. A fully equipped delivery room should be used if there is any doubt about the normality of the delivery or if there is a likelihood that forceps or a vacuum extractor will be needed.

A delivery room is set up with a full range of emergency equipment. There is an anesthesia machine to make it possible to give a general anesthetic quickly. An instrument table is ready with items such as a clamp for the cord, scissors with which to cut it, other scissors for an episiotomy, needle holders for repair of the episiotomy or vaginal lacerations, syringes for drawing blood samples from the umbilical cord, and a variety of basins and towels. In addition there is a warmer for receiving the newborn and apparatus for newborn resuscitation should that be necessary.

In the delivery room the patient ordinarily lies on her back with her legs lightly strapped into leg holders. Some sort of cleansing solution is then washed or sprayed over the area around the entrance to the vagina. This step is likely to be mildly uncomfortable, since the antiseptic solutions are cold.

After this preparation, sterile drapes are placed over the legs, under the buttocks and over the abdomen so that only the skin around the entrance to the vagina is exposed. The doctors wash their hands with antiseptic soap, and wear caps, masks, and sterile gowns and gloves. The delivery then proceeds under these aseptic precautions.

There is evidence that sterile precautions are not needed for a spontaneous delivery. Increasingly patients about to deliver under their own power are given the option of delivering in the bed in which they have been laboring, and many find this bed more comfortable than a delivery table. In the first place, the delivery table has a much thinner mattress than the bed. For another thing, the delivery room is intentionally set up with a sterile appearance and aseptic precautions and therefore lacks an atmosphere of warmth, however scientifically correct and however necessary it may be to cope with complications if they occur.

Should you decide to deliver in the labor room, most of the necessary equipment is readily brought in. If you wish to deliver in the labor bed and nevertheless need to be near all emergency equipment, it is possible to move you, in the labor bed, to the delivery room without putting you on the delivery table. It simply requires some flexibility on the part of the hospital staff who are providing you with care.

Wherever the patient delivers, if she is awake and alert we offer her the option of watching the childbirth in the mirror. I have even had women watch their own cesareans in this way.

At a time when all patients were taken to the delivery rooms with the expectation that they would be given general anesthetic, their feet were placed in stirrups, their knees were spread far apart, and their arms and legs were strapped down. At present, even though the great majority of patients are awake, some of these practices have persisted, but they are not of any medical value. Certainly a patient who is excited and delighted about the birth of her baby cannot be expected to maintain good aseptic discipline. She will not infrequently reach down and touch the sterile drapes which are covering her. Since the only contamination that comes from this is with the patient's own bacteria there is no reason to believe that this has anything to do with subsequent infection.

Cesareans, of course, are performed in operating rooms under full aseptic conditions, as with any major abdominal operation.

Fathers in the Delivery Room

For something like thirty-five years I have made the baby's father welcome in the delivery room if the mother wishes him to be present. In the last few years I have extended the invitation to lesbian partners as well. I have not encountered any difficulty resulting from this. I recall two occasions when a father felt somewhat faint and had to be asked to leave. I recall another father who infuriated his wife by spending his entire time with video and sound equipment and flood lights; she was understandably annoyed that he paid little attention to her. But by and large the experiences have been positive for all concerned and I think the practice is an essential part of family-centered obstetrics.

We are now routinely educating our patients' partners about decorum in a delivery room or an operating room and teaching them what to expect with a normal birth or a cesarean section. Some question has been raised as to whether her partner should be present when the mother is under a general anesthetic. As presence at the time of delivery allows the other parent an opportunity for early bonding, it seems to me that there is little to be lost by welcoming them. However, we usually wait until the anesthetic is in place and the patient has been draped for the operation.

When a patient delivers in a labor room under less formal and less aseptic circumstances, there is no longer any question whether members of the support system may be present at the time of delivery. The ultimate decision is always that of the mother, except that we make it clear that should an emergency arise the spectators will move into the background.

After the Baby Is Born

Evaluation of the Infant's Condition at Birth

A fetus inside the uterus is actually blue even when it is in what could facetiously be called the pink of condition. Its blood count is very high and the pressure of oxygen is comparatively low. As a consequence, although the delivery of oxygen to the fetus's tissues is adequate, the amount of oxygen in each red blood cell is low and the blood therefore looks dark. Oxygen is being delivered in a great number of separate containers (the red blood cells), each of which is only about two-thirds full. This explains why it is normal for a baby to have a blue color at birth. Fetal pallor (paleness), on the other hand, is a danger sign, because it indicates failure of the circulation or hemorrhage.

The healthy newborn frequently urinates just after birth and the healthy male newborn very often has a penile erection.

A scoring system that nicely describes the condition of the newborn was developed by Dr. Virginia Apgar, at the time an anesthesiologist at Columbia Presbyterian Hospital in New York. One of the elements in the Apgar score is the color of the baby. Newborns are always blue at one minute after birth, and many are still blue at five minutes if they are gently handled. The element of color in Dr. Apgar's system does not correlate very well with the baby's actual condition. Our British colleagues have recognized this and now score babies on only four of the five features that Dr. Apgar used, omitting the color score.

Apgar Scoring System

Score	0	1	2
Heart Rate	Absent	Rate below 100/min.	Over 100
Respiratory rate	Absent	Slow, irregular	Good
Muscle tone	Flaccid	Some movement	Active motion
Cry	Absent	Poor	Vigorous
(Color)	(Deep blue)	(Body pink, extremities blue)	(Pink all over)

The baby is observed and the score at one minute and five minutes of age recorded by a trained person. A score of three or less indicates that the baby is in poor condition and its life is in jeopardy. Immediate efforts at resuscitation must be begun. On the other hand a score of 6, 7, and 8 (by the British system) confirms that the baby is in excellent condition. For babies whose five-minute Apgar score is low, it has become the practice to record a ten-minute Apgar score as well.

We have learned that babies who have very low one-minute Apgars but who are given prompt attention and have normal Apgars at five minutes seldom show evidence of any damage later in life. A low ten-minute Apgar (below 6) is ordinarily indicative of injury, which will become evident in the course of the baby's later development.

If the newborn needs resuscitation, this is done by the most experienced person present. Prudent management calls for anticipation of difficulty by having trained people on hand who can give the baby skilled care as early as possible.

Modern delivery rooms are equipped with suction devices to assist in sucking mucus, amniotic fluid, and meconium from the newborn's nose, throat, larynx, and trachea. Oxygen is available for continuous or interrupted administration under positive pressure. Tubes to be passed down into the baby's trachea are on hand in the event it becomes necessary to intubate and begin positive-pressure resuscitation. The baby is placed where it can be kept warm. This can be done with overhead heaters that radiate heat down toward the baby without interfering with the work of the medical personnel doing the emergency care.

If there is reason to think that the administration of narcotics to the mother during labor plays a role in depressing a newborn baby's ability to breathe, the child can be given Narcan (naloxone), a narcotic antagonist. Many other drugs have been advocated from time to time for injection into the newborn baby, most of them of dubious value. Vigorous slapping, immersing the baby in ice water, dangling it by the feet, and similar measures are no particular help, and may be harmful. Patience, imperturbability, and gentleness will resuscitate more babies than all the strenuous methods combined.

Tending to the Baby

There are several kinds of cord clamps. The metal and plastic ones are shaped like a bobby pin and snap into place. They remain on the cord for twenty-four to forty-eight hours, giving it time to shrivel, and are then removed. It is probably unnecessary to put a bandage on the umbilical cord, as it dries much better when exposed to the air. No other attention is required.

A small amount of some antibiotic ointment is ordinarily put into each eye of the baby as a preventive against gonorrheal ophthalmia (conjunctivitis), an infection of the anterior chamber of the eye (behind the eyelids) due to gonorrhea, which can be contracted from the mother's vagina. We have now begun to see a similar kind of conjunctivitis that turns up at a week or ten days of life due to chlamydia infection. If the original antibiotic ointment has not succeeded in preventing this condition, repeat antibiotic therapy can be administered.

Before the newborn leaves the delivery room in most hospitals, its footprints are imprinted on a hospital form along with a fingerprint of the mother. An identifying band is placed on the mother's wrist and a duplicate of the band is placed around the baby's ankles. Another copy of the same band may be attached to the mother's chart.

Delivery of the Placenta

The attention next turns to the delivery of the placenta. It is attached firmly to the uterus over an area about eight inches in diameter. After the child's birth the elastic uterus retracts and becomes much smaller, since it is no longer ballooned out by the fetus. Soft, its muscle fibers uncontracted, the uterus rests, following the strenuous work. In a variable number of minutes—usually just a few—it begins to contract again. The placenta is spongy, noncontractile tissue; the uterus, pure contracting muscle. With the further contractions of the undistended uterus, the area to which the placenta is attached diminishes marvelously. Since the placenta cannot contract and remains the same size, the flimsy attachment between the two is torn through, leaving the placenta free in the cavity of the uterus. With additional contractions of ever-increasing magnitude, the uterus obliterates its cavity by squeezing the free placenta downward into the capacious vagina.

Once this has occurred, the mother is able to push the placenta out of her vagina simply by further bearing-down. She can be assisted in this effort by gentle traction on the umbilical cord. There is no need to hurry the birth of the placenta in the absence of bleeding. The natural birth of the placenta is quite painless.

The uterus, after separating the placenta and expelling it into the vagina, assumes a different shape and position. When this occurs the uterus can be grasped through the abdominal wall and pushed downward toward the pelvis. The firm mass of muscle acts as a piston and thrusts the placenta halfway out; then the obstetrician gently pulls and twists the partially extruded afterbirth from the vagina. The membranes, being joined to the placenta, come away with it.

At some time shortly after the birth of the placenta, it is examined carefully to see that it is completely delivered. A placenta is formed by the fusion of twenty or so cotyledons, each of which is actually a small placenta. Each is a complete circulatory unit, and they are crowded compactly together. The placenta is like a mosaic of smooth, even tiles, each tile being a cotyledon. If the mosaic is complete it can be concluded that the placenta has been born intact. If there is a defect, and one or more of the cotyledons is missing, the remaining placenta can be removed by putting a hand into the uterus. However, when I have been delayed in examining the placenta and later have found a portion missing, if the patient was not bleeding I have left it to nature to complete the delivery.

Failure to Separate

Occasionally the normal mechanism of placental separation and expulsion does not function and the placenta has to be peeled away from the uterine wall. If this is done very shortly after the birth of the baby or the patient is still under anesthesia, no further anesthetic is required. When the decision to do this is delayed until the cervix has had time to start to close, the procedure is quite uncomfortable and calls for anesthesia. The operator puts a hand into the vagina, and with it follows the umbilical cord through the cervix and up into the uterus. If the cervix has begun to close, the hand may meet some resistance, but this will yield to firm, gentle pressure. With the hand in the uterus, the operator feels for the plane of separation between the placenta and the uterine wall, sweeps around through this plane, and separates the placenta, takes hold of it, and withdraws the hand. This is a simple and safe procedure if it is done early, before serious hemorrhage can take place, by one who has had experience with the operation. Many doctors, knowing it is a benign operation, wait only a brief period of time for the normal separation of the placenta, before delivering it manually. Certainly everyone intervenes quickly if the placenta has partly separated and hemorrhage is taking place.

At the site where the placenta was attached, pencil-thick blood vessels are torn across. The reason women do not ordinarily bleed from this wound is that the uterus is specifically constructed to meet the situation. Its muscle fibers run crisscross, that is, they interlace and the blood vessels run in the spaces between. It is like fitting the fingers of one hand between the fingers of the other. When the fingers are loosely fitted and held before the window, light comes through the web; but if they are tightly fitted, not even the tiniest beam filters past. In the same way as the light, the blood vessels of the placental site are shut off, the walls of the vessels squeezed together by the tightly contracted, interwoven muscle bundles surrounding them on all sides.

Because of the possibility of hemorrhage, it is important that the uterus remain firmly contracted after the birth of the placenta. If the uterus does not do this it can be encouraged to contract by massaging it gently through the abdominal wall. Nursing the baby, which results in the release of oxytocin from the pituitary, will assist in this process. If, after these measures, the uterus continues to relax and bleed, the patient is given either oxytocin or ergonovine. The latter drug has been synthesized in the laboratory in the form of methylergonovine (Methergine). Either of these drugs, given intravenously or injected into a muscle, stimulates powerful uterine contraction.

In addition to these drugs we now have a prostaglandin compound, 15-methyl prostaglandin, which can be injected directly into the uterus through the lower abdominal wall or into the cervix through the vagina. By either route it produces well-sustained uterine contractions and can stem a serious hemorrhage. The side effects from prostaglandin under these circumstances are mild.

The blood loss at delivery may be virtually nil but can be as much as several quarts. Since women come to term with a markedly expanded blood volume, they often can tolerate a blood loss of up to two quarts without suffering much more than an increase in the pulse rate. So massive a sudden blood loss would throw a nonpregnant adult into shock. However, when blood loss after childbirth approaches two quarts and the volume amounts to a hemorrhage, the attendants have to consider whether to replace the loss by blood transfusion. The indications for transfusion are a progressively rising pulse rate and dropping blood pressure, clear evidence of inadequate volume of blood in the arteries. It is reassuring that in recent years the incidence of postpartum hemorrhage has considerably decreased, largely because we are no longer anesthesizing women for delivery with drugs like ether and chloroform, which cause relaxation of the uterus and thereby weaken the contractions that would stop the bleeding.

Repair of the Vagina and the Perineum

Repair of an episiotomy or a perineal laceration can be carried out either in the delivery room or in the labor bed. This is now done with fine absorbable sutures, composed either of catgut or of polyglycolic synthetics. The latter are absorbed with little or no residual scarring. The sutures are all buried in the tissues and there is no need to remove them. They vanish rapidly along with the discomforts of the repair.

My own preference is to sew up with continuous lengths of suture material that comes already attached to the needle and need not be threaded through an eye. The repair is made at more than one level of tissue; how often the needle goes in and out depends upon the length of the laceration or episiotomy. I do not, therefore, count the number of "bites" I have taken with the needle, overall, and am generally unable to give an exact answer to the patient who asks, as many do, "How many stitches did I have?" My usual reply is that I have put in enough sutures to close the defect and no more.

The Immediate Postdelivery Care of the Mother

If the birth has taken place under general anesthesia, the mother usually remains on the delivery table or the operating table until she has awakened and is breathing without a tracheal tube. She is then transferred to a recovery room for further observation. The patient's partner and her newborn can join her there as soon as she is alert enough to hold the baby. The mother who has delivered under conduction anesthesia or with no anesthetic at all can go immediately to the recovery room, accompanied by the baby and the mother's partner.

The principal role of the recovery room is to check the mother's pulse and blood pressure and to observe her carefully for evidence of bleeding. If the delivery has been by cesarean the abdominal incision has to be inspected from time to time, but with any kind of delivery, watch has to be kept on the amount of bleeding from the vagina. The most significant immediate danger to a newly delivered woman is hemorrhage. Nine times out of ten this bleeding is from the uterus and is due to failure of the uterus to continue to contract adequately. After a difficult delivery there may be unrecognized lacerations, either at the site of the incision for a cesarean or in the upper vagina and cervix. If bleeding continues despite the fact that the uterus remains firm, further investigation must be undertaken promptly to find out whether such a laceration is present. The relaxed uterus, as mentioned above, can be treated medically; lacerations require meticulous surgical repair.

The length of time the mother is kept under observation in the recovery room depends upon whether the labor and delivery have been uneventful and the recovery from anesthesia smooth. If an epidural anesthetic or a general anesthetic has been employed the patient is ordinarily not transferred until any aftereffects have completely worn off. Women who have delivered in the labor bed without anesthesia are perfectly able to be up and about within the next few minutes, and require only a brief stay in a recovery room.

It is perfectly safe for women who have not been anesthetized and have a normal recovery to get up and walk to the postpartum unit. Hospital routine, however, may call for all patients to make the journey on wheels; either in a recovery room bed or a wheelchair, depending on circumstances.

When my first two children were born in the 1940's, all women were required to stay in bed for the first seven days after delivery, no matter how healthy they were. After so long a stay in bed, they practically had to relearn how to walk without losing their balance. But we learned a dramatic lesson from the experience evacuating maternity wards during air raids in World War II. These were life-threatening emergencies, and with a need to hurry and a shortage of wheeled equipment and of personnel, hospital staffs made the decision that healthy women should walk out of the wards, so that the available equipment could be reserved for the more disabled. To everyone's surprise, those who had got up and walked did better in the recovery period than did patients, equally healthy, who had spent the first seven postpartum days in bed.

The lesson has not been lost. We now take it for granted that a woman who has had a normal birth can get up and walk away from the delivery room, or labor bed, without suffering any ill effects; indeed, it may be beneficial. This is not to say that you may not be tired after being in labor all night and may much prefer to lie down and be waited upon. But it is the case that normal labor and delivery are superbly handled by healthy women.

Postpartum Chills

Women who deliver without having received any pain relief medication frequently experience severe shaking chills. They start several minutes after delivery and may last for as much as half an hour. We do not know their cause. We do know that they are harmless, although very unsettling. The best guess is that, since the fetus is a heat producer, the mother reacts to losing that source of heat much as she would the removal of an electric blanket in a chilly room. We keep warm blankets in the recovery area as the ideal treatment for postpartum chills.

The Postdelivery Care of the Baby

As soon as the baby is born, it can be given to the mother, who can survey it and satisfy herself that it is normal. Right after this, the professionals make their own inspection for abnormalities not immediately visible to the untrained eye. It is rare, however, to find any such thing in babies who act normally in the newborn period. At some later time, and this varies considerably from hospital to hospital, the newborn is taken to the nursery. There the baby has an extensive, detailed examination by a member of the staff in a careful search for abnormalities. Babies who are the product of a normal pregnancy and a normal labor, whose newborn score, either by the

Apgar or the British system, is high and who are of normal external body build are rarely found to have significant problems. In the detailed initial examination the examiner looks for rarities. In the overwhelming proportion of cases the baby gets a completely clean bill of health. This is promptly communicated to the mother.

14

Seven Births

A friend of mine, herself a mother, commented to me about
this book that it is written from the point of view of an observer,
the doctor. She felt sure that women who are pregnant or expect
to be so would react differently to descriptions of labor by
women who had recently experienced it. This seemed emi-
nently sensible to me. I therefore asked five women to describe
their labors for use in this book. They are not average women.
Each has writing ability although none is a professional writer.
All had strongly supportive partners and elegant babies. They
describe four normal labors and three cesareans. I have edited
their essays only enough to protect their privacy.

A First Labor for H. J.

I woke up at 2:30 A.M. (on my due date!), feeling a small gush
of liquid. Thinking my membranes had ruptured (they hadn't,
what I felt was probably just mucus), I woke my husband,
Wayne. Within half an hour, I started feeling contractions. They
were not at all painful, but came every ten minutes or less.
We were too excited to sleep (a mistake), so I took a shower
and just relaxed at home.

By morning, I noticed a bloody show, and we went to the

doctor's office to find out how far along my labor was. My regular obstetrician was, unfortunately, unavailable, so I saw Gloria, one of the certified nurse midwives who works in the same practice. She was wonderful throughout the labor and delivery. An exam revealed that I was three centimeters dilated, 50 percent effaced, and in early labor. Gloria expected the baby to be born sometime in the next two days, depending on how long this latent phase of labor lasted.

By early evening, contractions were coming four to five, and then three minutes apart. The answering service was slow in reaching the midwife, so I panicked, and insisted on going to the hospital. The fetal monitor (a half-hour hookup upon arrival is routine at this hospital) showed contractions every four minutes. When examined by a resident, I was still only three to three and a half centimeters dilated, though 90 percent effaced. Our choices were to go home, or to walk around for a few hours and return for another exam. It was pouring rain outside, so we decided to stay at the hospital and see whether I would progress. When we returned to the maternity floor, I found out that I had gone nowhere in three hours. The only thing that had changed was that the contractions were now starting to hurt. After some pleading, we were allowed to remain at the hospital. While we did go to the hospital much earlier than we probably should have, I felt more comfortable remaining there. Had I been home, I would have constantly worried about when to leave. At the hospital, I didn't have to worry about anything. There were plenty of people around whose job it was to do all the worrying for me.

We spent the night walking the corridors of the labor and postpartum floor. A nurse would occasionally call us in to the labor room to check my blood pressure, and listen to the fetal heart, but otherwise we were left pretty much alone. Whenever I felt a contraction, I would lean against a wall, or against Wayne, and do my Lamaze breathing. The contractions were momentarily painful, but still quite bearable. However, as the night wore on, I began to get scared, tired, and just plain miserable. There were women screaming in all the adjacent rooms, and the new babies in the nursery (Wayne thought that showing me the babies would encourage me) looked as large as elephants. Surely nothing that big could ever get out of me!

I didn't want to wake Gloria (the midwife), who was sleeping at the hospital, so I walked up to the resident and said, "I need moral support." She just mumbled something in response, barely looking up from her desk. The nurses, though, were very helpful, and kept telling me that all the screaming ladies were in situations different from my own. Many were alone in labor, without their husbands; others had attended no childbirth preparation classes, and had no idea what was happening to them.

At about 7:00 A.M., Gloria came in to examine me again. I was only five centimeters dilated, but she assured me that things would now speed up. (She was right, the baby was born about five hours later.) Gloria ruptured my membranes (to help speed labor) and I asked for some Demerol. The Demerol had some effect on the pain, but more importantly, allowed me to sleep between contractions, giving me a badly needed vacation from labor. Wayne woke me each time a contraction began, so that I could start to do the breathing rather than wake up at the peak of a contraction, totally out of control.

The Demerol wore off while I was in transition. I tried to do the special Lamaze breathing for this stage of labor, but got totally confused. Wayne and Gloria finally convinced me to switch back to the previous breathing technique, and it worked fine. (Moral: Learn everything in natural childbirth class, but once in labor, do what works best for you.) I kept begging them to "cancel" or postpone just one contraction so that I could rest. This was followed by the sinking realization that no one could control my contractions—begging would get me nowhere. At nine and a half centimeters, I really wanted to push, but a small lip of cervix stood between me and full dilation. "So, cut it off!" I said. Everyone in the room, but me, laughed. Gloria said I could push after eight more contractions, I bargained for four, we compromised with six.

As the second, or pushing stage of labor progressed, I became more aware of my surroundings. The residual effects of the Demerol had worn off entirely. I finally felt that I had some control over my body, and I could see the baby's head begin to crown. I noticed that Wayne had put on blue surgical coveralls. Gloria was joined by a nurse and by another midwife who came in to visit during her lunch hour. The atmosphere was pleasant and relaxed, but businesslike.

I delivered in the labor room. Wayne held my head forward to get me into a better position to really push, and he and the nurse each supported one of my legs. After a couple of hours of pushing, the baby came out quite easily, with just a small episiotomy. I cut the cord, and then Wayne held the baby while Gloria delivered the placenta (what a bloody, messy thing), repaired the episiotomy, and cleaned me up. The baby (later to be known as Arthur) seemed not the least bit traumatized by the day's events, and just looked around his new world. I made an inept attempt at nursing. My lack of milk was matched only by Arthur's lack of appetite.

And that was the end, and the beginning. I was taken to a hospital room, and the baby to the nursery. Wayne went home to get some sleep. I managed to take a quick shower (clinging to the walls for support) before being besieged by well-wishing visitors and phone calls. By evening, I had forgotten all the pain, and was telling anyone who would listen that I couldn't wait to do it all again.

H. J.'s Second Labor

There is much less to say about a second labor than a first. The birth of a second child, besides being quicker and easier than the first, is simply no longer a unique experience. Exciting as it was, I knew I had done it before. In addition, this idea of a new baby was a much more real rather than abstract concept this time. Labor was simply a means to a desirable end.

My labor began early in the evening, a few days after my due date, with mild, irregular contractions, and a bloody show. My husband, Wayne, and I decided to sleep for as long as we could, taking the precaution of having my mother stay over to babysit our two-year-old son. By 2:30 A.M., the contractions were strong enough to wake me, and about five minutes apart. Our son, Arthur, had insisted that night on sleeping in our bed, and my mother was sleeping in the living room, so there was simply no place in our apartment for us to labor in peace. We therefore left for the hospital by about 4:00 A.M., though I realized that I still had plenty of time.

Upon admission exam, I was about three centimeters dilated and in the early stages of active labor. We spent the next few hours walking the halls, stopping whenever I had a contraction to do Lamaze breathing. By then, my obstetrician had arrived, and offered to rupture my membranes in the hope of speeding the pace of labor. Wayne and I continued walking for a while, as the contractions became decidedly stronger. My doctor stayed available to us, on the labor floor the entire time, coming in to examine me, lend moral support, or tell jokes whenever I felt I needed him. Labor was progressing fairly rapidly. I was in control of the contractions, and it never occurred to me to ask for any pain medication.

I stopped coping well during the last half hour of the first stage of labor. I was no longer able to breathe quietly during contractions and spent them moaning, complaining, and saying, "It didn't hurt so much last time." I wasn't feeling particularly heroic that morning, and when things hurt, I expressed my displeasure. During one particularly painful contraction, I hurled wet paper towels, with perfect aim, at a picture on the wall of the labor room. Wayne said all the correct-but-useless things like "Helen, you're doing so well, just a little bit longer," and fed me ice chips and cherry soda (beats an IV any day). In between contractions I was fairly lucid, and carried on a somewhat coherent conversation with Wayne and my doctor.

I had been pushing to relieve strong back pressure during the last of the dilation contractions, but when I reached the expulsive stage, the urge to push was uncontrollable. In a few minutes, the baby's head was crowning, and it only took a couple of pushes more for our second baby boy to be born. I watched in the mirror as a cute little head started to scream, even before the rest of his body had fully emerged. Wayne cut the cord, and we took turns holding the baby and taking pictures while the doctor delivered the placenta and repaired a small episiotomy. While the thrill may have been more subdued this time, I haven't enjoyed the experience any less, and the real exciting part, getting to know this new little person, has barely begun.

A. S.'s First Labor—A Cesarean

It's been fifteen months since the birth of my son, Alexander; yet it seems like yesterday.

Like all expectant mothers, I had a lot of fears and apprehensions concerning my pregnancy; my biggest one being, Will my baby be normal and healthy? To ensure a good beginning, I ate well, drank plenty of milk, restricted my caffeine and alcohol intake, and took my vitamins every day.

The beginning of my pregnancy was marked with a minimal amount of morning sickness. In general, I felt good. My problems began when I went into premature labor in my fifth month. I was hospitalized for four days, at which time I was 50 percent effaced. The days and weeks went by, and I was thankful that I was still pregnant.

As my due date approached, I began to think about the delivery. My husband, Stanley, and I signed up for childbirth classes. By the end of the tenth week of classes, we knew how we wanted labor and delivery to proceed. We had a birth plan that we wanted to follow as much as possible during labor, which included Stanley being present throughout labor and delivery, walking instead of being confined to a lying-down position, no intravenous, no drugs for pain relief, only an external fetal monitor, and a delivery in the labor room instead of the delivery room. I had my heart set on following this plan. I left no room for deviation.

My due date came and passed. I was already 50 percent effaced and approximately two centimeters dilated. I was delighted that I was able to carry my baby a full nine months.

I went into labor six days after my due date. My water broke at about 7 P.M., just before Stanley and I were going out to eat. It was a slight trickle of water and I wasn't sure at the time if my water had actually broken or I had urinated. This would be the last meal before the baby would be born. I went to sleep as soon as we came home, as I was anticipating being awake for a long time.

I was awakened by contractions at about 1 A.M. By the time we got to the hospital, between 2 and 3 A.M., my contractions were two to three minutes apart and lasting thirty to forty-five seconds. I thought for sure I was at least six or seven centimeters dilated. When I was examined, I had only dilated to four centimeters. I was hoping that since I had been 50 percent effaced and two centimeters dilated before going into labor, I would have a shorter labor. I was examined again between 7 and 8 A.M. and I was only six centimeters dilated.

Since I was dilating at such a slow rate, my obstetrician suggested the administration of Pitocin.* Up until this point, I felt I was dealing with the pain well. I had not taken any pain medication and I was following my breathing techniques. When I heard the word Pitocin, it was as if my whole line of defense broke down. I had been told from a few friends how unbearable the pain was when they were given Pitocin, and there was no way I wanted to be subject to more pain. Being given Pitocin also meant that I had to have an intravenous, which I hated, and I would be restricted to a lying-down position in bed. I also had to have an internal fetal monitor. I couldn't believe this was happening to me. I had my birth plan prepared and this was not a scheduled part of it. After an hour or so on the Pitocin, I broke down and agreed to have an epidural. The doctor had increased the dosage of Pitocin and I couldn't deal with the pain any longer. The epidural relieved the pain only on the right side of my body, and I had as much pain on the left side as if they hadn't given me anything. I was given more pain reliever through the epidural about an hour later. When I was examined again at about 11 A.M., I was still only six to seven centimeters dilated. I was no longer in control of the pain, partially because I knew I was not progressing as rapidly as I wanted to and should have. I was given Demerol in the hope I would relax more and my labor would progress faster. I dozed on and off during contractions. It was as if I was aware of what was going on around me but I wasn't an active participant. The Demerol wore off about an hour later and I was then seven to eight centimeters dilated. The baby's head had not engaged and his heart rate seemed to almost stop during contractions. I was even given oxygen because they were afraid he wasn't getting enough.

It was at this time that another obstetrician was consulted for a second opinion. The final decision in view of how poorly I had dilated, the baby's head not being engaged, and my vaginal tissue being very swollen, was to do a section. Panic set in. I looked at my husband with tears in my eyes. Maybe

*A.S. is referring to oxytocin.

if I had tried a little harder I wouldn't have to have a section. I didn't want a section. I couldn't even watch the film during the Bradley classes when they showed a woman having a section. Besides, I already had a scar from an appendectomy and I didn't want another one.

After a while, I resigned myself to the fact that I had to have the surgery. I was worried about the baby being subject to a long labor and the different drugs. I felt a lot of pain and I was tired. I then thought of the section as a sign of relief.

It seemed like an eternity from the time the doctor decided to do the section until they actually did it. Stanley waited outside the delivery room while they prepped me. I chose to have a spinal instead of a general anesthesia. I definitely wanted to be awake for the birth of my child, the most unforgettable experience of my life. We had both gone through a lot during labor and I wanted to see him as soon as he was born.

The delivery room was cold and within minutes after the spinal, I couldn't feel anything from my waist down. It's a scary feeling to actively try to move your toes and not be able to do so. I couldn't help but think that this is how people who are paralyzed feel: The only difference is that I will get my feeling back and they won't.

When I was ready, the doctor draped a sheet over a frame over my chest so I wouldn't be able to see the surgery. This was fine with me because I probably would have fainted. I felt pressure on my abdomen as they pushed to get the baby from my uterus, but no pain. I couldn't believe my ears when I heard the doctor say "It looks like a big one, about nine pounds." I was expecting his weight to be about seven pounds.

The first question in my mind was, "Was the baby normal and healthy?" but because I was afraid that the answer might be "no," I asked, "Was it a boy or a girl?" I had been taking medication to prevent contractions from my fifth month into my eighth month, and I didn't know what effect this would have on the baby.

I was expecting a lot of crying when Alex was born, but I only heard one little cry. I thought for sure something was wrong. His umbilical cord was clamped, he was wiped off, and the pediatrician examined him briefly. When I looked to my side, tears came to my eyes as I saw Stanley holding this precious new life who was just looking around at his new world. Indeed Alex was a healthy baby who had scored a nine on his Apgar test. He was then placed by my side.

I was sewed up and taken to the recovery room. A short time later, Alex was brought to me. I was relieved and happy the delivery was over, yet I felt I was a failure. I was angry with myself about the course of events during my labor. Everything I didn't want to happen, happened. Not only did I take pain relievers, I took almost everything a pregnant woman could have during labor and delivery, short of being given a general anesthesia. How ironic the whole situation was. When I was five and a half months pregnant, I almost delivered the baby. I had to take medication into my eighth month to prevent contractions. I carried the baby past my due date, and now I wasn't able to deliver him. I started to wonder if something was wrong with my body. Women all over the world have normal pregnancies and deliveries; why wasn't I one of them?

I began to have feelings back in my toes about an hour or so after I was given the spinal. I had no other side effects, not even a headache.

I was up and walking around the next morning. Since I had difficulty getting up and down and in and out of bed, the nurses would bring Alex to my arms to nurse and put him back in the bassinet when he was finished. I took pain medication only the first two nights before I went to sleep, nothing during the day. I was recuperating so well that my obstetrician let me go home on the fourth day after my section. I was looking forward to sleeping in my own bed again.

As I look back on my pregnancy, I can't help but think that Alex is a product of twentieth-century medicine. There are now medications to help sustain a pregnancy and doctors have become skilled at performing sections. Tears still come to my eyes to think that if it wasn't for this twentieth-century medicine, Alex might not be here today . . . and what a loss it would be.

A Second Labor for R. R.

I was cranky and unsociable all day Monday, but forced myself to take my two-year-old son, David, to his playgroup, trying to have pleasant conversation with the other mothers but just feeling that I was tired of being pregnant. While David napped that afternoon, I wandered around the house, too hyped-up to nap myself, but no energy to actually do anything constructive. By the time I got to sleep (around 10 P.M.) I was exhausted and fell into a deep sleep. I had been having intermittent contractions for the past few weeks, like intense menstrual cramps, but the contraction that woke me up at 1 A.M. was different; it was more emphatic. I waited fifteen minutes and there was another one, rolled over toward my husband, Richard, and whispered, "This is it." What a difference from my first onset of labor; then, not knowing what to expect, I had a day of feeling "crampy" and another day of intermittent contractions, and a long actual labor with slow dilation and difficult delivery. This time there was no question about it, I was in labor. I watched the time tick away on the clock, sometimes dozing off, but always being awakened by the contraction. Richard and I talked about what to do. I got out of bed at 5 A.M. (by now the contractions were more frequent) and took a long hot shower. Meanwhile, Richard called my sister and told her to forget about going to work, she was on call to stay with David. At 6 we called the doctor's service and spoke to the on-call doctor who suggested we wait a little longer and then call my own doctor at home. The contractions were five to seven minutes apart, but there was little discomfort in between each contraction. When I spoke to my doctor (around 6:45 A.M.) I said, "I'm in labor"; there was no question about it, no "I think I'm in labor" or "I'm not sure about this." There was no question about it in my mind, and he suggested that we start out for the hospital (an hour's drive for us). Unfortunately, it was rush hour and we had to cross the George Washington Bridge. The radio reported a fifteen-minute delay at the tollbooths and when we got there, we decided to take advantage of the exceptional circumstances. Richard flagged down a policeman, told him I was in labor, and we went through the toll plaza on a stopped lane of oncoming traffic, much to the surprise and anger of all those other motorists who were patiently lining up. We reached admitting at 8:30 A.M. and went straight to the labor room, spent a half hour watching the fetal monitor and seeing what my contractions looked like on paper. When

I was finally examined by the resident and told I was six centimeters dilated, I was surprised; my mind was set on another long labor. My doctor arrived at 9:30 and told Richard to change his clothes; then I really knew that things were progressing. The labor nurse was encouraging, and whenever she checked the fetal heartbeats, she noted that the baby had moved lower and lower down the birth canal. I was getting scared. The contractions were more intense and I didn't want to lose control. Richard and the nurse were coaching me, I was using my Lamaze breathing and then my doctor asked if I wanted to deliver in the labor room; it's not easy to make decisions in a state of pain but he was so reassuring about the lack of risk and kept on saying how "normal" this labor was. He and the nurse talked about breaking my membranes, and after that, things are a blur. I believe there was a quick progression to feeling like pushing, I screamed that I felt like pushing, and suddenly all these faces were surrounding me— boy, did I scream. It felt like the only way to relieve the pressure and sensation that a large loglike object was slowly moving out of my vagina, and then, there she was. I had expected another boy, and what a surprise, a daughter. The rest of the experience has been described so often, the wonder of this new person lying on my chest, watching and examining her while busy hands were removing the placenta, sewing up the episiotomy, and generally attending to the lower half of my body, Richard and I were staring at Nanette, our new person.

One day after my first delivery, if you had asked me whether I would willingly go through the labor and delivery experience again, I would have been negative, or noncommittal (at best). Ask me that question today and I'd say yes enthusiastically.

J. B., Who Had Two Cesareans

I was the last woman in the world I thought would have to have a cesarean. My mother had eight healthy children, no misses. Her mother bore seven, *her* mother had twelve. Healthy as a horse, I figured I was born to breed.

Eighteen months apart, I have had two babies by cesarean section. My firstborn was three weeks late and born in forty minutes, an emergency under general anesthesia. Because his trouble was a fluke (wrapped cord) and not a recurring condition, all of us—myself and my husband, the midwives and doctor—were hoping our second born would enter the world ordinarily.

My forty-fourth week of pregnancy started and so did my labor. It lasted five days, never too insistent, but persistent. Defying the laws of nature, it would slow down when I was active and intensify if I tried to rest or eat. On Day 4 I checked into the hospital for an IV for dehydration and Demerol for sleep. Rested, labor stopped, me and the baby checked out fine, and we went home.

We returned to the hospital about midnight. Labor slowed again about five centimeters, at six centimeters signs of fetal distress worsened, near dawn I signed on the line for a second cesarean.

My husband will tell you the difference between our son's birth and our daughter's is that when they rolled me out of the room the first time he was sure he'd lost us both. With my daughter, he came along and could see that I never missed a breath.

The biggest difference to me was that instant the doctor pulled her head out, before she took a breath, she looked me square in the eye, and I knew she was mine. This feat was accomplished by my being conscious, my doctor persuading the anesthesiologist that if she could work without a drape he could too, and by being allowed to keep my glasses on.

When my son was born, I missed his first day. Our get-acquainted banter was "Are you my baby? . . . Yes, you're my baby boy!" which I thought was typical to all new babies. With my daughter I could see, hear, smell, touch, and know that she was my Helen, and never have to ask.

My recovery was quicker, too, the second time. I got unplugged from the catheter and IV before I left recovery, was on my feet by the afternoon, and showered before breakfast the next morning. My incision was so small that the residents would come and wonder at how a seven-pound one-ounce baby ever wriggled out. I was ready to go home in four days, and everybody lived happily ever after.

A Third Labor for M. N.

To my mind, there is no exact "due date," rather an approximate one give or take two weeks. Our two older children had each been born two weeks "early" and I was prepared for our third child to be born anywhere from November 28 to December 12. On the morning of November 27, as I was making the beds prior to leaving for an obstetrical appointment, I felt something warm and wet drip down between my legs. I examined the liquid and concluded that it was my water breaking. However, as I was not having contractions and as I am by nature both cautious and careful, I decided to continue getting dressed and doing the household chores before organizing myself for the birth of our baby. When these were completed, my physical situation had not altered radically: intermittent spurts of liquid, pressed out on bending or squeezing, and lots of pressure in the pelvic area.

At this point, mostly because I had been advised that third labors are fast, I phoned my husband at work. In the half hour that it took him to arrive home, I initiated the arrangements for the care of our two older children and packed my hospital bag. When we arrived at the hospital, thirty-five minutes later, my physical condition was relatively unchanged. I admitted myself while my husband parked the car (urban hospital), rode up to the maternity floor standing and unaided, and met my obstetrician there. I told him my symptoms and he suggested that we obtain a reading on the fetal monitor. He indicated that if no strong contractions were evident by that time, we would undoubtedly be better off returning home. One hour and a half and two monitors later, we finally had a legible and continuous reading. It was not yet 2 P.M. and my labor had settled down to contractions five minutes apart. With my husband doing the timing, I was doing my breathing exercises and keeping up with the contractions. At two minutes apart I was still doing O. K.

Although I had been informed by many people that third babies are born fast and easy, I still had difficulty coping with this last phase of labor. The intensity of the pain seemed no less than in my previous two birthing experiences. This, coupled with the lack of respite between contractions, made me increasingly irritable until I started to panic. I guess the purpose of the coach and obstetrician is to break through the panic and organize the effort into the birth of the baby. Fortunately, both my husband and obstetrician had been through this with me before and were able to help me regain control. Mercifully, labor was very short, and with lots of encouragement I was able to push the baby out. The physical relief was unbelievable and the mental relief followed immediately. Our daughter was born at 3:30 P.M.

15

Difficult Labor

Thirty years ago it was clear that a change was taking place in our approach to the management of difficult labor. Cesarean section, an operation that a hundred years earlier was a death sentence, had become so safe that it was no longer a common cause of maternal mortality. Contraction of the pelvis, once the usual cause of obstructed labor, had been virtually eliminated by improvements in nutrition. We developed more effective methods for augmenting the natural forces of labor, since we had less to fear from pelvic obstruction and could now resort to cesarean even late in labor should augmentation of labor fail. Our attention turned to the quality of the newborn rather than simply its survival.

All this has resulted in an increase in the frequency of delivery by cesarean. I believe, however, that the pendulum has swung too far in that direction. Now, for each increase in the rate of section deliveries, there is no longer proportional gain for either mother or baby. It therefore behooves us to maintain all our skills in the management of difficult labor by vaginal as well as by abdominal delivery.

Dystocia (from the Greek, meaning "difficult birth") is due to three principal causes: Inadequate uterine contractions, excessive size or awkward position of the fetus, and birth canal narrowing.

In the treatment of dystocia, there are general measures that apply to every patient. Adequate rest in labor increases the ability of the mother to cooperate. Anesthesia can play a role by reducing the pain, which itself may become a barrier to the efficiency of the process. We maintain the mother's caloric intake by giving her fruit juice or intravenous glucose solution. Adequate amounts of fluid and such electrolytes as sodium, potassium, and chloride are also provided to replace losses in perspiration, urine, and amniotic fluid. Antibiotics are used for patients who show evidence of infection.

Inadequate Contractions

We do not have any accurate measure of the effectiveness of labor. In one patient, what seem to be strong and frequent contractions may accomplish little in the progress of labor. In another patient, contractions that appear mild to moderate and cause little discomfort may produce rapid progress in labor. Observing the frequency of contractions and the pain they create tells something about the efficiency of labor, but in an individual patient the observation is of only limited value. We can use electronic equipment to record uterine contractions and to estimate their force either with external electric fingers or with internal pressure gauges. These devices tell us about relationships of contractions to the progress of labor in large groups of patients but cannot predict the progress of an individual patient. The final criteria for the adequacy of uterine force are the two factors we observe in following a labor: the descent of the presenting part and the progressive dilation of the cervix.

As observed by vaginal examinations in a first labor, the cervix once it is more than 3 to 4 centimeters dilated, opens at about 1.2 centimeters (one half-inch) an hour. For second and later labors the rate is about 1.5 centimeters an hour. The pace tends to increase as the first stage continues. Labor is not mechanical and this rate of progress does not occur in a clock-like manner every hour. There are starts and stops in progress. If, however, there is a failure of the cervix to dilate over a period of two to three hours, we must consider the diagnosis of inadequate contractions. It is essential to look for the other causes of delay in progress listed below. Unless contractions have become infrequent or weak, the final diagnosis of inadequate contractions is necessarily based on the exclusion of other factors.

The uterus is a smooth muscle, and is therefore not subject to fatigue in the same way that the muscles of the skeleton can become tired. Thus, the first stage of labor will go forward despite fatigue and serious illness in the mother. It is not unusual to blame premature or excessive use of pain medications for prolongation of the first stage of labor. I doubt the validity of this. In the first place, none of the drugs ordinarily used for pain relief has any effect on the contractions of the uterus. There are reasons to believe that epidural block may actually shorten the first stage of labor. When the drugs are given before the woman has gone into progressive labor, that is before the cervix is three to four centimeters dilated, it is tempting to think that any subsequent delay is due to the drugs. Actually, the diagnosis of labor has been made prematurely.

Prolongation of the first stage of labor is considered an indication for intervention. Under these circumstances, if the duration of the first stage of labor is measured from the time pain relief is initiated, steps to intervene with surgery or oxytocin may be undertaken even before true labor has begun. Premature administration of analgesia may therefore be a problem.

Use of Oxytocin (Pitocin)

The chief mode of treatment of inadequate contractions at the present time is the use of oxytocin. This hormone is a product of the hypothalamus, that portion of the brain which is responsible for the general regulation of most hormonal functions. Oxytocin is stored in the pituitary gland. It has powerful effects on the uterus at term, and for this reason is given in dilute solution intravenously. The drug is supplied in one-milliliter ampules containing ten International Units of the hormone. This is then diluted for intravenous use. The diluted hormone is administered either by a continuous electric pump or by a controlled drip, which can be adjusted to give slow rates of flow. There is no consensus as to the ideal rate for administering oxytocin intravenously to augment labor. Some students of the drug recommend that it be started at one to two milliunits (thousandths of a unit) a minute and doubled every fifteen minutes until a change in the cervix occurs and the presenting part descends. Thereafter the drip is continued at that level. Other equally competent observers recommend increases every forty minutes, from one to two to four to six to eight and so forth milliunits per minute, a much slower increase than doubling. The most recent opinion, as yet incompletely confirmed, is that it is even more effective to give the oxytocin in pulses eight to ten minutes apart rather than by continuous flow.

Practitioners generally agree on the conditions that should be met while any woman is treated with intravenous oxytocin for inadequate progress in labor. One is that the patient be under continuous professional observation. Another is that there be continuous monitoring of both the uterine contractions and the fetal response to the oxytocin to be certain that excessive doses are not being used. The cervix and the station of the presenting part should be examined frequently during this period to find out whether the hormone is working.

Just how long to continue oxytocin augmentation of labor is a matter of judgment. If it is having an adverse effect on the fetus, the administration of the drug must be decreased or stopped. My conviction is that active labor should not last more than twelve hours. Stimulation of labor should not be employed until a delay of two or more hours has been demonstrated, after labor has begun. In practical terms this means that even though both mother and baby are in excellent condition, administration of the drug should not continue for more than six hours unless it is clear then that delivery is imminent.

Giving the oxytocin intravenously has an important safety feature. If the patient's response to it suddenly becomes excessive, the administration can be stopped abruptly. Enzymes present in the mother's blood stream inactivate the hormone rapidly and the overstimulation ceases.

Rupturing the Membranes

A word of comment on the fetal membranes. If labor is progressing normally, it is a matter of indifference whether membranes are intact or ruptured. However, there is an association between prolongation of labor and failure of the membranes to rupture. This may be because the contractions are too weak to achieve the rupture. It may also result from the fact that the uterus is overdistended with amniotic fluid and baby. Artificial rupture of the membranes, by decreasing that volume, may make the uterus more efficient. For that reason it is the practice to rupture membranes artificially when a decision is made to augment the labor with oxytocin, unless the membranes have already ruptured by themselves.

In some hospitals, when they monitor the fetus, it is the practice to apply an electrode through the cervix to the baby's skin for a direct record of fetal heart activity. This produces a more reliable tracing than the recording of the fetal heart by external ultrasound. It also ruptures the membranes if they are not already ruptured.

Before this occurs, the amniotic fluid cushions the baby's head against the force of the uterine contractions. When the membranes rupture, fluid flows out and the cushioning effect is lost. Slowing of the fetal heart may then be greater when contractions compress the head. These decelerations should not be confused with fetal distress.

There is no such thing as dry labor, even with prolonged periods of membrane rupture, despite rumors to the contrary. The baby and mother between them can maintain an adequate amount of amniotic fluid in the uterine cavity for many weeks. If however the membranes rupture more than twelve weeks before term and the pregnancy continues to close to term, this may adversely affect the development of the baby's lungs.

Oxytocin in the Second Stage

It may happen that labor needs augmentation in the second stage. A uterus that has functioned efficiently during the first stage changes its pattern in the second stage. Particularly with first labors, the contractions of the uterus and the voluntary effort by the patient added together may not be adequate to maintain progress. If the mother has failed to bring the presenting part down after one hour in the second stage, she may be helped with oxytocin stimulation given in the same way as it is used in the first stage of labor, and with the same precautions. The time limit on this is a few hours at most. The goal is to try to achieve a normal birth, or to make forceps or vacuum extraction easy.

Abnormalities in Fetal Size and Position

Labor at term lasts longer with bigger babies than with smaller ones. This is only partly due to a tight fit with larger infants. The other factor is that with very large fetuses, especially in first labors, the uterine muscle is overstretched; this reduces its efficiency. It is seen most dramatically with twins and when the uterus is distended by excessive amniotic fluid (polyhydramnios).

When all else is normal a healthy woman having her first baby can expect to have an uneventful birth of any baby up to four thousand grams (approximately nine pounds). Above this weight, mechanical difficulties in birth become more frequent, so that when we are certain that the baby is over ten pounds (forty-five hundred grams), we opt for abdominal delivery. The largest baby I have seen deliver uneventfully through the vagina weighed about twelve and a half pounds. However, when the first stage of labor is prolonged and the descent of a baby of this size is delayed in the second stage of labor, cesarean would be the choice as a method of delivery.

As suggested above, the problem with fetuses of excessive size in the first stage is delay in dilation of the cervix, and indeed the failure of the cervix to dilate may occasion the diagnosis that the baby is very large. Second-stage problems are much more serious. If the head is too large to fit properly through the birth canal, it does not descend and it becomes obvious that cesarean is required. But often the shoulders of a very big baby are relatively larger than its head; the reverse of the case with a baby of normal size. As a result, even after the easy birth of a large head, severe difficulty may be encountered in delivering the shoulders. It is now too late to do a cesarean. The necessary efforts to complete the delivery may damage the nerves to the baby's arm or fracture its collarbone. The fracture heals well, but the nerve injury may be lasting. As I mentioned in regard to the world's largest baby (page 83), we have become more alert to these problems and are saving these massive babies by timely cesarean.

Hydrocephalus

Other size difficulties may be due to local abnormalities. The commonest of these is hydrocephalus (Greek for "water in the head"). In this condition the drainage of the fluid that is normally inside the brain fails, but the formation of the fluid continues. The brain steadily swells, spreading the movable plates composing the skull to a size that cannot fit through the birth canal. The diagnosis of hydrocephalus can now be made with considerable accuracy by sonography of the fetus, and plans for management can be made in advance of labor. In a high proportion of these cases there is also polyhydramnios, which itself may call attention to the presence of the anomaly.

There has recently been an intense effort to save these babies, either by draining the fluid from the baby's head prior to birth or by delivering the baby early and treating it with neurosurgery. Thus far the results have been disappointing. Most of these babies have other serious abnormalities that limit their ability to survive. We can and should study them by sonography to identify these other defects, and we can measure their brains to determine how much brain tissue survives. Still, many of these unfortunate fetuses die during labor despite all efforts.

If the diagnosis of hydrocephalus is not made until labor, or treatment is deliberately postponed until that time, proper management is to drain the excess fluid from the baby's head in order to decompress it to a size that will pass through the birth canal. This is done during labor, with a long needle passed through the vagina and open cervix or by puncture of the head through the mother's lower abdominal wall.

If a hydrocephalic fetus presents by the breech, the head is drained after the trunk has been born. A small-diameter catheter is passed up the spinal canal into the head and the excess fluid drained off. The head then shrinks to a size that readily permits delivery. So far as I know, there is neither ethical nor religious objection to this operation on the fetus.

Delivery of a hydrocephalic fetus by cesarean requires an enormous uterine incision because of the size of the head, unless drainage can be done at the time of the cesarean. Under such circumstances, therefore, the cesarean is of no benefit to the mother or the fetus. Cesarean is indicated only on good evidence that the newborn can be expected to survive.

On rare occasions, tumors of the infant reach great size and obstruct delivery. There have recently been reports of the survival of such fetuses with appropriate surgical intervention when the correct diagnosis has been made by the sonography.

Much more common, however, is an abnormality of the position of the baby. The diagnosis of an abnormal lie prior to the onset of labor is not an indication for elective cesarean, as fetal position is not fixed until labor has started. If, after the onset of labor, the lie is such that the baby must be delivered abdominally, the operation is regarded as an emergency.

Transverse Presentation

When the fetus lies with its long axis (the line of its spinal column) at right angles to that of the mother, the position is called a transverse lie. If the fetus is transverse when labor starts, normal birth is not safe for either the mother or the baby. For the infant the risk is that the cord may prolapse, or fall past the baby, who, under these conditions, does not fill the lowermost part of the uterus. The cord thus becomes obstructed, endangering fetal circulation. The risk to the mother is that a live term infant in transverse position cannot move through the birth canal, because it will not fit without turning. The incidence of rupture of the uterus in such a case, if labor continues, is prohibitively high. Vaginal birth is a rare event unless the fetus dies first. The treatment for transverse lie in labor, with very few exceptions, is cesarean.

Breech

It is not unusual for a fetus to be in a breech position (the buttocks down into the pelvis and the head up toward the ribs) from time to time until the last four to six weeks of pregnancy, at which time most fetuses settle down into a head-down position. Left to their own devices, however, about 3.5 percent of all babies come to rest as breeches and remain so at the onset of labor. The latest I have seen a baby turn from breech to vertex was on the expected date of confinement.

There is no particular cause for most breech presentations. As a rule, they are simply accidents of posture of the baby. When a woman with a normal uterus has had a delivery by the breech, there is a slightly increased likelihood, above the general rate, that she will have another breech. A woman with one of the partial or complete duplications of the body of the uterus, itself an unusual event, may have all her babies by the breech.

In breech presentation, most commonly the legs are alongside the baby's trunk, with the feet near the face and the baby presenting by its buttocks. This is a frank breech, and the likelihood of normal birth in this position is very close to that of the baby presenting by the vertex. Labor is usually normal. Less frequently the baby sits in the yoga position, with buttocks and feet presenting: This is a complete breech. In other cases one or both of the legs may be extended so that the lowermost portion of the uterus is occupied by the feet and the breech is relatively high. This is called either a single- or double-footling breech. The problems with this kind of breech are very similar to those encountered with the vertex position, in which the head is very high in the pelvis. These conditions may be related to inefficiency of uterine contractions, and there is a tendency to prolongation of the first stage of labor. How far down in the birth canal the feet come during the labor is probably a matter of no importance. They may in fact fall through the cervix well before it is fully dilated. What matters to the progress of labor is the level of the buttocks.

The principal problem with breech presentation is the risk of umbilical cord obstruction, which can result in stillbirth.

This is not a danger to the mother. If you visualize a newborn baby you will realize that the navel, which is the point of origin of the umbilical cord from the abdominal wall, is very much closer to the buttocks than it is to the head. With a vertex presentation the head and the shoulders are ordinarily born before the naval itself enters the pelvis. At this moment cord blood flow may be obstructed, but since the head is born, the baby can breathe.

With a breech presentation the cord necessarily is relatively low in the uterus. Indeed, with footling breeches, about one time out of eight the cord falls through the cervix into the vagina. When this occurs early in labor the likelihood of the vaginal birth of a healthy baby is remote. Even if the cord behaves well and remains up in the uterus, as the breech descends through the pelvis the likelihood of cord obstruction remains greater than with a vertex presentation. Many of my colleagues believe that the risk of cord obstruction is such that almost all babies presenting by the breech should be born abdominally.

Labor with a breech is in no way different from that with a vertex, although the actual delivery is different. It is no more painful and exposes the mother to no greater risks.

Occiput Posterior

On occasion a fetus of ordinary size is found in labor to be in the occiput posterior position. Such a baby lies with its occiput at the six o'clock position, its face toward the mother's pubis. As I have mentioned, this is a mechanically difficult position. The combination of a very large baby with an occiput posterior may seriously delay progress in labor. For this reason, many physicians regard it as an indication for oxytocin stimulation, forceps, or cesarean, particularly in first labors.

Most of the abnormalities of position can be adequately diagnosed by sonography in labor. However, when it is not possible by this means to be certain about the position of the fetus, the use of X-ray examination is justified, both to pin down the diagnosis of position and to screen for fetal anomalies.

Diminished Pelvic Capacity

The bony pelvis is a complex structure, made up of seven bones: the sacrum, the two iliums, the two ischiums, and the two pubic bones, joined together to form a ring. The sacrum consists of the lowermost five segments of the spinal column, different from the vertebrae above because they are fused together to form a solid bone. Attached to the lower end of the sacrum with a flexible joint is the three-segment coccyx, a remnant of the tail and quite without function. It is not of any obstetrical importance.

The iliums are the major bones of the side walls of the pelvis. They attach to the sacrum on either side at the sacroiliac joints, and the bones of the legs fit into them at the acetabulums, the ball and socket joints that permit the motion of the thigh. The iliums are also fixed firmly to both the pubic bones and the ischiums. The pubic bones meet each other behind the skin that bears the pubic hair and, with the ilium, form the ring of the pelvic inlet. The ischiums attach to the ilium and to the pubic bones. We sit down on the most prominent protrusions of the ischiums. With the pubic bones, they form the front arch of the pelvic outlet. The lower end of the sacrum is the back boundary of the outlet.

Taken together then, these seven bones make up the bony passage through which the fetus passes in the course of labor.

When we stand erect the weight of the trunk is borne by the sacroiliac joints and the hip joints. It is not surprising that a good deal of backache is attributable to stress and injury to these joints, which are not ideally constructed to carry the strain.

At the joint where the pubic bones meet there is a cartilage, the symphysis pubis, which occasionally loosens in pregnancy. But for practical purposes the bony pelvis remains fixed in size and the attachment of the bones to one another does not change.

A hundred years ago rickets was a common childhood disease. It resulted in a softening of the bones, which allowed them to bend and to move in relation to one another. In the first and second year of life, when children began to get up and walk around and thereby put the weight of the trunk on the sacrum, the effect of the rickets was to allow the sacrum to push forward toward the symphysis pubis. This narrowed the front-to-back space of the inlet of the pelvis, sometimes enough to form an obstruction to the vaginal birth of a live baby, although the narrowing was not such as to preclude sexual intercourse. This kind of pelvic contraction has vanished with the disappearance of rickets.

The bony problems that we see now are observed in little people when they are fertile; we also see them in connection with severe pelvic fractures, and with congenital abnormalities of the pelvis, a rare condition.

The little people present an interesting obstetrical problem. Medically we identify two types of inherited dwarfism: the true ateliotic (from the Greek, "incomplete") dwarf who has normal proportions but miniature size, and the chondrodystrophic (from the Greek, "cartilage" plus "ill" plus "nutrition") dwarf, the individual with a normal-sized head and trunk but unusually short arms and legs. The body build of the chondrodystrophic dwarfs results from the failure of the long bones of the arms and legs to achieve normal length.

The ateliotic little people rarely have children, but the chondrodystrophic ones are normally fertile. The appearance of these latter dwarfs may be familiar to you from the paintings of the brilliant Spanish painter Velazquez, in which they are shown at the royal court. With this type of dwarfism the pelvic inlet is frequently narrowed, and since the fetuses are of normal size obstruction results. The treatment of course is abdominal delivery.

Pelvic congenital anomalies, all of them extremely rare, are due to failures of normal shape and formation of the sacrum. This distorts the pelvis and narrows the inlet from side to side.

The final group of abnormalities are the consequence of pelvic fractures, commonly due to falls from extreme heights or to automobile accidents. The orthopedic management of these abnormalities has improved greatly in recent years, so that it is now unusual to see a woman whose pelvis has been distorted by such an accident. With severe deformity the obstetrical treatment is cesarean.

Soft-Tissue Obstruction

Soft-tissue obstruction as a cause of difficulty is an unusual event. On occasion a fibroid (myoma or leiomyoma) may lodge between the presenting part and the bony pelvis. This may occur with fibroids that grow within the cervix or within the uterine wall. Even fibroids that have grown out from the body of the uterus itself can drop into the pelvis below the presenting part and cause obstruction. Whether this will be an obstacle to delivery cannot be decided before labor begins.

The same is true of large ovarian cysts and the even less common pelvic kidney, either of which may be felt in the pelvis below the presenting part. In this event the proper treatment is cesarean section. An ovarian cyst can be removed at the time of section; a kidney is left undisturbed.

If ovarian tumors that warrant removal are found early in pregnancy, it is wise to remove them promptly to avoid the possibility that they will later obstruct labor.

It is generally agreed that it is unwise to undertake removal of myomas at any time during pregnancy. The risk of hemorrhage is considerable, due to the richness of their blood supply, a consequence of the hormone effect of the pregnancy.

The uterus and vagina form at first from paired tubes, which later, in the embryo, fuse together in the midline. Occasionally this junction is not perfectly accomplished and the wall between the right and the left sides does not vanish entirely. Such a wall, called a septum, may narrow the cervix and form an obstruction to labor.

Occasionally previous surgery to the cervix results in scarring such that normal dilation of the cervix cannot occur without extensive tears. For that reason any patient who has a history of prior surgery in the upper vagina and the cervix should be carefully examined in early pregnancy and again when she reaches term, to be sure that tissues have softened under the influence of the hormonal effects of pregnancy, eliminating any difficulty. Extensive cancer of the cervix is another condition that can prevent normal dilation of the cervix, with a chance of tears and bleeding.

There may be a septum across the upper vagina at the junction between the upper and middle third of the vagina; these septa are necessarily incomplete and do not obstruct either the outflow of menstrual blood or the access of sperm to the uterus and tubes above. However, they may provide a serious obstruction to normal birth. If such a septum is found early in pregnancy it should probably be surgically removed. If it is encountered for the first time in labor, abdominal delivery is advisable.

The concept of cervical dystocia, in which unusual rigidity of the cervix prevents it from dilating despite what seems to be strong labor, has been very difficult to verify. The management is no different from that of inadequate uterine action.

Some practitioners have thought that there is rigidity of the soft tissues in older women having babies for the first time. It has also been suggested that strenuous sports tend to toughen the perineum and to form an obstruction to the final stages of labor. I seriously doubt that either of these concepts has any reality. If there actually is a thickening of the soft tissues around the lower vagina or the perineum, it can readily be dealt with by episiotomy.

When a woman in labor has difficulty in urinating, her bladder fills and eventually becomes obvious as a bulge in the lower abdomen. This is more likely to occur in a prolonged labor, giving rise to the impression that a full bladder obstructs the labor. However, when the fetal head or breech is down in the pelvis, the bladder becomes an abdominal and not a pelvic organ. It is above the presenting part and it can hardly obstruct labor in that position. I believe therefore that a full bladder in labor is a sign of dystocia, and not a cause.

16

Fetal Monitoring

The first observation that a fetus in its mother's uterus was alive and well was made early in the nineteenth century by François Mayor, a Swiss surgeon, who reported that he could identify fetal life by placing his ear on a mother's abdomen and hearing the fetal heartbeat. This unmistakable sound can be heard as early as the eighteenth week of pregnancy in slender women.

At the beginning of the twentieth century it was already known that very rapid and very slow heart rates were signs of trouble. But it was not until the development of reliable means of recording fetal heart rates in the 1950's that it became possible to relate changes in them dependably to the diagnosis of fetal welfare. The next step was taken when we realized that, in labor, with the cervix partially open, we could obtain blood samples for biochemical study from the skin of the presenting part of the fetus.

The addition of ultrasound and sonographic techniques more recently has made possible improved predictability prior to labor. At present we are confident that we can decide, by making use of these methods of fetal monitoring, whether or not the fetus, still inside the mother, is in good condition.

The Purpose of Fetal Monitoring

Some fetuses encounter difficulty before they are born. When factors such as previous stillbirth, blood group incompatibility, or severe toxemia are identified in the mother's history by laboratory tests or by physical examination before labor, the pregnancy is considered at high risk. In rare cases, trouble appears for the first time in labor, when it may be caused by excessive uterine contractions or by obstruction of the umbilical cord, either of which can block the baby's access to support across the placenta.

Our goal is to find the evidence of fetal distress early enough to prevent lasting damage to the fetus. The earlier we try to do this, however, the harder it is to be certain of the diagnosis and of the correctness of a decision to act upon it.

A concept of fetal rescue has taken shape. Some causes of fetal distress respond to treatments that allow the pregnancy to continue. An example of a slowly progressing risk is Rh disease, which can be treated by *in utero* transfusion. Another is the abnormality of fetal heart rate due to defects in electrical conduction in the heart and for which cardiac drugs can be given. When distress appears in labor, we can give oxygen to the mother, who then passes it on to the fetus; we can shift the mother's position in the hope of relieving the pressure of the fetus on the cord; and we can give drugs to reduce the force of labor.

In some situations these measures do not suffice to relieve the distress. We then decide whether the situation is hazardous enough to require immediate delivery to give us direct access to treating the baby. If the mother is late in the second stage of labor, prompt delivery by the vacuum extractor or forceps may be the method of choice. If she is in early labor or not in labor yet, the recourse must be to cesarean.

Has Fetal Monitoring Increased the Number of Cesareans?

There is little question that it has. It is not a major factor, as it accounts at most for no more than 15 percent of the increase since 1970. Those who feel that this is too great an increase argue that borderline monitor findings are used to justify operations that were not done in the past and are not needed now. They believe that outcomes among the babies are not improved by the operations.

It is not necessary to treat every case of fetal distress hurriedly by surgery. I advocate fetal monitoring among high-risk patients in labor because careful monitoring can often provide the assurance of fetal safety that will allow awaiting a normal vaginal birth or a forceps delivery.

The central issue is whether the increased number of cesareans reduces the number of damaged babies. That some cesareans do this is beyond question. I have done such operations, but a cesarean is not a guarantee of a good baby if damage has already taken place.

Cesareans exact a toll on the mothers. Despite its astonishing safety, it is still a major operation with attendant risks of anesthesia, hemorrhage, and poor healing of the abdominal wound.

There is no test we can make of the value of cesarean section in reducing the number of babies damaged by fetal distress that does not incur an unacceptable level of risk to mothers or babies. Following the usual experimental design, by operating on alternate mothers with distressed fetuses and treating the others nonsurgically, we would inevitably cause injury to some fetuses who could have been helped by timely operation and expose some mothers to an unnecessary surgical risk. In addition, a meaningful experiment would have to be done on hundreds of cases, and in any one maternity service this would take years to complete. Survival of mother and baby is much too crude a standard. The quality of the baby and its freedom from injury cannot be decided for at least six years after birth.

So I think we must continue to treat before we can achieve absolute diagnostic certainty, knowing that in individual cases it will appear that we might have stayed our hands.

338 PREGNANCY, BIRTH AND FAMILY PLANNING

Abnormalities of the Fetal Heart Rate

The normal fetal heart rate is between 120 and 160 beats per minute. There are commonly variations of 10 to 15 beats per minute, usually in response to fetal movements. A normal recording is readily recognized.

When a fetus is depressed the fluctuations become less. This also occurs when the baby falls asleep and becomes less active, but these periods tend to last about only half an hour. The use of sedative and narcotic drugs such as phenobarbital and Demerol can have the same quieting effect. Loss of variation over a period of several hours, however, is a sign of serious difficulty.

When membranes have ruptured and labor pushes the head into the pelvis, there may be slowing of the fetal heart. This deceleration begins with the uterine contraction and ends as the uterus relaxes. The slowing is due to compression of the head and is a normal response. More marked decelerations may be due to interference with umbilical blood flow because the cord is either around the baby's neck or trunk, or caught against the bony pelvis. So long as recovery is rapid the fetus is not injured.

Late decelerations—starting well after a contraction has begun and persisting after the uterus has relaxed, while membranes may still be intact—are evidence of fetal distress. A third pattern of deceleration is occasionally seen, quite unrelated to contractions and thought to be due to transitory episodes of compression as the fetus moves against the umbilical cord.

On occasion mixtures of these deceleration patterns are observed and present serious difficulty in diagnosis. Additional clinical and laboratory data must then be considered.

Periods of speeding up (tachycardia) or slowing down (bradycardia) that last for several minutes at a time are of more serious import. Tachycardia is usually due to fever in fetus or mother. If the fever is due to intrauterine infection, prompt treatment with antibiotics and delivery is required. If the fever is due to an incidental infection outside the uterus, it must be treated vigorously to reduce the fever. Such treatment is not called for when the tachycardia results from an abnormality of electrical control of the fetal heart rate, with a rate of 200 or higher. The cause is best diagnosed by echocardiography, a type of ultrasound. The treatment for this condition consists of giving cardiac drugs to the fetus by administering them to the mother.

Bradycardia, a slowing of the heart rate below 110 beats per minute, can be evidence of severe fetal distress if it persists for more than a minute. The cause is usually a failure of placental exchange, due either to uterine contractions interfering with the maternal circulation of the placenta or to severe cord obstruction. The heart rate may drop from normal to rates as low as 50 and 60. If this persists for more than a few minutes the fetus is often damaged and prompt delivery is therefore urgent. While the preparations for delivery are being made, the immediate steps are to change the mother's position, give her oxygen, and, if the uterus is being stimulated, to stop the drug.

A rare condition, congenital heart block, is manifested by a fetal heart rate of 50 to 60 beats per minute for weeks or months prior to delivery. It does not result in brain damage to the fetus.

An unusual pattern is a fluctuation of rate of about 15 beats per minute every twelve to fifteen seconds. This is called a sinusoidal pattern and may be seen before labor. It is most often associated with severe fetal anemia in which case it is a grave sign.

What Does Fetal Monitoring Consist Of?

Fetal Monitoring before Labor

Fetal monitoring prior to labor is recommended in all patients with a high-risk pregnancy, such as women with diabetes or long-standing high blood pressure, those with previous still-births or other unfortunate outcomes of pregnancy, those whose pregnancies have lasted longer than forty-one weeks, and women with Rh isoimmunization. The duration of pregnancy at which these studies are carried out depends upon the patient's history and the severity of the complication.

Fetal Activity Records

The mother can record fetal movements by herself, taking a pad of paper and a pencil and, for several one-hour periods during the day, writing down how often the baby moves. Each baby has its own habits in this regard. A sudden drop in activity is a dangerous sign, and should be reported promptly to your care provider.

Electronic Monitoring

This is begun by placing the patient comfortably on her back or left side and applying a gauge to record uterine contractions and fetal movements and an ultrasound unit to register the fetal heart rate. The information from these gauges is fed into a printing recorder that continuously registers the frequency and strength of the contractions and the rate of the fetal heart. This record may take 20 to 120 minutes. It is called a non-stress test or NST.

Recent improvements in non-stress testing have made it possible to attach gauges to the mother for hours, or even days, in such a way that the information is broadcast by lightweight transmitters to a nearby recorder and the patients need not remain in bed. A few investigators have even gone further by developing an over-the-shoulder container for tapes to record the data. The patient can take this unit with her and transmit the taped information to the physician by telephone without the need to go to a hospital or clinic for frequent recording.

If the NST recording is not clearly normal the next step is to obtain a contraction stress test (CST). If uterine contractions are not already occurring, they can be induced by the administration of oxytocin in a dilute intravenous drip. The goal is to produce about three contractions in a ten-minute period and to observe the response of the fetal heart rate. This amount of uterine activity can be induced as well by stimulation of the mother's breasts and nipples. The nervous system reflex in response to such stimulation releases the mother's own oxytocin. This is the same reflex that results in milk let-down in nursing mothers.

The occurrence of late decelerations with these contractions may be a sign of severe fetal stress and an indication for prompt delivery. If labor can be induced, this is ideal, since in a certain percentage of women the decelerations abate when labor ensues. If labor cannot be induced, cesarean may be necessary for the safety of the baby.

Sonographic Studies

Estimations of the size of the fetus and of the volume of amniotic fluid can be made by the examiner's hand. If more accurate information is needed, it is obtained by ultrasound examination. If the fetus is in good health there are ample pockets of amniotic fluid. When excess fluid is present, further study is needed.

When fetal growth retardation is suspected, ultrasound is used to get accurate measurements of the head and abdomen. A series of such measurements might show the growth of the head (biparietal diameter, or BPD) to be greater than that of the abdomen (transabdominal diameter, or TAD). Such a finding would indicate less retardation of growth in the head. If both diameters grow equally but more slowly than normal, it is an ominous sign. In normal fetuses the BPD is greater than the TAD up to about the thirty-sixth week of pregnancy; thereafter the TAD becomes larger and can be used to estimate fetal size.

In the presence of medical complications and twin pregnancies, sonographic measurements are now being made of the blood flow in umbilical arteries and veins and in the uterine arteries. This technique is called velocimetry (Latin: *velox*, fast; *meter*, measure). A careful interpretation of the flow rates can give information about fetal welfare.

Further Studies of Fetal Welfare

Biochemical testing of the fetus prior to labor is possible by study of amniotic fluid obtained by amniocentesis. This is of great value in deciding the severity of fetal anemia in instances of isoimmunization. It is also possible to study the fluid for the amount of several fatlike chemicals (phospholipids, such as phosphatidyl glycerol, sphingomyelin, and lecithin) whose presence is closely related to the maturity of the fetal lung. These data can be used to predict how well the baby will be able to breathe should it become necessary to deliver it prematurely. They are reported as the L/S ratio (L for lecithin and S for sphingomyelin) and as the fraction of phosphatidyl glycerol. An L/S ratio of 2 or greater usually predicts that the baby will not develop respiratory distress syndrome after birth. Similarly, if more than 2 percent of the fatlike chemicals consists of phosphatidyl glycerol, the newborn is not likely to have respiratory difficulty.

Interpretation of all these laboratory studies requires skill and experience to make a decision when to deliver the high-risk fetus and, perhaps more importantly, when not to.

Fetal Monitoring during Labor

Fetal monitoring during labor is carried out by all the techniques mentioned above. Once the head or the breech of the fetus has descended into the pelvis and the cervix has begun to dilate it becomes possible to attach fine wires to its skin. The recordings of fetal heart rate are thus obtained with less "noise" in them than with external ultrasound.

Occasionally, when membranes rupture in labor, meconium appears in the amniotic fluid. Meconium is the dark-green normal content of the fetus's large bowel. The fetus passes it in response to stress. If there is ample amniotic fluid the mixture tends to be thin. Where there is diminished amniotic fluid the meconium is dense and thick and this probably has a much more serious prognostic significance. The appearance of meconium is an indication for fetal monitoring.

Further information as to the condition of the fetus can be obtained by study of a few drops of blood from the skin of the presenting part. If the cervix is adequately dilated, a plastic cone, open at both ends and fitted with a light, is passed into the mother's vagina and pushed up against the baby's skin. The skin is then pricked so that it will bleed. The shed blood is collected in a long thin tube, about the thickness of the needles used to give intravenous fluids. This blood sample is then studied for its acid-base balance, expressed in numerical form as pH.

The normal fetal skin blood pH is about 7.32, depending a bit on the mother's pH. As labor progresses and mother and baby are stressed, the value tends to fall. At the end of normal labor it may be as low as 7.22. When distress is suspected from fetal heart rate abnormalities or passage of meconium, it adds information to obtain a fetal pH, which in severe distress can fall as low as 7.05.

We now have devices which, when attached to the baby's skin, will yield information about the concentration of oxygen and carbon dioxide in fetal blood, but this information does not, in the present state of our knowledge, add much to what we can learn of the condition of the fetus from pH studies alone.

Should Fetal Monitoring Be Routine?

This has been a matter of controversy for at least a decade. Among normal women with known normal fetuses the likelihood of unexpected fetal distress in labor is about one instance in a thousand. Furthermore, most of these abnormalities can be detected by listening to the fetal heart every fifteen minutes in labor. It may well be excessive to subject thousands of normal women to continuous electronic monitoring in labor to diagnose the rare instances of fetal difficulty that cannot be found by simpler means.

Fetal monitoring is not a substitute for personal attention during labor. It may be argued that the cost of the electronic equipment involved is less than the salaries of skilled people. However, the output of the fetal monitors has to be studied by people with clinical experience; the machines do not interpret themselves. There is no disagreement that in high-risk situations fetal monitoring during labor is an asset. I believe that the universal application of fetal monitoring should await the perfection of noninvasive techniques that will not significantly diminish the comfort of women during normal labor.

17

Obstetrical Operations

When I first entered obstetrics, most babies were being born in hospitals and home deliveries were vanishing. There was considerable use of general anesthesia and of forceps operations. Cesareans accounted for no more than 5 percent of births, even among those patients we would now classify as high risk.

These relative proportions have shifted radically over the past generation. The trend toward prepared natural childbirth and away from general and even regional anesthesia has almost eliminated the use of elective forceps delivery. Simultaneously, families are becoming smaller and women are having their children later in life. As a result, not just the survival but also the quality of each infant is now receiving increased emphasis.

The persistent thought, not entirely based on fact, has been that cesarean birth spares the fetus all the trauma attributed to vaginal birth. Cesarean has therefore been increasingly chosen by doctors in situations in which increased fetal risk may be present in labor. Fetal monitoring, providing information about fetal condition that we simply did not have a generation ago, can be skillfully used to make certain that the fetus is not in jeopardy. In the hands of inexperienced attendants, however, the evidence it produces can be wrongly interpreted as predictive of impending disaster, and on this basis the patient is often treated by cesarean.

The availability of trained anesthesiologists and capable pediatricians has given assurance of improved outcomes for mother and newborn in the event of section. Awareness of this must play a role in the doctor's evaluation of the gain-risk ratio. The risk of maternal death from cesarean, even though it is several times that of vaginal birth, is extremely small—perhaps less than 1 in 10,000 births. If this is weighed against the chance of fetal injury from a delay in delivery or a difficult birth— both events avoidable by section—the decision in equivocal situations is likely to be in favor of cesarean. Furthermore, in the event of a poor outcome for the fetus, we are all aware that doctors will more probably be forgiven if they have intervened surgically, particularly if they have done a cesarean, than if they have refrained from such intervention.

One of my respected friends insists that it is the right of the infant to be well born; the idea persists that somehow this can be more certainly guaranteed by cesarean birth. It appeals to common sense that abdominal delivery eliminates the hazards of labor and vaginal birth. Nevertheless, given competent fetal monitoring, the risks of fetal injury in labor are remarkably small among normal women. Certainly much less than one infant in a thousand is exposed to the risk of any damage, great or small.

The hazards of actual delivery, late in the second stage of labor, are increased in cases of breech births and in forceps deliveries. Cesarean will eliminate these risks. However, cesarean birth does incur significantly increased risks to the mother: discomfort; fever due to infection and an abdominal operation; the need for more extensive anesthesia; hemorrhage from unavoidable surgical accidents; and the likelihood that cesarean will be the method chosen for all her subsequent deliveries. These factors do not apply to every cesarean birth, nor do risks of injury in vaginal birth exist in most vaginal deliveries. Furthermore, in many conditions where risk to the fetus of continuing the pregnancy is the reason for delivery, cesarean does not necessarily result in a better outcome for the newborn than does vaginal birth.

Another factor in the increase in operative obstetrics is the understandable desire of pregnant women to have brief and relatively painless labors. This has produced an increasing use of conduction anesthesia, which in its turn has brought about an increasing use of operative intervention in delivery, by forceps and the vacuum extractor as well as by cesarean. The decision how to deliver a woman in a particular labor must, of course, be made on an individual basis, carefully weighing the risks against the benefits of each of the proposed methods before settling on one.

A generation ago it was accepted that treatment which benefited the mother also benefited the fetus. It was also acceptable to expose the fetus to the chance of some trauma for the sake of minimizing damage to the mother. These attitudes appear to be changing. Injury to the fetus is no longer considered an appropriate consequence of pregnancy complications. With this in mind, obstetricians in several states have asked courts to order women to submit to cesarean in cases where the only predicted danger was to the fetus. Such orders have been issued, apparently placing the welfare of the baby before that of the mother.

Good obstetrics cannot condone more complex operative procedures done solely to shorten labor, for under these circumstances delivery is carried out before the patient is ready, thus substituting a needless and dangerous procedure for one which would be simple and safe minutes or hours later. The obstetrician whose inexperience or excessive sympathy prompts him to make undue haste because of the importunings of an overanxious family or patient has frequent cause for regret.

It is impossible to fix the optimum obstetrical operative rate, for it depends on many variables. The type of clientele a particular doctor or hospital draws affects it; the greater the reputation of either, the larger the proportion of problem cases. As previously stated, analgesia and anesthesia are also important factors, as is parity (the number of previous deliveries). More important than the gross operative rate are the types of operations and particularly the obstetrical end result. Are the mothers left healthy and well, with future childbearing unprejudiced? Are the babies vigorous and uninjured?

Under these circumstances it is essential that everyone concerned have a clear understanding what obstetrical operations consist of and when and how they are properly done.

The significant interventions in contemporary obstetrics are as follows: forceps; vacuum extraction; breech delivery and version; episiotomy; induction of labor; and cesarean section.

Forceps Delivery

Most operative vaginal deliveries are done by means of a special instrument, the forceps. This consists of two separate thin steel blades with inner surfaces curved to fit the sides of the infant's head. The blades are inserted separately into the vagina, opposite each other, and when their handles are articulated, the child's head is securely grasped between the blades. With moderate traction on the handles, exerted in the axis of the vagina, the head is extracted.

The word *forceps* in Latin means "a pair of tongs." It is said to have been derived from the earlier Latin words *fornus* ("oven") and *capere* ("to take"). The obstetric forceps in its modern form, an instrument capable of extracting a living child without injury to it or to the mother, is an invention of the early seventeenth century. Previous to this, single-bladed and even double-bladed instruments, called hooks, were in use, but probably only for the extraction of a dead child. The old double-bladed instruments had a permanent articulation so that each blade could not be inserted separately; they looked like the once-familiar ice tongs.

The inventors of the modern obstetrical forceps were a singular medical family—the Chamberlens. In 1569 the first of the English line, William, emigrated from France to England to escape the persecution of the Huguenots. Most of the Chamberlens were Royal Surgeons or Physicians, and several English queens were delivered by them. This obstetrical dynasty of Chamberlen extended uninterruptedly from Peter the Elder's admission to the Guild of Barber-Surgeons in about 1596 to the death of Hugh, Junior, in 1728. They were no ordinary men; they lived hard and tempestuously, unwilling to confine their energies within the narrow scope of their professions.

History of the Forceps

The forceps was probably invented in about 1600 by Peter the Elder and kept as a hereditary family secret to be buried with Hugh, Junior, in 1728. According to modern medical standards, such conduct was wholly unethical, and any twentieth-century doctor who would dare a similar practice would find himself ostracized, read out of all medical societies, and anathema to decent people. However, it is obviously unfair to judge the behavior of one century by the standards of another.

How was the secret finally revealed? The existence of the forceps was hinted at as early as 1616 at a meeting of the Royal College when a slurring reference was made to the boast of Peter Chamberlen the Younger "that he and his brother, and none others, excelled in the management of difficult labors."

Hugh, Senior, emigrated to Holland in 1699 under suspicion of debt. While there he appears to have obtained some money, for he returned to England for two years before settling permanently in Amsterdam. While in Holland, probably at the time of his supposed flight, he sold the secret of the forceps to Hendrik Van Roonhuyze, the leader of Dutch obstetrics. During the succeeding years of the early eighteenth century the secret oozed out in England and on the Continent. William Giffard of London used the forceps openly on April 6, 1726, calling it "extractors." He is generally considered "the altruistic and honorable physician who should receive full credit for introducing the forceps into general use in England." By 1733, when Edmund Chapman published the very first account of the forceps, there were already several models, and their use "was well known to all the principal men of the profession, both in town and country."

The retention of an important medical secret transmitted from generation to generation for a century and a quarter is unique in history. The Chamberlens were crafty enough to exclude all others from the room when they operated; they used the forceps unassisted.

Not because of its antiquity—for other obstetrical operative procedures antedated it—but because of its importance, delivery by forceps merits first place in the discussion of obstetrical operations.

Types of Forceps

For several decades every skilled obstetrician felt obligated to design his own forceps and to name them after himself. However, only a few basic types have survived to present-day use. All forceps have two blades that are readily separated from one another but can be joined together, much as the two blades of a pair of kitchen scissors are joined. The length of the handles varies, and the lengths of blades as well, and there are varieties of curvature. Some of the blades are solid where they wrap around the baby's head and some have windows.

All forceps have two curves—one to fit the curve of the birth canal and the other to allow the blades to wrap properly around the baby's head. These curves vary slightly from one forceps to another. Most commonly in use in the United States are the Simpson forceps, the Tucker-McLane forceps, the Luikart forceps, an instrument more slender and delicate than the first two, and the Kielland forceps, the most delicate of all. The experience of an individual operator with a particular pair of forceps is probably more important to successful use than the particular variety of instrument used for a given delivery.

Indications for a Forceps Delivery

Delivery by forceps is safe only if specific conditions have been met. The head of the child must fit deeply into the pelvis without serious bony obstruction, the membranes must be ruptured, and the cervix completely dilated. A forceps operation cannot be done prior to the second stage of labor except as an emergency when the cord has prolapsed, late in the first stage of labor, in a woman who has previously delivered large babies. In such a situation immediate extraction of the fetus—rather than waiting to carry out a cesarean—may save the fetus's life.

Indications for forceps delivery are properly divided into two broad classes, the fetal and the maternal.

One fetal indication is the appearance or worsening of evidence of fetal distress late in labor. The methods that we use in identifying this are described in the section on fetal monitoring. Severe fetal distress prior to the second stage of labor is necessarily dealt with by cesarean. In the second stage of labor, as the head descends through the pelvis, the forces imposed upon it may cause slowing of the fetal heart rate. When this slowing begins and ends simultaneous with a contraction it is probably well within the baby's ability to adapt to it.

On the other hand, slowing down that begins late in the course of the contraction and persists well beyond the end of it is evidence of chronic stress. This may be accompanied by the appearance of meconium in the amniotic fluid. The presence of meconium is not proof of stress but an indication that fetal difficulty must be considered. When a fetus reaches the limits of its ability to adapt to stress the muscles around its anus may relax, and meconium, which is the normal content of the fetus's large intestine, will then be expelled into the amniotic fluid. The appearance of meconium in a breech presentation may not be abnormal at all. Since the breech is down deep in the pelvis, meconium may be squeezed out much like toothpaste out of a tube.

When there is evidence of stress it is usual to take a measurement of the fetal pH. The evidence is that when the early signs of fetal distress appear and are corroborated by slightly reduced pH measurements, the fetal outcome is not adversely affected if delivery is achieved within one hour. The attendants must keep in mind that the fetus in distress does not tolerate a difficult delivery as well as does the normal fetus. The appearance of prolonged periods of fetal heart slowing (bradycardia with or without a contraction lasting longer than a minute) immediately raises the question of prompt delivery. If the presenting part is well down in the pelvis, particularly if it can be seen at the entrance to the vagina, forceps intervention is clearly indicated.

Some of these bradycardias are occasioned by accidents to the umbilical cord in which the cord is compressed between the child's body and the rigid walls of the pelvis. The umbilical cord may be looped around the child's neck or over the body and be adequate in length until the baby descends in the birth canal and pulls the cord tight.

The decision as to whether to intervene necessarily involves the experience, skill, and judgment of the attendants.

Maternal Reasons for Forceps

Maternal indications for forceps in the absence of any evidence of fetal distress are less clear-cut. Sometimes a patient, in bringing the vertex down through the pelvis, simply does not make the progress needed to rotate it to the ideal position, occiput anterior (OA). A delay of this sort may occur with very large infants and with those presenting in the occiput posterior (OP). Or a patient who goes rapidly and efficiently through the first stage of labor has much less effective contractions in the second stage of labor. It is usual to treat delays of this sort with intravenous oxytocin, but this does not always succeed in bringing about a spontaneous delivery, and forceps may be needed.

As has been mentioned, conduction anesthesia may sometimes be responsible for prolongation of the second stage of labor. One of the solutions is to allow the anesthesia to wear off, with the hope that the bearing-down efforts of the mother will be improved when she can more intensely feel the urge to push. However, it is not inappropriate, when it appears that forceps delivery will be without difficulty, to carry out the forceps while the anesthesia is still effective.

Occasionally, a patient finds it possible to bring the baby's head into view at the entrance to the vagina but somehow lacks the strength for the final push. Women who are unfortunate enough to have had a long latent labor, during which they have gone without solid food and sleep, may finally reach the second stage of labor too fatigued and distraught to push well.

For a long time it has been believed that, if the second stage of labor is prolonged beyond two hours, there will be a steadily increasing morbidity for both mother and baby. In general, there is merit to this position, and forceps intervention has been undertaken for this reason. However, as long as the mother is making progress in the second stage and monitoring indicates that she and the fetus are in good condition, there is probably no need for intervention simply because of elapsed time.

Classification of Forceps Operations

Outlet forceps are done when the baby's head has bulged in the entrance to the vagina but has failed to deliver, either because of resistance by the perineum or inadequacy of the bearing-down. This may be solved by an incision in the perineum, the episiotomy, but if this in turn fails to facilitate the normal birth, forceps can be applied and the head readily delivered by the obstetrician.

Low forceps is the term used to describe a delivery initiated after the baby's head has become visible at the entrance of the vagina at the peak of the contraction, in the OA position or only very slightly deviated from that. By this time the head has traversed the narrowest portions of the maternal bony pelvis and has been at least partially molded to a shape that will permit easy delivery.

Mid-forceps includes all forceps operations that do not meet the criteria for low or outlet forceps. The leading point of the infant's head must be well down into the pelvis so that it can be certain that the obstruction to delivery is not at the pelvic inlet. However, the head may not have rotated into the OA but may be in one of the transverse or oblique positions. Under these circumstances it is necessary to rotate the head into an occiput anterior to deliver it. This risks injuring the maternal soft tissues. The considerable force necessary in some instances to rotate the head and then pull it the remaining distance through the birth canal can be sufficiently great to do injury to the fetal brain. It is therefore important to know that the pelvic capacity is adequate and the metabolic status of the fetus normal before undertaking to deliver by mid-forceps. Fewer and fewer mid-forceps operations are being done in the United States.

A significant variable in the outcome from mid-forceps deliveries is the experience and skill of the operator, both in deciding when to deliver and how to do it. There is a most interesting study among the twenty-odd obstetrical units run under careful supervision by the United States Navy. The proportion of mid-forceps deliveries to total deliveries in these hospitals varies over a considerable range but there seems to be no relationship between fetal outcomes and the incidence of mid-forceps.

Another variable affecting forceps operations is that outlet forceps can easily be done under pudendal block or even with local infiltration of the perineum or as low forceps. Mid-forceps calls for somewhat more potent anesthesia, not only to relieve the pain of the operation but also to relax the muscle tissues of the mother and facilitate the extraction.

High Forceps

The forceps was originally invented in the seventeenth and eighteenth centuries, when rickets was a common complication in urban obstetrics. It was intended to solve the problem created by the failure of the head to come through the inlet of the pelvis, an inlet narrowed because of the disease. Such high forceps operations were not expected to deliver a live child. These procedures are now a thing of the past.

Performance of a Forceps Delivery

Before anything more formidable than outlet forceps, anesthesia is administered to the mother. This may be a general anesthetic, but a conduction anesthetic is more commonly used. The usual types are low epidural, saddle block, and pudendal block. The pudendal block is given through the skin of the perineum or through the vaginal mucosa and is therefore put into place after the patient has been prepared for delivery. The conduction anesthetics that depend upon injection of drugs into the spinal canal are put into place before the patient is put into position for the forceps operation on the delivery table. For delivery, the patient lies on her back, knees apart, with her legs supported in that position either by stirrups or by the hands of members of the support team.

The vaginal area receives the customary antiseptic preparation, and the patient is draped with sterile towels or paper drapes. The operator then performs a careful vaginal examination to determine the position of the head by feeling for the two soft spots (fontanels) at the front and back of the child's head. The front fontanel, where four bones join, is relatively large and diamond-shaped, whereas the one in back where three bones join is much smaller and triangular. Sometimes, because of the way in which the bones have shifted against one another in the course of labor (molding) or because of the caput succedaneum (a normal swelling of the baby's scalp), it is difficult to identify these landmarks reliably. The operator can then slide fingers alongside the baby's head and feel for an ear. Since the front of the ear is fixed and the back of the ear is loose and floppy, it is possible to tell the direction in which the occiput is pointing.

After determining the position of the head the operator picks up one blade of the forceps and slides it into the vagina alongside the baby's head in such a way that when the two blades of the forceps are brought together the maternal (pelvic) curve of the forceps will be in the same direction as the curve of the vagina. Minor adjustments are occasionally needed in the position of this first blade of the forceps against the baby's head. When application of the forceps is completed, each blade should be resting over an ear of the baby. This is especially important when the baby is presenting in the occiput transverse (OT), the position in which the back of the baby's head is pointing toward the mother's side. It may be necessary with OT to introduce the first blade of the forceps over the baby's face and then jiggle it around (a technique called wandering) until it falls over the side of the baby's head. When the first blade is properly in place the second blade can then be readily applied and the forceps brought together (articulated). If the application of the forceps is not correct the blades do not lock properly. This is an indication to remove and adjust them. Once the operator is satisfied with a proper application, extraction of the baby can begin.

If the baby's head is not in the occiput anterior, where it should be as the head is being born, efforts are made to rotate the baby into that position. Some operators prefer to pull the baby's head down as they accomplish this rotation, and others rotate the baby's head before pulling. Once the baby's head is in the appropriate position, the operator exerts traction on the forceps: that is, pulls it down in the direction of the birth canal. Exactly how this extraction is done varies from operator to operator. I do what I can to mimic the forces of labor. If it is possible to feel the uterus I make traction when the uterus is contracting. If the patient can cooperate I ask her to bear down along with my pulling. If this is not feasible due to anesthesia I generally pull for about ten or fifteen seconds, release for a moment, then pull again, and then pull a third time trying to simulate the three maximum bearing-down efforts that occur with a uterine contraction. I try to pull for something under a minute at a time, at intervals of about a minute and a half, and repeat this kind of cycle as often as necessary to achieve delivery. Most forceps operations last no more than five to ten minutes. If the obstruction to birth is so severe as to require more time or greater force, the operator should seriously consider abandoning the effort and delivering the baby abdominally.

Finally, within the forceps, the baby's head appears in the outlet and crowns. From that point on the mother can usually push the baby's head out by herself.

Most operators perform an episiotomy, since more space is required in the outlet when the baby is born inside forceps and therefore lacerations of the vagina are more common. The remainder of the birth of the child is exactly the same as it is with a spontaneous birth.

The force necessary to carry out a forceps operation depends upon the station of the pelvis to which the head has descended and on the size of the baby. The quality of contractions and of bearing down in the second stage also play a role. An outlet forceps requires very little force, but mid-forceps can require a good deal of exertion on the part of both the operator and the mother.

"Prophylactic" Forceps

From the 1920's to the 1960's the concept of "prophylactic forceps operations" had considerable acceptance. The thought was that the baby would be spared the stress of the last half hour or so of labor and, being delivered in forceps, would be born under complete control of the operator. The mother was also spared a period of hard work in bearing down. It was also thought that if a large episiotomy was done, the mother would be spared difficulties related to vaginal relaxation later in life.

In retrospect there seems to be very little to support these arguments for prophylactic forceps. We have evidence that the stress of half an hour of labor on the head of the fetus is no greater than that produced by a forceps operation.

In addition, an episiotomy is an incision principally in the skin and some of the muscle tissues that surround the entrance to the vagina and the anus itself. It is not this area which creates the problems with vaginal relaxation in later life. The connective tissue that supports the bladder and the rectum is located higher in the vagina. If childbirth does injury to those structures it does so early in the second stage of labor. If we wished to prevent all cases of vaginal relaxation due to pregnancy it would be necessary to deliver all babies abdominally. The continuing trend toward natural childbirth and avoidance of intervention has markedly diminished the frequency with which obstetrical attendants choose to do elective forceps operations and episiotomies.

Incidence of Forceps Operations

At present, the incidence of forceps operations in major teaching hospitals ranges from 1 percent to 8 percent, depending upon the training and expectations of the physicians and of the patients, upon the relative proportion of women having a first baby, and upon their social status. It also depends upon the extent to which patients are educated for natural childbirth and whether the physicians in a given institution generally practice prophylactic forceps deliveries. It is not possible to say that a given rate is either good or bad.

Complications of Forceps

Pressure injuries where forceps are applied to the fetus's head usually are limited to simple abrasions of the skin. When the orientation of the forceps on the skull is not ideal there may be a bruise over an ear. If the tip of the forceps makes pressure on the cheek just ahead of the ear it can produce a temporary paralysis of the muscles served by the seventh cranial nerve. In that case the baby's mouth will be pulled away to the other side and the baby will blink inadequately on the side of the paralysis. This injury clears up quickly, within the first few days after birth. Forceps applications that are badly done, particularly if excessive force is added, have been known to produce skull fractures. Fortunately, these ordinarily heal without doing any injury to the baby's brain and without leaving any later evidence of the event.

Vacuum Extraction

Many efforts have been made over the years to replace the steel forceps with a gentler instrument that can extract the baby without putting as much pressure as do the forceps on the sides of the baby's head. The first such instrument to gain widespread use was the vacuum extractor introduced in Sweden in 1954. It consists of a metal cup about three inches in diameter and about one inch deep. This is placed over the baby's scalp and a carefully controlled vacuum is created inside the cup with a pump. This gradually sucks the baby's scalp into the cup and holds it there, forming an artificial caput succedaneum. The operator, by maintaining this hold on the scalp, can use the instrument as a handle on the baby's head. The scalp is quite loosely applied to the skull, and the artificial caput is just as harmless as the caput that normally forms on the head of most babies. With this handle, the operator can rotate the head into a more favorable position and then make traction by pulling on the suction cup with a chain attached for that purpose. The Swedish instrument is now being replaced to some extent in the United States by a soft cone-shaped cup of a synthetic material, which works on the same principle. Negative pressure is made in the same way as with the metal cup, and the operator waits a few minutes for swelling of the scalp to make an adequate handle. It is important to palpate around the edges of the cup to be certain that no vaginal tissue has been sucked into it along with the baby's scalp.

Once the cup is in place traction can be made in nearly the same way as traction on the forceps. An advantage of the vacuum extractor is that it is attached at the leading part of the baby's head, and thus does not use any space in the vagina or pelvis. The significance of this is that the baby's head can adapt itself to the pelvis instead of adapting to the forceps.

The vacuum extractor has not had widespread use in the United States. In some countries in Europe it has virtually replaced forceps, and obstetricians there are quite satisfied as to its safety and efficiency. It does produce a conspicuous purple bruise on the top of the baby's head at the site of the artificial caput, but it has not been responsible for any of the injuries that have been observed with forceps. When it is particularly difficult to be sure of the position of the baby's head, the vacuum extractor can be applied to the lowest part of the head. Traction then may bring the baby's head down to a point where it is possible to see or feel its position. Then, if need be, forceps can be applied.

Bearing down by the mother facilitates progress during traction with the vacuum extractor. For that reason, I prefer to use it with local anesthetic infiltration of the perineum, pudendal block, or a low epidural block, any of which allows the mother to bear down in cooperation with the traction made by the obstetrician. Since, as I have said, the instrument itself uses no space alongside or above the head of the fetus in the vagina, it can be applied with less discomfort than the forceps. It can in fact mimic spontaneous birth. An episiotomy can be done but may not be needed.

Breech Birth

Breech presentations are classified in terms of the parts of the fetus which present. Frank breeches present by the buttocks, with the baby's legs along its trunk. Cord prolapse, the condition in which the umbilical cord falls into the cervix or vagina below the presenting part, occurs with frank breech about 4 times in 1,000 cases as compared with 3 times in 1,000 with vertex presentation. When the buttocks and feet present together, a complete breech, the chance of cord prolapse rises to about 40 in 1,000. When only feet present—a single or double footling breech—the cord prolapses 120 times in 1,000 cases. Cord prolapse can only take place after rupture of the membranes. When the breech descends, the cord may become obstructed, whether or not it has prolapsed.

The Course of Breech Labor

The first stage of labor with the breech is the same as that with the vertex presentation. The same rules of patient care and monitoring apply. If cord prolapse occurs before vaginal delivery is immediately possible the baby should be delivered abdominally. When membranes rupture an immediate vaginal examination is done to screen for prolapse.

While membranes are intact fetal monitoring is done in the same circumstances with the breech as it is with the vertex. After membranes rupture and late in the first stage of labor, continuous monitoring is our best reliance for early diagnosis of cord obstruction.

When the patient enters the second stage of labor I prefer to transfer her to the delivery room. Since the breech is slightly smaller than the head the second stage may be briefer than it is with the vertex presentation. With a frank breech presentation the buttocks gradually bulge through the introitus in just the same way as a vertex does. With footling breeches and complete breeches, where the baby's legs are down lower than the buttocks the baby's feet may well deliver first.

As long as progress continues and the fetal heart remains good, the best management is to encourage the mother to bear down, unaided, until the baby has delivered to the navel. From this point the operator can safely be of some assistance to the mother.

Ideally, two other trained people in sterile gowns and gloves should be prepared to assist with the delivery. The baby's trunk, hips, and feet, being very slippery, are wrapped in a towel. The baby's trunk is rotated so as to turn its back toward one side of the mother. The trunk can now be pulled gently downward toward the floor or gently upward toward the ceiling in such a way as to assist an arm, preferably the anterior arm, to deliver. The trunk is then rotated 180 degrees to make the other arm the anterior arm, and deliver it. With the aid of bearing down, this goes quite rapidly. The baby is now lying with its back toward the mother's abdomen. The operator can support the baby's prone body on an arm and with that hand reach into the vagina, over the baby's face. By putting pressure on the bones in the baby's cheeks with a finger on either side of the nose, the head is flexed to bring the face out over the perineum. This is assisted by making pressure over the back of the baby's head through the mother's lower abdomen. Once the baby's mouth and nose have come through the introitus sufficiently for the baby to breathe, it can cough and cry, even though the entire head is not yet born.

These maneuvers in the birth of the breech are readily carried out without instruments. Some operators do an episiotomy early to facilitate the birth of the head. Vaginal lacerations are exceedingly unlikely. Breech delivery in no way alters the birth of the placenta, nor does it make any maternal complications any more likely.

There are, however, some increased hazards for the fetus in breech birth that are not present in vertex presentation. One already mentioned is the possibility of cord prolapse. Another risk is delay in the birth of the head. This occurs because, after the navel is delivered, circulation through the umbilical cord either is markedly slowed down or comes to a complete halt. It will be obvious if the cord has collapsed.

At this stage the baby must depend on its own respirations for gas exchange. The head therefore has to be delivered within a few minutes. Delay can occur because the head is the largest part of the baby. If the simple maneuvers described above fail to deliver the head the next step is the application of forceps for the delivery. As I mentioned, the Piper forceps was especially designed for this purpose and is the most commonly used instrument. I personally prefer to use the Simpson forceps. Whichever forceps one uses, the help of a second operator is needed to hold the baby's trunk in position while the forceps is being applied. Once the baby's mouth is brought down low enough in the birth canal to allow the baby to breathe, the rest of the forceps delivery can be done slowly and deliberately.

Breech Extraction

If the breech is high when evidence of cord obstruction appears, abdominal delivery is the treatment of choice. However, if the breech is already low in the pelvis, a breech extraction can be undertaken. The mother will need to be adequately anesthesized; she may already have been given an epidural or a saddle block, or a brief general anesthetic may be required. The operator puts a hand up alongside the breech and into the upper vagina or the lower uterus, and grasps one of the baby's feet. This foot is then brought down and wrapped in a towel; the operator can then exert traction on it. This will ordinarily bring the breech down and the remainder of the delivery proceeds as has been described above.

Commonly when the mother has not been able to deliver the breech baby by her own efforts, and it has had to be extracted as here described, one or both arms, instead of being folded over the baby's chest, may be swept up behind the baby's head. It may then be difficult to bring the baby's arm out simply by making traction on the trunk. The solution is to rotate the baby's trunk in the direction of the arm behind the head. This will often allow the arm to deliver. Otherwise the operator's hand can bring it out from this position. The baby's other arm may have to be delivered by the same maneuvers.

Careful studies of many breech deliveries have shown that, when labor and delivery are managed by skilled and experienced operators helping the mother, the outcomes for breech babies by vaginal birth are not sufficiently less favorable than cesarean outcomes to justify delivering all breeches abdominally. The incidence of cesarean section will, under the best circumstances, be greater for breech presentation than it is for vertex presentations because of the potential complications that I have described. On the other hand, the great majority of breech deliveries will proceed to an excellent outcome, given monitoring in labor and meticulous attention during the second stage.

External and Internal Version

In a patient with ample amniotic fluid and a nicely relaxed uterus it is possible to turn the baby in the uterus from one position to another. This is most readily done between the twenty-fourth and thirtieth week, when the baby itself is freely moving around. There is almost as much amniotic fluid as there is baby and there is very little to confine the fetus in any one position.

Closer to term there is relatively less amniotic fluid and the lie of the baby tends to become more stable. However, a baby can still be turned by external pressure from the breech to the vertex in a high proportion of cases. Clearly, the earlier that this is done in pregnancy the more likely it is to be successful and the less likely it is to be necessary. The goal is to reduce the number of cesareans done solely for breech presentation.

Sometimes in the last few weeks external version is very easily done and the baby remains in a vertex presentation thereafter. Studies have recently been reported of trials at version late in pregnancy, in which the mother has been admitted into the hospital and been given drugs to relax the uterus so that uterine tone (the resting contraction force) will not impede the performance of version. Using this technique it is possible to turn enough babies to reduce the incidence of breech presentation from 3.5 percent down to about 2 percent. This procedure has to be done gently and with care because it is possible, in turning the baby, to produce cord obstruction or cause partial placental separation. The fetal heart therefore has to be observed carefully during and immediately after the procedure to detect ill effects if there are any. The operator must be fully prepared to carry out an immediate cesarean if evidence of persistent fetal distress appears.

There is some thought that the mother's position has an influence on the fetal presentation. Recommendations have been made to patients to spend some time in the knee-chest position in the hope this will assist the baby in converting from a breech to a vertex. I do not know of any controlled studies to indicate whether or not this works.

Internal Version

Internal version is correctly termed internal podalic (Greek: *pous*, "foot") version because the operator inserts a hand into the uterus and grasps the fetus by one or both feet, to turn the baby from a vertex (head down) or a transverse presentation into a footling breech. The name "internal podalic version" is commonly abbreviated to "version." Except for assistance with a breech birth, version is the earliest known obstetrical operation. It was used in antiquity, lost for intervening centuries, and reintroduced in 1550, prior to the development of forceps. At that time, if labor was obstructed, the only way to extract the baby without using hooks was pulling it out by its feet. Cesareans were not done because mothers were not expected to survive major surgery.

Version should only be done by those experienced in its performance. Nowadays, the indication for it is the extraction of a second twin, soon after the birth of the first child, when this twin is not in a breech or vertex presentation. If a second twin presents in a transverse lie, internal podalic version is ordinarily relatively simple. The uterus is relaxed since the first twin has recently been delivered. Twins are usually smaller than other term babies and the foot or feet are readily grasped. The mother must be given appropriate anesthesia, but profound general anesthesia is usually not needed.

Induction of Labor

By induction of labor we mean bringing on labor before it has begun of its own accord. The reasons for doing this include conditions related to the mother's health, those related to the fetus, and sometimes reasons of convenience.

The commonest maternal reason for inducing labor is toxemia of pregnancy (high blood pressure with liver and kidney complications). When maternal blood pressure has been elevated for a considerable period of time and is not satisfactorily controlled, safety for the mother may require bringing the pregnancy to a close as soon as possible. When membranes rupture prematurely the risk or presence of infection may be a reason for induction. The common fetal reasons are fetal distress related to maternal diabetes, toxemia, or excessive prolongation of pregnancy past the expected date of confinement. Fetal anemia related to isoimmunization has become less usual as an indication for induction, because the routine use of Rhogam forestalls the occurrence of the disease.

Induction for convenience falls into two categories. When a fetal death has occurred in the third trimester but labor has failed to ensue within the proper waiting period of ten days to two weeks, labor may be induced. The convenience of the mother is the other possibility in this category.

I have strong feelings that induction should not be done for the convenience of the doctor or the mother's partner. Conflicts with a doctor's social schedule are not a reason to induce labor. Not every induction goes smoothly; if induction is done for some trivial purpose without the mother's full enthusiasm, there are sometimes reasons to be sorry.

I always plan to be present when my patients deliver. On occasion, however, I have other professional obligations that must be given priority, and when I do, I feel obliged to provide a proper alternate to take on my obstetrical responsibilities. I do not consider it justified to manipulate a patient's treatment to suit my personal convenience. The possibility that the patient's own attendant may be absent should always be explained early in the prenatal course so that the absence does not take her completely by surprise.

Necessary Conditions for Induction for Convenience

The baby must assuredly be at term and of term size. The pregnancy must be entirely normal. The infant should be presenting by the vertex with the head engaged in the pelvis and the membranes intact. The cervix should be soft and its opening in line with the vaginal axis. The cervix should be dilated to two to three centimeters so that there will be no difficulty in rupturing the membranes. When all these conditions have been met induction is begun by simply puncturing the membranes with an appropriate instrument and allowing labor to start.

When the conditions listed above are met, induced labor is in no way different from labor that has begun on its own. Completely normal patients on the brink of going into labor rarely require any assistance outside of rupture of the membranes. Labor may even be induced by introducing one finger into the cervical os, between the membranes and the inner lining of the cervix, and separating the membranes away from the cervix. This probably works by inducing the patient's own cervical production of prostaglandin; this is part of the onset of spontaneous labor.

Induction on Indication

It happens sometimes that there are medical reasons for induction of labor although all the ideal conditions for induction have not yet been met. One way to deal with this is to induce uterine contractions. The simplest method is breast stimulation, which results in the release of oxytocin and may induce sufficient contractions to tip the woman into labor. The same effect can be achieved by giving the patient oxytocin intravenously in minute but increasing amounts to bring about effective uterine contractions.

For reasons that I do not understand, induction of labor has become synonymous in the mind of the American lay public with the aggressive administration of oxytocin. There is no question that oxytocin is a potent drug and when used in excess can produce very painful contractions. On the other hand, large doses are certainly not essential to the success of induction. Indeed, a well-managed induction should in fact be no more uncomfortable than a spontaneous labor.

Labor can also be induced by the insertion of suppositories of prostaglandin PGE_2 into the vagina. A vaginal gel, containing the same prostaglandin, is in the final phases of study for induction purposes. This preparation softens the cervix and tends to encourage its dilation at the same time that it induces uterine contractions. A substantial portion of the patients treated with prostaglandin PGE_2 goes into labor. Others may become more prepared for an induction by rupture of the membranes. Other prostaglandin preparations for this purpose are under investigation.

On occasion there is reason to induce while the cervix is still less than one centimeter dilated, a rather unfavorable condition. Under those circumstances it may be possible to rupture membranes and wait twelve to eighteen hours in the expectation that spontaneous labor will follow. This method of inducing labor should not be undertaken if it is not possible to follow it up by cesarean if the induction fails.

We generally make our decisions on inducibility by pelvic examination and palpation of the cervix to establish what is called a Bishop score, which is derived from observations on the length of the cervix, its dilation, and the level of the presenting part.

Cesarean Section

Cesarean section is done by making an incision in the lower abdomen, exposing and cutting into the uterus, and removing a child who is mature enough to survive. The uterus and the abdominal wall are then repaired.

Origin of Name

Pliny the Elder (A.D. 23–79) mentions the operation and states that it is the source of the surname of the Roman emperors, since "Caesar" is related to the Latin word for "cut," and it is romantically assumed that Julius Caesar (c. 100–44 B.C.) was "cut" from his mother's womb. It seems highly improbable that he was born in this way: first, because his mother survived his birth for many years, and cesareans at this time were almost certainly never done on living women; and, second, because the ancients favored a very different origin for the name of their emperors. In the Punic language, *caesar* meant elephant, and since Julius once slew an elephant he was probably given this heroic sobriquet, which passed on to his successors.

Another improbable derivation for the term "cesarean section" is the claim that at about 750 B.C., during the reign of Numa Pompilius, a law was passed which made it obligatory to open the belly of any woman who died near term in order to rescue the infant from its uterine grave. Originally codified as *lex regia*, under the emperors it became *lex caesarea*. It would have been a most remarkable law if it had been enacted in this, the earliest period of Roman history; however, its authenticity is highly questionable. And so it remains totally uncertain as to how the operation got its name.

History of the Operation

The early history of the operation is equally vague. What did Pliny know about it? Was it ever done in his day? Was there a law in antiquity in regard to post-mortem cesarean sections? There are uncertain references to cesarean sections in the Talmud, the book of Jewish post-Biblical law and lore written between A.D. 76 and about A.D. 200. Do these references in the Talmud to women who survived after being delivered by *"yoze dofan,"* a "cut in the side," mean that women actually lived after cesarean section almost two thousand years ago?

It is somewhat apocryphally reported that in 1500 Jacob Nufer, a swine-gelder, wiped his butcher's knife on his Swiss Alpine trousers and before a gallery of thirteen midwives delivered his own wife by cesarean section. Frau Nufer is said to have survived the operation and subsequently presented the bold Jacob with two more children, born normally.

Postmortem (Latin: "afterdeath") cesarean was probably freely practiced in antiquity; unquestionably it was widely used in the late medieval period and the early Renaissance.

The first detailed report of a cesarean on a living woman was the account of an operation done in Germany in 1610.

Of the thirty-eight cesarean operations performed in Great Britain from 1739 to 1845, a period of more than a century, but four women recovered.

According to the researches of the preeminent medical historian, the late Colonel Fielding H. Garrison, the first cesarean in this country was performed by Dr. Jessee Bennett in rural Virginia. The surgeon-husband did not publish a report of the remarkable feat, and several years later, when asked why, he replied that no doctor with any feelings of delicacy would report an operation that he had done on his own wife, and added that no strange doctors would believe that operations could be done in the Virginia backwoods and the mother live, and he'd be damned if he would give them a chance to call him a liar.

On January 14, 1794, in a frontier settlement of the Shenandoah Valley, Mrs. Bennett was confined in her first pregnancy. Labor was difficult because of a contracted pelvis, and neither her husband nor the consulting doctor was successful in the attempt at delivery by forceps. The choice lay between a destructive operation on the child, its death and piecemeal removal, and a cesarean section. The patient chose the latter and, since the other doctor firmly refused to have anything to do with so dangerous a procedure, the unpleasant task fell to the husband. The patient, stretched on a crude plank table, was put under the influence of a large dose of opium. Assisted by two women, Dr. Bennett laid open the abdomen and uterus with a single, reckless stroke of the knife and rapidly delivered his daughter, who was still alive. He paused long enough to remove both of his wife's ovaries. As one of the witnesses declared, "He spayed her, remarking as he did so, 'This shall be the last one.'" The wound was closed with stout linen thread and, contrary to expectation, mother and child did well. The first cesarean-section baby in this country lived to be seventy-three.

Before 1876 few women survived a cesarean birth by many days, partly because of the crude surgery of that period and partly because the operation was reserved for desperately ill women—women who had labored for days and who were already profoundly infected. In that year Professor Edoardo Porro of Pavia contended that it would be best to remove the whole uterus at the time of the operation, for with the removal of the large wounded organ the chance for postoperative hemorrhage and inflammation would be lessened. The wisdom of Porro's teaching soon became obvious; however, the great drawback to his technique was the fact that it rendered the woman permanently sterile. Today this type of cesarean section, removal of the uterus after its incision to deliver the baby, is referred to as a cesarean hysterectomy.

In 1882, twenty-nine-year-old, red-headed Max Sänger, then a lowly *Privatdozent* in Leipzig, published an epoch-making two-hundred-page treatise on *Der Kaiserschnitt* (The Cesarean Section). He called attention to the importance of sewing the uterine incision firmly together again after cutting open the uterus to deliver the baby. Of course it had always been customary to suture (sew) the wound in the abdomen, but previous to Sänger's contribution the unsutured uterus was dropped back in the abdomen, to remain there a constant source of danger— danger from hemorrhage and danger from growth of bacteria out of the open uterine wound into the abdominal cavity. An American, Harris, and others too, had suggested stitching the uterine incision together, but they did not suggest the orderly and thorough way that Sänger evolved and published. Since Sänger's operation was only a refinement of the old type of cesarean, and since it did not remove the uterus, it is referred to as either the classical or the conservative cesarean section.

Because of dissatisfaction with the results of Sänger's operation if performed on women who had been in labor for several hours, Frank of Cologne brought forth the low cervical cesarean in 1907. Frank's new technique consisted of freeing the bladder from its filmy attachment to the lower portion of the uterus (the low cervical segment), then pushing the bladder out of the way, down in the pelvis, and incising the uterus through the area from which the bladder had just been dissected free. After child and placenta are removed, the wound in the uterus is sewn together, and then the bladder drawn up and tacked by sutures in its original position. This seals off the uterine wound from the abdominal cavity by plastering the bladder entirely over it. It is like putting a large rubber patch over an inflated ball whose edges had previously been cemented together.

Modern Results

The results of cesarean section at the present day are a far cry from those of eighty and even twenty years ago. We no longer wait to operate until all else has failed, and cesarean is no longer being done as part of the treatment for medical conditions in the mother. Most (though not all) operations are done to protect the welfare of the fetus. Most of the mothers are in excellent condition and well prepared to stand the rigors of a major operation. The use of blood transfusion, improved techniques of anesthesia, and antibiotics have all done much to reduce the serious risks of section.

Another significant feature contributing substantially to the present safety of cesarean section is the use of a uterine incision in the thin, lowermost portion of the uterus, commonly called a cervical or lower-segment cesarean section. This operation has almost completely replaced the classical section, in which the incision is made in the muscular, thicker body of the uterus. The bleeding and the likelihood of uterine infection are greater with a classical incision, and disruption of the uterine incision in a subsequent pregnancy is much more of a threat than when the incision is made in the lower segment of the uterus. Finally, the recovery from a lower-segment section is much quicker and smoother than with the classical section.

The lower-segment operation is done through either a longitudinal skin incision (lengthwise from the pubic area to the navel) or a transverse incision (from side to side across the lowermost portion of the abdomen). What is really of importance is not the skin incision but the incision in the uterus itself. I have never managed to get used to calling the transverse incision the "Bikini cut." This overemphasizes the cosmetic aspects of the incision and tends to reduce the mother to the status of a sex object. Nevertheless, I do strongly prefer the transverse (Pfannenstiehl) skin incision, because it hurts less and heals more dependably.

Cesarean offers the baby as good a chance as a normal vaginal delivery and a better chance of uncomplicated survival than does a difficult vaginal delivery.

The Operation

It requires about three-quarters of an hour to perform a cesarean section. A longitudinal (lengthwise) skin incision takes a few minutes less than the preferable low-transverse incision. In either event, the operator makes an incision with a knife through the skin and the fat down to the glistening tough white connective tissue of the abdominal wall, called the fascia. In a longitudinal incision the fascia is then divided from a point slightly below the navel down to the pubic bone. The muscles beneath this incision are pulled apart gently. Using scissors, the operator divides the peritoneum longitudinally in the midline, exposing the uterus.

Prior to cleansing the skin of the abdominal wall and placing sterile drapes over it, a catheter is inserted into the bladder to keep it empty and out of the way during the operation. The catheter may or may not be removed at the conclusion of the cesarean.

With a transverse incision the skin is incised at the upper margin of the pubic hair. Your doctor may wish to have the hair shaved or clipped with clippers before doing the surgery. I am satisfied that this step is unnecessary, and I simply make the incision just a little bit below the upper limits of the hairline.

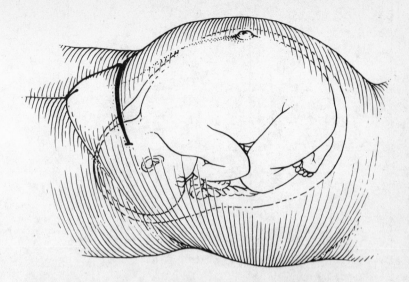

A semitransparent sketch of mother and fetus on the operating table to show the location of a transverse skin incision for cesarean. The mother's head is to the right. Sometimes the incision in the skin is lengthwise, from the mother's navel (seen in the drawing over the baby's back) down to the level of the mother's pubic hair line.

If the incision is transverse the tough fascia is divided with scissors to either side. Then the muscles are loosened from their attachment to the fascia and pulled apart, much as with the longitudinal incision. The peritoneum is then opened, exposing the uterus.

If a classical incision is to be done the operator cuts the uterine wall longitudinally with scalpel or the scissors for a distance of about six inches. If this incision comes down on the placenta the placenta is either pushed out of the way or cut.

With the lower-segment incision the operator identifies the point where the bladder lies loosely low down over the uterine wall. The flimsy attachment makes it possible for the bladder to fill and empty. The thin peritoneal covering of the uterus just above the bladder attachment is then incised and opened with scissors in a transverse direction. The bladder can easily

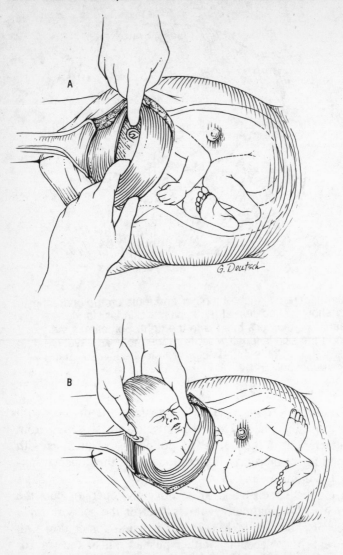

In these two illustrations, the mother is on the operating table in the same position and her navel is shown. The abdominal wall has been cut and is held out of the way by the instrument seen inside and low in the mother's abdominal cavity. The bladder has been pushed down off the uterus, and in A the surgeon's fingers are enlarging the uterine incision by stretching it to the right and left. In B the baby is being delivered through the uterine opening thus created.

be pushed off the wall of the uterus, down into the pelvis, and tucked away behind a retractor. In the area cleared of the bladder, an incision approximately six inches in length is made transversely in the lower segment. If the membranes are still intact, they will bulge into the incision. If necessary, the incision can be enlarged with the operator's fingers or with scissors, to make it large enough to bring the baby through.

When membranes have previously been ruptured there may not be much fluid. Intact membranes are incised with a gentle flick of the scalpel and the fluid allowed to drain.

Delivery of the Baby

The operator, using a hand or a single blade of a forceps, gently shoehorns the infant's head out of the incision and then delivers the rest of the child.

If the baby's head is deep in the pelvis because the cesarean is being done when labor is well advanced, it may be necessary for an assistant to reach into the vagina and push the baby's head up from below, to facilitate its delivery.

If the baby presents as a transverse or a breech it is delivered by breech extraction or partial internal version and breech extraction through the incision in the lower segment.

The baby's umbilical cord ordinarily is clamped and cut promptly and the baby handed to a pediatrician, so that the operating team can devote its attention to the uterine incision, which commonly bleeds quite profusely at this time. Clamps are placed on the edges to limit the bleeding. The placenta is removed from the opened uterus through the incision from which the baby has just come. Oxytocin is usually administered at this time, either intramuscularly or intravenously, to enhance uterine contraction.

Closing the Incision

The wound in the uterus is ordinarily closed with two rows of sutures to bring the raw edges of the uterine incision together and thereby to stop the bleeding. There are almost as many ways of repairing the uterus as there are surgeons who know how to do cesareans, and no one way is known to be superior to any other. My own choice is for the simplest possible repair. Since I have only infrequently done repeat sections for patients on whom I have previously operated, I cannot bear competent witness as to whether the technique of repair that I have described works better than other, more complicated ones.

The incision made in the peritoneum to push the bladder off the uterus is then closed with the simplest kind of sewing. The operator next inspects the fallopian tubes and ovaries to be certain they are normal.

Closure of the abdominal wall is done in the same way as in other abdominal surgery. I use a simple suture in the peritoneal layer of the abdominal wall, although this step may be unnecessary. I let the muscles fall together, and carefully repair the fascia with sutures. The skin can be closed with a layer of stitches, which are subsequently removed, or with a fine suture, which remains and is absorbed. Some surgeons use stainless-steel staples. Healing is extraordinarily rapid in the absence of infection. Sutures and staples can be removed in a few days after the completion of the operation.

At present, anesthesia for cesarean is most frequently epidural; spinal anesthesia is also suitable for cesarean section. General anesthesia is equally satisfactory. Both conduction and general anesthesia produce the needed relaxation of the mother's abdominal wall. When general anesthesia is used, the mother is put to sleep for only a brief interval. The medicines next used to paralyze her muscles do not cross the placenta to the fetus. Thus the baby gets minimal exposure to the drugs. There is virtually no perceptible effect of the general anesthesia on the newborn. This is also true with epidural and spinal. Traces of the anesthetic agents can later be found in the baby's blood but they produce no clinical effect.

The blood loss at cesarean is between a pint and a quart. Pregnant women tolerate blood loss of this magnitude remarkably well and ordinarily do not require blood transfusion. When the operation is done for a bleeding problem such as placenta previa or premature separation of the placenta, blood loss may be much greater and it then may be necessary to give blood. Our anesthetists usually administer a quart of intravenous solution rapidly to the mother prior to section as a preventive measure. This helps to assure an adequate volume of maternal blood.

Complications Due to Cesarean

Cesarean is a major abdominal operation; the usual complications of such surgery may occur, but since almost all mothers
are young and healthy, these difficulties are infrequently encountered.

The most common worries are infection of the uterus and
of the incision in the abdominal wall. These are usually due
to the mother's own bacteria. They are more frequent when
the cesarean is done to treat intrauterine infection (chorioamnionitis) or when labor is advanced. Response to antibiotics is
ordinarily prompt and recovery hardly delayed. Breast feeding
is not interfered with.

As noted, there is substantial blood loss at cesarean. This
results in anemia, which is best treated by oral iron tablets and
a good diet.

Recovery from Cesarean

Now that we have learned the virtues of early ambulation, if
the section is done early in the day the patients are encouraged
to get up out of bed and move around on the same day. If the
operation is done late in the day or at the end of a long and
uncomfortable labor the ambulation may be postponed until
the next day. Abdominal dressings have become smaller and
smaller. I myself have not used any at all for thirty-five years.
This makes it possible for the patient to take a shower the day
after the operation. If she is not ill, the mother can take a
regular diet as soon as she has an appetite.

The patient can care for her baby and can begin breast-
feeding whenever she feels up to it. The stay in the hospital
has become shorter following a cesarean just as it has done
following normal birth. For those patients motivated to do so,
who feel well and have recovered rapidly, I have seen no harm
come from having them go home as early as the third day after
cesarean. However, if the patient is anemic following a cesarean and requires additional bed rest before going home to
take on household tasks and the feeding of a new baby, she
should stay longer and regain her strength.

Advice on activity, exercises, and resumption of sexual activity are exactly the same for a patient following a cesarean as they are for a normal birth.

There is no medical reason now known to delay starting a new pregnancy following a cesarean birth. The uterine wound will have plenty of time to heal, and will do so quickly enough. I am speaking now of the incision in the uterus since this, and not the skin incision, will determine how the uterus fares in the next pregnancy.

Indications for Cesarean

The commonest reason for cesarean at present is the failure of the labor to make normal progress despite appropriate treatment. Until recently this failure was believed to be almost entirely due to inadequate space in the pelvis for the baby's head, but this explanation is no longer generally accepted. Sometimes, indeed, a baby of prodigious size fails to fit, but even in this case the diagnosis is not simple, because large babies stretch the uterus to the point where it is inefficient. The commonest reason for failure to progress in labor is in fact insufficient uterine action, which may persist even when the uterus is stimulated with intravenous oxytocin. If the cervix fails to achieve full dilation and medical stimulation and hopeful procrastination do not bring about delivery within a reasonable time, it is wise simply to terminate the labor abdominally. I am convinced that good labor should result in delivery in a matter of twelve hours and that labor longer than this is likely to be associated with poor maternal and fetal outcomes.

Cesarean sections are also done for abnormal presentations of the fetus. In the most striking form, the long axis of the baby is at right angles to the long axis of the mother, a transverse lie. With this lie, the mechanics of labor are such that a term baby is unlikely to be born alive not only because it does not fit through the pelvis when it is lying in this way but because in this position accidents to the umbilical cord are very common. As I have mentioned, in a breech presentation with the breech out of the pelvis, and an increased likelihood of cord prolapse, the decision is frequently made to deliver the baby abdominally.

Another reason for doing a cesarean is obstruction to the birth canal by maternal soft tissues. This may be due to an ovarian or uterine tumor that has dropped into the pelvis below the presenting part. Abnormalities of uterine and vaginal development can result in midline walls in the uterus and vagina that obstruct passage of the fetus.

Severe toxemia of pregnancy and other forms of pregnancy-induced hypertension may imperil the mother's health unless it is possible to accomplish medical control. It may be necessary to deliver the mother to eliminate the stress of pregnancy on her cardiovascular system and prevent a stroke.

Approximately once in every two hundred deliveries the placenta is located in the lower segment and over the cervix, preceding the presenting part and resulting in inevitable hemorrhage when the cervix dilates. This is often treated by abdominal delivery. Another abnormality, the premature separation of a normally implanted placenta, may result in reduction in the exchange of gases and transfer of nutrients to the fetus on such a scale that the delivery should be hastened.

Fetal Reasons for Cesarean

Another group of indications for cesarean section are those situations where disease of the mother secondarily results in problems for the baby. Examples of this are: inadequately controlled diabetes; active herpes type II infections, so situated that delivery of the baby past an infected area may infect the baby; an infection in the uterine cavity, usually as a result of premature rupture of the membranes.

Idiopathic thrombocytopenic purpura (*idiopathic*, "of unknown cause"; *thrombocytopenic*, "reduced number of platelets in the blood"; *purpura*, "purplish spots due to bleeding under the skin") may be a reason for section. ITP is an autoimmune disease, in which the mother's blood contains an antibody that damages her platelets and interferes with normal clotting of her blood. This antibody can cross the placenta and affect the baby similarly, in which case the stresses of labor may cause fetal bleeding. If it can be shown that the baby is likely to have ITP, then cesarean delivery is chosen.

In some instances of severe isoimmunization there is strong evidence that the baby is profoundly anemic and needs to be delivered well in advance of term. If the mother is not suitable for induction of labor, the delivery may have to be carried out abdominally.

When a mother's pregnancy has gone two or more weeks past full term there may be evidence of fetal stress, which can be so serious as to contraindicate labor. In this case induction of labor is inappropriate and the baby should be delivered by cesarean after adequate proof of the diagnosis by sonographic study.

The commonest fetal indication for cesarean at present is fetal distress. This diagnosis is usually made after the patient has fallen into labor and monitoring has demonstrated an abnormal and steadily worsening fetal heart rate pattern. This diagnosis is not easy to make with certainty except in extreme cases. When the diagnosis is difficult to establish by monitoring, sonography may be helpful, and a blood sample from the baby's scalp can be analyzed to determine whether or not it is developing acidosis.

Studies are presently underway to learn whether stopping labor when early signs of fetal distress appear will allow the baby figuratively to catch its breath and recover. The great majority of these babies are subsequently born by section and emerge in good condition. Not enough such cases have thus far been studied to allow us to judge whether there is actually benefit to the fetus from arresting the labor in these circumstances.

Cesarean for Previous Cesarean

Finally, one of the commoner reasons for cesarean at present is that the last delivery was by section. Certainly if the condition that necessitated the previous cesarean section is still present the operation should be repeated. On the other hand, a brief review of the indications for section I have just listed will show that most of them are present only for that pregnancy and are not likely to recur.

Seventy years ago cesarean sections were done under very

different conditions from those at present. Virtually all those cesareans were done through a classical incision. The threat of disruption of the uterus at the site of the classical scar in a subsequent labor was considered so great that labor following previous section was not allowed.

The likelihood that the uterine scar of a previous cesarean incision will rupture during a subsequent pregnancy, either before or during labor, is about 2 per 100, whether the prior section was classical or lower-segment transverse. The significant differences between the two are in the consequences of a rupture should it occur.

The classical scar in the upper muscular body of the uterus can tear directly into the peritoneal cavity. About 40 percent of the time the placenta is implanted on the front wall of the uterus under the scar and the rupture therefore initiates placental separation and consequent hemorrhage. Contractions of the uterus tend to push placenta and baby out through the defect— much like squirting the seeds out of a grape—whether or not the patient is in labor. If the placenta is on the back wall of the uterus, the baby is delivered into the peritoneal cavity and the placenta follows. The separation of the placenta cuts the baby off from its maternal support system and the fetus is likely to die of asphyxia before it can be rescued by an abdominal operation. The inevitable serious hemorrhage in the mother due to this calamity results in a hundredfold increase in the maternal death rate.

When a previous cervical scar ruptures, the body of the uterus remains intact. Its contractions, instead of causing the fetus to erupt into the peritoneal cavity, simply continue to push the baby down further into the birth canal. A cervical rupture is not into the peritoneal cavity but rather is located behind the bladder. Since the placenta and its blood supply are in the body of the uterus, placental separation does not take place and bleeding is usually negligible. The baby remains in a position from which it can readily be delivered. The risks to mother and baby are only slightly greater than those of a normal pregnancy.

I consider the risks to mother and fetus from the rupture of a classical section incision to exceed by far what is acceptable in present-day obstetrics. I therefore do a repeat section seven to ten days before term, or, if necessary, when labor begins. Almost half of the ruptures occur during labor.

It used also to be accepted as a truism that a mother who had had a cesarean section could not be allowed to have more than two more sections. This has also turned out to be a superstitious belief. Nor is the previous incision likely to be disrupted by a later twin pregnancy, by the presence of hydramnios, or by the stretching of the uterus to accommodate a baby much larger than the previous one. With proper precautions, too, stimulating labor does not increase the likelihood of disrupting the scar.

In most of the studies in which patients with previous cervical sections have gone into labor, 60 to 70 percent deliver normally and uneventfully, provided the reason for the previous section no longer exists. When I deliver a patient who has previously been sectioned, I make it a point to feel the scar inside the uterus immediately after the birth of the baby, to be certain that it has remained intact. This information is of value in deciding the route of delivery in the next pregnancy.

Disruptions of lower segment scars are rarely responsible for maternal bleeding. The fetus seldom experiences any difficulty due to its mother's previous cesarean.

Labor Following Previous Section

Under all these circumstances my management of patients with previous cervical section is to await the onset of labor and to expect the labor to be completed normally. If the woman, for example, repeats a previous pattern of failure to progress and again does not respond to treatment then I do not hesitate to repeat the section.

Previous cesarean is associated with an increased incidence of placenta previa, in which the placenta descends ahead of the baby; this may then be an independent indication for section. Patients who have previously delivered only by section and who then deliver normally are naturally pleased to find that the recovery from a normal birth is more comfortable and speedier than recovery from an abdominal delivery.

An organization using the acronym of VBAC (Vaginal Birth After Cesarean) has undertaken a vigorous educational campaign to persuade women to seek care from hospitals and physicians who are prepared to supervise a normal birth following previous cesarean section. This management has been a standard practice in Europe for the last generation, so that we do have ample information as to its safety. It is nevertheless still true that in the United States, nine out of ten women with previous sections are delivered by section again.

Elective and Emergency Sections

Cesareans that can be planned in advance and done by appointment are referred to as elective sections. Those that are decided upon after the patient has gone into labor or done without advance plan, for such events as hemorrhage from placenta previa or prolapse of the umbilical cord, are classified as emergency sections.

Elective section should be done as late as possible, either at term or as close as can be managed, to give the infant a chance to achieve maximum maturity. For this purpose we need as accurate a reading as we can get of the duration of the pregnancy. This is not too difficult if we have been following the patient from the early stages and recording the findings as we go along. Sonography also is a useful and accurate tool for establishing the duration of pregnancy. But if we are not able to determine the duration of pregnancy by any kind of physical observation, doing the cesarean should wait until the patient goes into labor; then we know that the pregnancy has gone as far as it can go.

How Many Cesarean Sections Can a Woman Have?

At present there is no limit to the number of cervical cesarean sections that can be done with safety to the mother. The operation generally heals so well that on occasion it is difficult at repeat operation to find a scar in the uterus. The abdominal wall withstands repeated incisions remarkably well. The limiting factor on the number of cesareans therefore now appears to be the mother's willingness to experience repeated operations.

Many people without training tend to think that a new incision is made with each cesarean section. This is not the case.

We usually go through the site of the previous incision and, if there is a substantial skin scar, remove it. There is therefore no external evidence of the number of cesareans that have been done.

On the other hand, cesarean is a major operation and my own conviction is that the patient has a perfect right to decide how many such operations she will have. There is no added risk to sterilizing the patient at the time of cesarean, if she decides she wants it done, although the state where she lives may require specific procedures to be followed as a condition to elective sterilization.

Incidence of Cesarean Section

Cesarean section incidence has risen gradually over the last decade. For the entire United States it is now about 15 percent of all births, and in many obstetrical hospitals it now exceeds 25 percent of all deliveries. In light of our knowledge that it is not mandatory to repeat all cesarean sections, the rate of the repeat operation should decline but the incidence of first cesareans—called primary sections—continues slowly to increase.

A substantial argument for this increased incidence of cesarean is the observation that it has been associated with a steady decrease in the rate of fetal loss in the perinatal period. There is accumulating evidence, however, that the matter is not as simple as it would seem. A large maternity hospital in Indianapolis has reported that, over the period of nine years, from 1973 to 1982, its rate of primary cesarean section has remained at less than 5 percent. The uncorrected fetal loss rate (which includes the cases of congenital defect that would have succumbed regardless of the route of delivery) decreased from 35 per 1,000 to 18 per 1,000. The authors of this study attribute the improvement in outcomes to better neonatal care, a factor entirely independent of any change in the rate of primary cesarean section.

A similar experience has been reported by a large maternity hospital in Dublin, where the cesarean section rate has also remained under 5 percent from 1965 to 1980. Considering all babies born weighing more than one pound in that hospital, the perinatal loss rate dropped from approximately 42 in 1965 to about 17 in 1980. In close to 9,000 births in 1980 the cesarean section rate was 4.8 percent. These authors only encountered four cases of what they considered obstructed labor, all with very large infants.

It has been suggested that birth by cesarean is of particular benefit to premature babies in view of their relative fragility. Two fairly large studies have been reported in which the babies were sorted out by birth weight, mode of presentation, and type of delivery. It emerged that there was no real difference in the outcome between vaginal birth and cesarean for either vertex presentations or breeches in any weight group. What seems to make the major difference to the baby's prospects is its maturity, and not the route by which it is delivered.

Incidence of Obstetrical Interventions in Other Countries

We have recently had the results of a large-scale survey of obstetrical interventions in the major countries of Western Europe. The incidence of cesarean section varies from 3.6 percent in Holland to 11.9 percent in Finland, and comparable rates in the other Scandinavian countries. The rates of operative vaginal deliveries (forceps and vacuum extraction) in contrast were highest in France and in the United Kingdom. Among operative vaginal deliveries, forceps were twice as frequent as vacuum extractions in France. Vacuum extractions were more than ten times more frequent than forceps operations in Denmark, and in Sweden the ratio was more than twenty to one. In Norway, however, the rates for forceps and vacuum extractions were about equal.

Overall, the rate of total interventions in most of the countries in Western Europe ranged from 10 to 20 percent. Poland, The Netherlands, and Czechoslovakia were the only countries with the rates of total interventions less than 10 percent. West Germany had a 25.6 percent rate of total intervention: the highest among the countries surveyed. This consisted of 12.7 percent cesarean sections and 12.9 percent of operative vaginal deliveries, the greatest proportion of the latter being vacuum extractions.

In summary, then, the various countries of Europe do not show any uniformity in the use of operative delivery. Perinatal mortality appears to be somewhat lower in the countries with higher rates of cesarean section. There is a suggestion of a slight relationship between the frequency of operative vaginal deliveries and of cesarean section, in that the two rates seem to rise together.

18

Convalescence after Childbirth

Physiological Changes

The puerperium (Latin: "having brought forth a child") is the period of several weeks that starts immediately after delivery and is completed when the reproductive tract has fully returned to its nonpregnant state. It is a period of rapid recuperation and readjustment from pregnancy to nonpregnancy. Physiologically it is distinguished by two conspicuous phenomena: the return of the uterus to its nongravid condition, and the appearance of milk in the breasts—though many less-obvious alterations occur, such as diminution in blood volume and the loss of excess tissue fluid.

The Uterus Shrinks to Nonpregnant Size

When the puerperium begins, the uterus is a two-pound mass of muscle, and by the end of six weeks it has shrunk to three ounces. During the first few days of the puerperium it is a smooth, hard, gourd-shaped organ with its apex a few inches below the navel. By the end of the first week it weighs one pound and has descended to two inches above the symphysis (the bone forming the front of the pelvic girdle). By the tenth day its top can just be felt above the symphysis, and after this it sinks within the pelvis and can no longer be felt in the abdomen. The process of shrinkage (involution) progresses more rapidly in a woman who nurses. The diminution in size and weight continues, and after five or six weeks the uterus is once more the size and weight of a pear. This cycle of growth followed by involution, which the uterus repetitively undergoes in each pregnancy and puerperium, is unique in physiology. No other organ multiplies itself more than tenfold and then regresses back to its basic size. The growth is caused by a vast increase in the size of each individual muscle fiber forming the uterus, not by an increase in the number of fibers, and involution involves divestment by each cell of the additional cytoplasmic material.

Puerperal Vaginal Discharge

The puerperal vaginal discharge, called lochia (Greek: "pertaining to childbirth"), has a bright-red blood color for the first three or four days; from the fourth to the tenth day it becomes paler and pinkish; and from about the tenth day on it is yellow-white, often with a little blood admixed. Ordinarily all discharge disappears between the third and fourth weeks. The total fluid and tissue lost through the lochia has been collected and weighs eight to nine ounces. The lochia is often incorrectly called menstruation; the origin and constitution of the two are very different.

For the first few days after delivery it is comfortable to wear a perineal pad; the amount of bleeding is likely to be such that you will need a large-size pad. Once the volume of lochia has decreased to that of an ordinary menstrual period it is safe to switch to vaginal tampons. But be warned that tampons should not be left in place for longer than six hours. There is strong evidence that the toxic shock syndrome associated with the use of high-absorbency tampons is really due to leaving the tampons in place long enough for bacteria to grow within the tampon, using for their nourishment the menstrual discharge itself.

Since the lochial discharge comes from the uterus there is nothing to be accomplished by using vaginal douches or deodorant sprays.

Return of Menstruation

True menstruation first returns at variable times after delivery. If the woman does not suckle her child, the menses usually reappear within four to eight weeks. In the woman who nurses there is the most extraordinary variability; the menses may return at any time from the second to the eighteenth month, the average being five months. One study found that 90 percent of nonlactating women and 30 percent of nursing mothers had a return of the menses within three months after childbirth. In both groups the amount of bleeding and the interval between the periods may be quite unusual for the first several months. In some, it appears that the rhythm-producing mechanism requires an adjustment period for complete regulation. Painful menstruation, dysmenorrhea, is almost always improved by a pregnancy; in many the pain, which may have been incapacitating, never returns.

Bleeding in the period before the resumption of real menstruation is sometimes erratic. Your postpartum bleeding may come to a quiet end, only to resume a few weeks later for a day or two. Even as late as six months after delivery brief periods of unusual bleeding may appear without warning. If the bleeding exceeds what you were accustomed to before delivery in the first two days of menses and persists, consult your doctor.

Increased Urination

One of the more striking phenomena of the puerperium is the marked increase in urinary output that commonly occurs somewhere between the second and the fifth day after delivery. Normal pregnancy is associated with a large increase of blood volume, consisting mostly of water. After delivery, the body acts to eliminate this excess water load. This does not actually result in a complete loss of edema in all patients. Sometimes a woman who has not noted any swelling of the ankles prior to delivery may be dismayed by having her feet puff up on the second or third day after the baby is born. It is not understood why this takes place but it certainly is both harmless and transient.

Lactation

During pregnancy breasts are prepared for the secretion of milk by the influence of the estrogen and progesterone produced by the placenta. These hormones inhibit the release of prolactin from the pituitary at the same time that they promote the growth and specialization of the breast tissue for the formation of milk. When the placental hormones are abruptly withdrawn as the placenta is delivered, there is a prompt release of prolactin. This results in an increase in the formation of colostrum, the thin, sticky, pale fluid which is the precursor of milk. Newborns obviously find it delicious. It has the immediate benefit to them that it contains maternal antibodies that the mother herself has formed in resistance to bacteria and viruses.

Within the next two days milk formation begins in earnest. The breasts tend to enlarge further and their veins become more prominent. A hungry baby who is nursing well will minimize engorgement, or overfilling, of the breasts but even so, some mothers produce much more milk than the baby can consume. The breasts then overfill and become tender. There may also be aberrant breast tissue in the armpits (axillae). In lactation this too fills with milk, and may form painful lumps, especially if the ducts in this tissue lack drainage because they are not connected with the nipple.

Suckling results in the reflex release of oxytocin from the pituitary gland into the mother's blood. The oxytocin stimulates contraction of the fine muscle fibers that surround the lacteal ducts in the breasts, pumping the milk into the lacteal sinuses (storage spaces) behind the nipple. This phenomenon is called let-down, and the mother can feel it happen. It makes the milk in the duct system readily available to the infant. The uterus also responds to the oxytocin with contractions.

Back pressure in overfilled areas of the breast suppresses the further formation of milk, and the discomfort of engorgement gradually decreases. Emptying the breasts only encourages increased milk formation, but there is a nice balance: As the infant increases its milk intake, the production increases, but overproduction is automatically suppressed. When the breasts are overfilled and uncomfortable a good supportive brassiere and local ice packs will produce relief. It is futile for the mother to reduce her fluid intake. Milk is a secretion that will persist despite everything other than life-threatening dehydration.

By the same token, increased fluid intake does not effectively improve lactation. There is a firmly established mythology that drinking large quantities of beer is of value in increasing milk production. The water in the beer is of no greater value than water from any other source. The alcohol, on the other hand, tends to block oxytocin release and may thereby trivially inhibit let-down. This might make the breasts feel fuller, but the effect has never been tested scientifically.

Certainly calm mothers produce more milk and the sedative effect of alcohol is probably of value in this respect, just as it is in treating the insomnia of late pregnancy. The Pet Milk Company was quite right in its radio slogan that "you get more milk from contented cows."

Mastitis (infection of the breast tissue) does not occur in the immediate puerperium. An elevated temperature on the third or fourth postpartum day invariably has its origin elsewhere than in the breasts. This does not mean that engorged breasts may not be quite painful. The cure includes good support of the breasts with an adequate brassiere, ice packs, analgesics, and continuation of nursing. I do not believe that there is such an entity as "milk fever."

It is not necessary for a nursing mother to drink cow's milk. Indeed, there is no other mammal that drinks milk during its adult life, and the most successful milk producers, specifically dairy cattle, drink no milk at all. Milk is a pleasant beverage, which I happen to like—a nicely balanced food—and it can be made part of a well-rounded diet, but you need feel no qualms of conscience if you prefer to omit it from yours.

A woman's ability to produce milk cannot be gauged by physical examination or by laboratory tests. The size of the breasts or the amount of breast tissue seems to bear no relationship to this particular gift. The only index is the test of performance. As a rule, placid, emotionally stable women are better able to nurse than those who are tense.

Many substances taken by the mother promptly appear in

the milk. This is true of vegetable cathartics, antibodies, tranquilizers, sedatives, and alcohol. It is also true of most narcotic and addictive drugs. If alcohol is taken by a nursing woman in large quantities the baby's behavior may be affected, since it appears in approximately the same concentration in the milk as in the mother's blood. Certain foods such as garlic have strong odors that may show up in the milk and subsequently appear in the baby's breath, but the objections to this are purely esthetic.

Advantages of Breast-feeding

Mother's milk is easier for a baby to digest than cow's milk, even in the absence of a specific intolerance for the latter. The protein, fats, and carbohydrates in cow's milk are similar to those in human milk; for this reason cow's milk is the basis of almost all artificial feeding preparations, but human milk contains antibodies and white blood cells, not present in cow's milk, that protect the newborn against bacterial and viral infections. Gastroenteritis, one of the major killers of babies in Third World countries with warm climates, is almost nonexistent among breast-fed babies.

Breast-feeding necessitates intimate contact between the baby and the mother. As discussed elsewhere, this facilitates early bonding, allowing the baby and the mother to become familiar with the smell and sound of each other. The physical act of nursing is found to be sensually pleasing by many women. It is of course also materially less expensive than artificial feeding.

In addition to providing the newborn with valuable immunities, breast-feeding has beneficial physiological effects on the mother. The suckling stimulates a nervous reflex that releases oxytocin from the pituitary. Oxytocin has the dual effect of making the milk ducts release their milk into the nipple and of causing the uterus to contract. These contractions may be uncomfortable in women having second or later babies. A further effect of breast-feeding is that the mother goes into a state of hormonal dormancy in which she does not menstruate.

The nursing mother's pelvic organs thus return quite rapidly to their nonpregnant state. It has been known for centuries that suckling helps to control postpartum hemorrhage by inducing uterine contractions. Now that the mechanism is understood and drugs that will cause contractions are available in ampoule form, they can be given if it is impractical to have the mother nurse her baby.

The La Leche League

The La Leche League's purpose is to promote breast-feeding by providing assistance to mothers from women who have been successful breast feeders. The organization has been in existence for a bit less than thirty years and now has more than four thousand chapters all over the world. They offer support through publications and through counseling by telephone or by personal visit. The League avoids giving medical advice, although if you intend to breast-feed or indeed if you have begun and are having problems, you would do well to consult your local La Leche League chapter. You may find it listed in your local telephone directory under its name. You can find out whether there is a chapter in your area by writing to the La Leche League International, 9616 Minneapolis Avenue, Franklin Park, IL 60131.

Advantages of Bottle-feeding

The new mother, particularly if she is unfamiliar with the sensations of breast-feeding, needs reassurance that her baby is getting sufficient nourishment. Feeding from a bottle makes it possible to see how much the baby is taking at each feeding. Since normal and healthy babies make a steady and rapid increase in their feeds in first few days of life, this provides a visible proof that things are working as they should. Further, the mother who is not breast-feeding can turn the responsibility of feeding the baby over to someone else and this may increase her opportunity to rest. Bottle-feeding avoids problems with raw and cracked nipples, and the likelihood of a breast infection is virtually nil.

Refraining from nursing may preserve the shape of the breast. Pregnancy itself softens the breast whether or not it is used for baby feeding. However, sagging of the breasts is more common among women who have nursed, but by no means is present in every such woman. It can probably be minimized by wearing a well-fitted brassiere.

The Quality of Milk

The quality of the milk is dependent in part upon the food taken by the mother: A diet rich in protein increases the proportion of fat. A nursing mother does not have to stuff herself to feed her child adequately, but her diet should be increased and varied. The Food and Nutrition Board of the National Research Council issued pertinent dietary recommendations in 1970. For a five-foot-four-inch woman weighing 128 pounds it recommends 2,000 calories per day when not pregnant, 2,200 when pregnant, and 3,000 calories while nursing. The daily grams of protein required are 55, 65, and 75 respectively. Calcium intake should be increased from 0.8 grams to 1.2 grams and 1.3 grams each day. Alcohol in small amounts has no injurious effects either on the mother's milk or on the infant. Menstruation, contrary to some old wives' tales, exerts no serious effect on the quality of the milk. Human milk changes constantly to match the growing infant's dietary requirements.

Suppression of Lactation

Since milk forms whether or not the mother intends to nurse, there has been a search for ways to suppress lactation. Mechanical measures such as binding the breasts and intense ice packing simply do not work. All hormonal measures, most of which are effective, unfortunately have undesirable side effects. The recently developed drug bromocriptine (Parlodel), which suppresses formation of prolactin, promised to be ideal for the purpose of suppressing lactation, but in its turn it has been observed to be responsible for high blood pressure, seizures, and strokes.

The safest and surest method of suppressing lactation is simply not to nurse, and to endure the eighteen to twenty-four hours of discomfort due to the engorgement of the breasts. This can be relieved by good support of the breasts in an adequate brassiere and by moderate analgesics and ice packs. For a few days after the immediate period of discomfort has abated your breasts will be full but no longer painful. During this period you should not manipulate them nor express milk from them.

Conception While Nursing

Conception becomes possible when a ripe egg is released from a graafian follicle in the ovary. A temporary hormone-producing gland, the corpus luteum, forms in the follicular cavity from which the egg was shed. These events take place in response to follicle-stimulating hormone (FSH) and luteinizing (corpus luteum forming) hormone (LH). FSH and LH, the gonadotropins (from the Greek *gonos*, "genitals" and *tropos*, "change") come from the pituitary gland, which secretes them into the blood stream in a neatly timed sequence. The pituitary in its turn is regulated by gonadotropin releasing hormone (GnRH), a secretion from the hypothalamus.

Nursing sends messages via the nervous system to the hypothalamus at the base of the brain not to release any GnRH. As a consequence the pituitary and ovary are not stimulated, and remain dormant; thus, pregnancy cannot take place. Fertile ova are not released from the ovary and the woman does not menstruate. She is in a very low state of sex hormone secretion, which accelerates the shrinkage of the uterus back to its nonpregnant size.

An American woman who is supplying the baby with all its fluids and calories can rely on the contraceptive effect of nursing for the first three months. The time when a nursing mother resumes ovulation depends largely on the adequacy of her diet. In sub-Saharan Africa and Bangladesh, where most women are in a state of severe chronic malnutrition, return to fertility may not occur for two to three years after the birth of a baby if that baby is consistently nursed. In the United States, however, the richness of the diet is such that the ovaries return to normal cyclic activity much earlier. By four months postpartum a small proportion of women have begun to ovulate and will subsequently menstruate. By six months, even if nursing has continued, as many as 50 to 60 percent of nursing women will have ovulated. By one year the number ovulating is close to 100 percent. It is important to remember that a woman may start to ovulate while nursing and before menstruation has appeared. In a study of five hundred pregnancies, 9 percent of them occurred postpartum before the patient had resumed uterine bleeding.

Mechanical contraceptive devices such as condoms and diaphragms are perfectly safe to use after delivery, and obviously have no effect upon nursing. The same is true of intrauterine devices, but these should not be inserted before the fourth postpartum week, and then only if the uterus is firm; a danger of too early insertion is that the device may fall out.

Hormonal contraception, on the other hand, may have an effect upon the milk supply, although not always of serious magnitude. Oral combined (estrogen and progestogen) contraceptives cause a reduction in milk output in about one-third of the women who use this method, but the reduction is likely to be only temporary, and continued nursing normally will replenish the supply. Some hormone gets into the milk and is consumed by the baby, but the amounts are insignificant. A woman who wishes to use a hormonal contraceptive without risking a lessening of milk supply can take low-dose pills containing only progestins in a cyclical program. However, these low-dose pills are less effective as contraceptives than the combined orals.

Weaning the Baby

When you decide to stop breast-feeding, if the infant has not already made the decision for you, weaning can be abrupt or gradual. In the case of the former you can expect engorgement and leakage of milk for a few days. Gradual weaning is accomplished by stepwise replacement of breast-feeds by cow's milk in a bottle, spread out over as long a time as is convenient for mother and child.

An occasional woman leaks milk, from time to time, for months and even years after weaning. This is a medical problem only if it is associated with an absence of menses.

Weaning is made easier if it is possible to add or increase other foods in addition to milk in the child's diet.

Weight Loss

The average patient one hour after delivery weighs about 13.5 pounds less than before. An additional 3.5 pounds is lost between the first postpartum hour and the twelfth day, much of it increased tissue water. At the sixth week postpartum the gain in total weight above the prepregnant figure is made up of fat and, in those who nurse, also of breast tissue.

Loss of Hair Postpartum

Body hair, particularly head hair, grows in two phases. The anagen phase lasts three years, and about 90 percent of scalp hair is in that phase at any one time. The telagen phase is a resting period and usually lasts three months, after which those hairs fall out. However, in pregnancy all hair may enter the telagen phase. For this reason, a few months after delivery there can be a period of increased hair loss, but this does not exceed a small fraction of all body or scalp hair.

Medical Care during the Early Puerperium

Getting Up

A woman who has had a normal labor and delivery is literally able to get up and walk away from it. No special medical measures are needed. The internal organs resume their appropriate relationship immediately. The new mother can consume a hearty meal a half an hour after delivery if she is not too excited to eat. In short, delivery is not a disease state.

If she has delivered in a hospital that provides family-centered care, the new mother's partner will have been present at the birth and may wish to stay at her side for the next few days. This can be arranged for patients who are in private rooms. It is certainly true that labor is hard work and that the new mother has earned a period of rest. If she happens to have spent a good part of the night awake and in labor, she may need privacy for catching up on sleep. On the other hand, the mother may wish to share her achievement with her other children or with her parents or her friends. There is no strong medical reason for rigid restrictions on visitors.

The results of early ambulation have been excellent. There is no reason why a woman cannot be up and about, and it does wonders for her sense of well-being. She can take a shower and wash her hair. Bowel and bladder function return rapidly to normal, especially if the new mother is active. Women are clearly able to leave the hospital shortly after delivery, and the return to the supportive and familiar home environment is good for them. There is no need to isolate the newborn from relatives and friends even though the mother may need some rest. With all this, we seem to have settled down to a postpartum stay of about three days, although exceptional women want to and can depart in eight hours. Those who have had sections generally stay for five to seven days but there are some who choose to leave as early as three days and do not seem to come to harm.

Women with medical complications will have to proceed more gradually. Other patients will need to recover from the effects of anesthesia employed at the time of delivery. Those who have delivered by section have to manage the discomforts of an abdominal incision, but there is no reason medically to restrict their activity.

There are, however, those patients with special needs who are best served by a longer stay postpartum, notwithstanding general enthusiasm for early activity and early discharge. For the mother, if the birth has been normal, and she has been observed to be healthy at the sixth or so hour postpartum, there is no risk in going home as early as she likes. With the baby, however, it may be another matter. Conservative pediatricians, for example, are concerned with the possibility of conditions which, though rare, may precipitate a baby who is only twelve to eighteen hours old into severe and unpredictable distress. The specter of "crib death," the sudden infant death syndrome, lurks in the background of all discussions of early discharge from the hospital. New parents must be clearly advised of the risks, however remote, of early discharge and taught the precautions needed to minimize them. Certainly the mother should not go home early in the sole interest of saving money on the hospital bill, if her safety or that of the baby requires a longer stay.

Diet

Women who have delivered without general anesthesia can resume eating a normal diet as soon as they are hungry. Women who have had difficult cesarean sections and those who have had general anesthetics may have to deal with some degree of stomach upset, which usually manifests itself by nausea and an absence of appetite. Such patients should simply refrain from eating until normal appetite returns.

Exercises

The woman who has had an uneventful delivery can resume exercises as soon as she feels motivated to do so. There are a number of books available that describe exercises to be practiced after delivery. The ones that are of actual medical benefit are the ones that exercise the muscles of the abdominal wall. These muscles are inevitably stretched and spread apart by the growth of the fetus in the uterus, so that the abdominal wall suffers substantial loss of strength in the midline immediately after birth. The new mother can demonstrate this for herself by lying flat in bed and raising both feet off the bed with the legs stiffly extended. The midline bulge will then be readily visible.

What I have just described is, in fact, one of the better exercises to reduce the extent of this muscle separation, which is technically known as a diastasis recti. Doing sit-ups exercises the same muscles. Any other exercises can also be done if the mother enjoys doing them. There is no urgent medical reason either to do them or not to do them.

Afterpains

During the first few days of the puerperium most multiparas and some primiparas complain of afterpains. These usually begin soon after delivery but seldom last more than three days. They consist of painful contractions of the uterus, recurring irregularly and lasting about a minute. Afterpains are often initiated by the act of sucking, as noted earlier; whenever the child is put to the breast the uterus reacts by contracting, and such contractions may cause a spurt of lochia or the passage of a small clot. In most patients no therapy is required, but others must be repeatedly given codeine or some other analgesic.

The "Blues"

The medical literature of a generation ago paid considerable attention to the phenomenon of postpartum blues. This was described as feelings of sadness and tearfulness, which occurred without explanation to new mothers who had every reason to be happy. My impression is that this phenomenon has lessened in frequency and severity. I think this may be in part a consequence of the availability of effective contraceptives combined with the opportunity to abort unwanted pregnancies, so that the babies being born at present are really wanted and are welcomed into the family. Another possibility is that the patients are going home from the hospital so early that I simply do not see the women when they have the blues: It is taking place in the supportive environment of the home, leaving me blissfully unaware of its occurrence. But this explanation does not account for the patients who have had cesareans and stay in long enough to exhibit this transitory postpartum depression, but only rarely experience it.

Despite what I have just said, if you find yourself having unexpected spells of depression and weeping, by all means bring this up promptly and frankly with your doctor. In most instances simply bringing it out in the open and being reassured that it is not a sign of serious difficulty or psychiatric illness will be sufficient to help you to deal with the problem.

Personal Cleanliness

There is no reason for a new mother not to take a shower or shampoo her hair as soon as she feels steady on her feet.

Patients who have had sections may have an abdominal dressing that should be protected from getting wet, but if the dressing has been taken off or none has been put on there is no reason not to shower.

Care of Special Areas

The Vulva

This is the term used to describe the area of skin surrounding the entrance to the vagina. It includes the lips of the vagina—the outer labia majora (Latin: "larger lips"), which are covered by hair-bearing skin, and the inner labia minora (Latin: "smaller lips"), covered by hairless skin. Both have sweat glands. It also includes the sexual hair and the relatively hairless skin found between the entrance to the vagina and the anus. After delivery, the only care the vulva requires is a simple washing, best done in the shower. After a bowel movement the area can be washed off with a soapy washcloth and patted dry with a towel. Antiseptic rinses, ointments, and creams are unnecessary. The care is the same whether or not there has been an episiotomy or the repair of a perineal tear. If you have unusual pain in these parts of your body, you should bring it to the attention of the nurses or doctors.

You can minimize the discomfort of perineal repairs by walking and sitting normally. This functions to squeeze some of the swelling out of the area and relieve the local tension. A sitz bath (sitting in hot water for ten to fifteen minutes) will add to local comfort and is absolutely harmless.

Abdomen

The skin and the muscles of the abdominal wall are considerably stretched by pregnancy. The larger the uterus and its contents—for example, twins, excessive amniotic fluid, or a very big baby—the greater the likelihood of permanent changes in the skin and the muscles. However, both of these have a built-in tendency to return to the condition they were in prior to the pregnancy. As stated above, the muscles usually require exercise, and this is particularly true when they have been severely stretched. The skin, being more elastic, has a tendency to snap back by itself sooner or later, although the stretch marks of pregnancy may never vanish. Girdles and corsets have fortunately gone entirely out of fashion for postpartum wear. They functioned only as crutches and perpetuated the muscle weakness, which is much better dealt with by a conscientious program of exercises.

The Bladder

An obstetrical complication that frequently occurred in the days when forceps deliveries were common and were done under spinal or general anesthesia was urinary retention. The new mother was unable to void, and her bladder became severely stretched out. It was in that era that hospitals instituted the routine, which most still follow, of measuring the amount of urine passed in the first one or two voidings immediately following childbirth, and keeping track of the output in the first twenty-four to forty-eight hours postpartum. However, with the switch to minimal and local anesthesias and away from operative vaginal deliveries, urinary retention as a problem following normal deliveries is an unusual event.

Among patients who have had surgical deliveries or difficulty in vaginal birth, however, it is still necessary to take measures to protect them against urinary retention. For this the treatment is to install a catheter in the bladder, to drain urine continuously until the patient has fully recovered from anesthesia or from the effects of a difficult delivery. After eighteen to twenty-four hours, the catheter comes out and the patient ordinarily has no further problem.

The same treatment would be used in case a patient is unexpectedly unable to void after delivery for some other reason. In these cases it may be necessary to keep the catheter in place for as much as forty-eight to seventy-two hours, to allow the bladder wall to recover from the stretching it has undergone. Then, when the catheter is removed and the bladder again begins to fill, the patient experiences the normal sensations associated with the urge to urinate, and will be able to do so without difficulty.

The presence of a foreign body such as a catheter in the urethra and the bladder sets the stage for a urinary tract infection. For this reason it is good preventive practice to administer an antibiotic or a sulfa drug.

Bowels

Much as with bladder care, early ambulation, minimal trauma, and minimal anesthesia have virtually eliminated the severe postpartum constipation of decades back. The fact that the patient can rapidly return to normal exercise and normal eating habits allows her to return to ordinary toilet habits. This is true even when the patient has had an abdominal delivery. Patients with abdominal incisions and episiotomies find it difficult to believe that they can move their bowels without aggravating pain in the incisions, but it is really the case. As with voiding, the hospital staff makes inquiries of patients as to whether they have had a bowel movement and tend to look somewhat askance at the patient who has not done so. But even though the patient may go several days without having a bowel movement, she will probably be able to have it easily and spontaneously, without any treatment, once her intestinal tract returns to its normal level of activity.

Women who have had a long history of difficulty with constipation, of course, may need some help postpartum, but it is hardly an emergency. The help when given may consist of a small enema or a suppository. Stool softeners are probably less useful than stimulating bowel activity by resuming normal activity and normal eating habits.

Care at Home after Leaving the Hospital

I consider that the question of when a patient is ready to go home is a highly individual decision, personal to her. When she indicates that she is ready, I sit down with her and go through a series of suggestions for her guidance in self-care for the next several weeks. This presentation sounds roughly like this:

"When you go home you can be active within the limits of common sense. There is no reason to feel you have to be confined indoors. You ought not to push your activity to the point of feeling fatigued, because this will interfere with your getting sufficient rest to recover from the work of being in labor. Also, fatigue will interfere with your pleasure of taking care of your baby. Especially if you are going to be nursing, rest and tranquility are tremendous assets. Moderation in activity to begin with is the best general principle.

"Your diet can be pretty much whatever you enjoy. If you are going to be nursing you have to take additional calories and this we have discussed already. If you can be sure you are taking a well-rounded diet there is probably no need to take supplemental vitamins. But it probably would be wise for you to continue taking iron, since if you can keep the iron in your blood up at a high level the milk that you provide for the baby will also be rich in iron.

"Recreation away from home should be worked into your activities. There is no reason why you have to be condemned to cabin fever. If you can eat out once in a while or get away to the movies and just get a change in scenery that is all to the good. If you are breast-feeding, early on you will have difficulty going far because of the frequency of baby feeds, but you know this will pretty well take care of itself after a few weeks. Besides, you will be able to substitute a bottle for the breast every once in a while, to give yourself a little more time off.

"You can take showers or tub baths, whichever you prefer. These will provide all the cleansing your vagina and perineal area will need, but you may like to take a sitz bath from time to time if you are feeling perineal discomfort. If it is your preference to do so you can certainly switch from perineal pads to tampons. Please remember, however, not to leave tampons in longer than six hours at a time or at most overnight. The likelihood of having toxic shock syndrome is very much increased by leaving tampons in the vagina for long periods of time.

"I would like you to continue with the exercises I have shown you, to restore the tone of your abdominal muscles. These are the ones that involve holding your legs stiff and straight and raising them up off the bed, and doing sit-ups by raising your head and trunk. Both these exercises work the same set of muscles, and you can start them immediately. Some patients come to their follow-up visits and tell me they have not exercised because they felt too tired. Of course there is no change, or hardly any, in their abdominal muscle tone or the separation of these muscles since they left the hospital. The irony is that the relaxed, flabby abdominal wall tends to increase the feeling of fatigue, while making yourself exercise regularly will, in the end, make you feel less tired. One trick you can use, if you are feeling weak and tired at the beginning, is to raise one leg at a time, a little more each day, until you can get them into the vertical position, and then begin with both legs together, again a little more each day. You can do the same with the sit-ups.

"You may have the feeling that the muscles of your perineum around your vagina have lost their normal sensation of tightness. You can exercise these muscles too, just as you do the abdominal muscles. The simplest form of the exercise is what you do when you wish to stop urinating, a reflex you have when you are suddenly interrupted while voiding. After you have done this perineal tightening deliberately a few times, you will know what it feels like. You can then do it frequently, whenever you like during the day. It is called the Kegel exercise, after the gynecologist who first recommended it.

"As for other physical exercise, you can and should continue with whatever you are accustomed to and enjoy, although you should wait with jogging or other exercises that may cause discomfort to an unhealed incision or episiotomy, until healing is more complete. There is no medical reason at all why you should not go swimming as soon as you like after delivery.

"I have no particular advice to give you on clothing, except that you should wear things that are comfortable. At first you will probably have to wear maternity dresses but with exercising and weight loss you can expect to get back into your ordinary clothing within three or four weeks. Do not be discouraged if it takes a little longer; people vary.

"Resumption of sexual relations is almost certainly safe once you have stopped having a bloody discharge. This should be somewhere in the neighborhood of three and a half to four weeks after the baby. An episiotomy repair or an abdominal incision may still be a bit uncomfortable at this time but you can't really do yourself any harm with sexual activity.

"Please remember that if you are not nursing you are probably fertile and that you had better use contraception unless you wish to have another baby very quickly. If you wish you can start almost immediately taking oral contraceptives. If you have used condoms or diaphragm in the past you can go right back to that. For most patients the diaphragm does not have to be changed as a consequence of childbirth, although you can have it checked if you have misgivings about the size. If in fact you are going to be nursing the baby and providing it with its fluids and its calories you will have built-in birth control for at least three months.

"I would like to see you sometime in the next four to eight weeks. If you are not nursing and need help with birth control by all means come in sooner. If you are nursing you can put off the decision to come in until some other time at your convenience. I enjoy it if you bring the baby with you, I enjoy seeing the product. If any problems arise, feel free to telephone me about them."

This pretty well covers what I discuss with the patients. However, please understand that not all care givers are in complete agreement with me on all of these recommendations. If your doctor or nurse midwife disagrees with my advice, please follow that of your accustomed and familiar attendants.

Complications after Delivery

Just as any disease can occur during pregnancy it can also occur in the puerperium. I have seen patients with mumps, measles, chicken pox, appendicitis, infectious jaundice, gall bladder disease, and on and on through the catalog of acute illnesses. The treatment of these diseases is the same in the puerperium as it would be at any other time in the patient's life and need not be discussed here. However, the commonest complications in the puerperium are: excessive bleeding after delivery (including postpartum hemorrhage and delayed vaginal bleeding); puerperal fever due to infection in the uterus; mastitis and breast infections; urinary tract infections; and anemia.

Postpartum Hemorrhage

Because the placenta in tearing away from the uterine wall leaves open blood vessels, severe hemorrhage can occur in the postpartum period. In addition, at this time, bleeding can come from tears in the uterus, the cervix, the vagina, and the perineum. The principal reason that patients are kept in recovery rooms for periods of time following childbirth, even when it appears to be completely uneventful, is to watch carefully for such hemorrhage.

When hemorrhage occurs, the first step is to put a hand on the abdominal wall to be certain that the uterus is contracting adequately. If it is not, we administer oxytocin or methergine to bring about forceful contractions, and we may employ a newer method, administration of prostaglandin either intravenously or injected directly into the uterus. If these drugs produce uterine contraction and thereby stop the bleeding, the problem is under control.

If good uterine contractions occur and the patient nevertheless continues to bleed, the next step is a careful examination of the reproductive tract. This is done in a systematic manner, starting with the perineum and lower vagina and proceeding to the upper portions of the vagina and the cervix. Some light anesthesia such as nitrous oxide, which wears off quickly, is generally helpful in carrying out this examination adequately. The cervix is brought down into view and inspected throughout its entire circumference to be certain whether it is the source of the continued bleeding. If the structures so far examined are not actively bleeding, and the blood is coming from the uterus, the examiner puts a hand into the uterus and palpates to determine whether there is a tear in the uterine wall or, more likely, a fragment of retained placenta. Such a placental remnant can prevent the uterine muscle from closing down on the blood vessels and halting the bleeding.

If tears are found to be bleeding, steps are taken immediately to sew them closed. If, however, there are no identifiable sources of the bleeding and the uterus continues to relax and bleed, the very bleeding process itself can begin to interfere with the ability of the body to form clots. This condition is generally referred as disseminated intravascular coagulation (DIC), which describes the fact that fibrinogen, platelets and other factors required for adequate clotting are depleted in the course of the hemorrhage and the patient loses the ability to clot the blood. Treatment consists of administration of the clotting factors and continued other efforts to stop the bleeding.

If uterine hemorrhage continues, the next move is abdominal surgery. If the patient wants the surgeon to preserve her ability to have additional children, the initial step consists of tying the major arteries supplying the uterus in order to cut down the force and rate of blood flow. This will occasionally allow clotting to take place. In any event, this form of blood vessel ligation does not reduce the blood supply to a point that the uterus will fail to function normally thereafter. Should tying off the blood supply not result in stanching the hemorrhage, the final recourse is removal of the uterus. The decision to carry out these procedures requires experience and good judgment. Undue procrastination in the care of postpartum hemorrhage can lead to a disastrous outcome.

Delayed Vaginal Bleeding

It is normal to have a bloody discharge for two to three weeks after childbirth. In the course of this period, the blood gradually becomes mixed with mucus and the debris coming from the healing of the placental site. As the now-useless blood vessels gradually shrink, they may bleed. Therefore in the first two or three weeks passage of an occasional clot about the size of a quarter in diameter is not abnormal. However, after the first few days, the rate of bleeding should equal that of normal menses. The amount of bleeding should gradually taper off.

Occasionally, a week or two after childbirth, the bleeding may unexpectedly increase markedly, and you may pass larger clots. If this occurs you should be seen by a professional. There are two possible causes for this condition. The first is called subinvolution of the placental site. The shrinkage and healing of the large placental blood vessels has not completed itself normally. This usually corrects itself with the passage of time. Immediate treatment may consist of nothing more than administration of tablets of methergine to cause increased uterine contraction for twenty-four hours. Heavy bleeding can be treated by suction curettage on an ambulatory basis.

The other cause of bleeding may be the delayed separation of a retained placental fragment. It occurs spontaneously when a cotyledon (a subdivision of the placenta) is more adherent to the uterine wall than the rest of the placenta, and therefore the placenta breaks apart and the cotyledon is retained at the time of placental separation. This does not result from the efforts of a practitioner to deliver the placenta. Careful inspection of the placenta after its birth can disclose that a cotyledon is missing, but unfortunately, in the excitement of a delivery, such inspection is sometimes overlooked. This accident can be responsible for serious hemorrhage.

Pelvic examination will demonstrate that the cervix is not closed and that the fragment may be seen or felt inside it. It is fairly easy to remove it without anesthesia by using a small grasping instrument or a suction catheter. Only if the hemorrhage has been heavy enough to require giving intravenous fluids or blood transfusion need the woman be hospitalized. In any case, the removal of the placental fragment cures the problem.

Puerperal Infection

This term includes those conditions caused by the introduction of harmful bacteria into the postpartum uterus. The raw area where the placenta was attached offers rich nourishment for any bacteria that may intrude. These bacteria ordinarily come from two sources. One is the outside world, introduced by doctors, nurse midwives, nurses, and anyone else who comes into intimate contact with the patient's reproductive tract either during labor or in the immediate postpartum period. More commonly however, the infections are due to the patient's own bacteria, which take advantage of any reduction in the patient's normal resistance to her own germs. Cesarean section, for example, establishes a wound in the uterine wall; difficult delivery may result in maternal tissue damage and retention of fragments of placenta or membranes in the uterus. Puerperal infection is thus most common after operative delivery and after prolonged labor.

Puerperal infection makes itself known by a general sensation of fatigue, headache, chills, and elevation of temperature. We consider it to be present whenever the patient's temperature reaches 38 degrees centigrade or 100.4 degrees Fahrenheit on two or more occasions after the completion of the first twenty-four hours postpartum. The fever can go substantially higher than this. Care for puerperal infection begins with a physical examination to search for sources of the infection. Added to this is a study of the white-blood-cell count, which normally is below 12,000 white blood cells for every cubic centimeter of blood. If it goes above that—even as high as 35,000—it confirms the diagnosis of infection, although we still may not know where the infection is located. Bacteriological cultures are obtained from the uterine cavity, the bladder, and the bloodstream in an effort to identify the causative bacteria.

If the physical examination confirms the diagnosis of puerperal infection, the physician should not wait for the results of the cultures to administer broad-spectrum antibiotic therapy. I do not have a specific recommendation for the choice of a drug. Rapid developments in this field are constantly producing safer and more effective antibiotics, so that your doctor may well have available excellent therapies not even known to me as I write this. Whatever drug is used, it should be given intravenously if the patient has more than a mild infection.

With proper treatment, puerperal infection should clear up promptly. If it does not, a suspicion arises that the infection is complicated by the formation of abscesses in the pelvis. This is most likely to occur following cesarean section. The diagnosis can be established by pelvic examination and ultrasound. A pelvic abscess may require surgical drainage.

An uncomplicated puerperal infection does not have any remote consequences in terms of future childbearing, nor is it likely to repeat itself in the future.

A significant factor in the control of puerperal infection caused by the patient's own bacteria is the avoidance of tissue injury at the time of delivery. Good prenatal care also plays a role, since the maintenance of adequate diet improves a woman's resistance to disease. As prenatal care and the management of labor and delivery have improved, we have seen a marked reduction in the incidence of puerperal infection from this source.

Even more spectacular is the reduction of infection from bacteria transmitted to the patient by those giving her care. It is to control this that we wear readily disposable caps, masks, shoe covers, suits, and sterile gowns when we enter a delivery room. Antibacterial preparations are used to wash off the mother's external genitalia prior to birth whenever any operative maneuver is contemplated. The lower genital tract is sturdily resistant to infection from its own bacteria, but it must be protected against infection with organisms foreign to the mother.

When patients deliver normally in a labor room, the likelihood of infection is exceedingly low and therefore the precautions need not be quite so strictly enforced as for more complicated deliveries in the delivery room.

Mastitis

Mastitis, the development of localized inflammation of the breasts, seldom occurs prior to delivery. In the puerperium, it occurs almost entirely among nursing women. It rarely occurs until the third or fourth week after delivery and may occur as late as when the baby is several months old.

There are three different and distinct conditions that can produce painful changes in the breasts. In the first and commonest of these, the lacteal ducts fill with milk and then, for whatever reason, do not empty, and the breasts become engorged. There is no sign of infection, and there are no bacteria and few white blood cells present in the milk. The patient feels diffuse discomfort in both breasts, with no signs of local inflammation. If she receives local treatment, as described on page 389, the condition does not last long and has no further complications.

The second condition is noninfectious inflammation of the breast. One or two areas in one breast are tender and exhibit reddening of the skin over them. Chills do not occur and fever is not high. Under the microscope the milk of these women shows a moderate increase in the number of white blood cells, but few bacteria.

This type of inflammation should be promptly treated with antibiotics, and the breasts should be regularly emptied by nursing or pumping or both. Unlike simple engorgement, the symptoms of noninfectious inflammation are likely to continue for at least three or four days. Untreated, the condition will last seven or eight days and in 50 percent of the cases, the untreated patient goes on to develop frank infectious mastitis.

The third condition is infectious mastitis. This is due ordinarily to Staphylococcus aureus bacteria, which are found in the nose and throat and on the skin of apparently normal people. In a typical case, the nursing mother develops sudden and unexplained lassitude and aching of the joints, sometimes with chills and almost always with an elevation of temperature that may go as high as 40 degrees centigrade or 104 degrees Fahrenheit. There is an obvious local tenderness in the breast and on examination this tender area is found firm and the skin overlying it is red and hot. These areas commonly occur in the outer and lower quadrants of a breast. The Staphylococcus is probably transmitted to the mother from the baby, through some crack or abrasion of the nipple, a lesion that may be so small as not to be noticeable.

The baby is not sick with the bacteria but may have patches of skin infection, also due to the same organisms. In hospitals, nursery personnel are required to wash their hands frequently to minimize the transfer of these organisms from one baby to another. At home, where public bacteria do not intrude, it is not necessary for the family to follow this rigid cleanliness discipline.

In cases of infectious mastitis the milk contains many inflammatory cells and large numbers of bacteria. Ideally it would be desirable to culture the milk from such patients in order to get absolute proof of the bacteriologic diagnosis. The clinical diagnosis, however, is usually quite unmistakable even without laboratory findings.

With aggressive therapy, mastitis can be cleared up in two to three days. The treatment includes frequent nursing to empty the breasts and the administration of antibiotics that are effective against the Staphylococcus. At present the drug of choice is dicloxacillin. Small doses of antibiotic will get into the milk, but these will not do anything much more than change the odor of the baby's stool.

Untreated, mastitis continues for long periods of time. In the breast as elsewhere infections with Staphylococcus tend to produce abscesses, which may appear as early as a few days after the onset of the mastitis. For this reason infectious mastitis should come under vigorous antibiotic therapy quite early. If it does not, and an abscess does form, breast-feeding is seriously prejudiced and surgical drainage of the abscess may become necessary. The process then is prolonged considerably and recurrences are not at all uncommon. The likelihood of infectious mastitis can be reduced by observing the simple precautions described elsewhere in this book in the section, "More About Breast-feeding," page 546.

Urinary Tract Infection

Cystitis, an inflammation of the bladder, generally makes itself known by an urgency to urinate frequently in small amounts and severe sensation of pain in the bladder area on the completion of urination. The discomfort is not generalized and there is no fever, although it is a genuine infection, most commonly due to the colon bacillus. In its severe forms it can be responsible for the presence of blood in the urine, resulting from the opening up of small blood vessels in the wall of the bladder, which is part of the body's effort to combat the infection.

Prompt treatment of cystitis with sulfisoxazole (Gantrisin) or ampicillin, either of which can be given by mouth, will ordinarily clear up initial attacks of cystitis quite reliably. The drug should be given for seven days. It is desirable to obtain urine culture studies at the time of the initial infection and again a few weeks later when the patient no longer has symptoms in order to be certain that the harmful bacteria are not still a silent presence in the bladder.

The organism responsible for cystitis may also produce infection of the collecting systems of the upper urinary tract: the kidney pelvis, where urine briefly collects; and the ureter, which is the conduit from the kidney pelvis to the bladder. Infection in this location is called pyelonephritis (*pyelos*, "pelvis"; *nephritis*, "inflammation of the kidney"). It is usually accompanied by bacterial cystitis, but the infection of the upper tract dominates the clinical picture. Its effects include back pain over the kidney area on one side or both, chills, fever up to 40 degrees centigrade or 104 degrees Fahrenheit, and a general sensation of being ill. There is also burning on urination and loss of appetite. Prompt diagnosis is established by obtaining a urine culture and making a microscopic examination of the urine for pus cells and bacteria.

The patient usually responds quickly to treatment with Gantrisin or ampicillin, given in larger doses for pyelonephritis than for a simple bladder infection. Treatment should in any event be continued for seven to ten days, and a follow-up culture of the urine is imperative, to detect the continuing presence of the organism even after symptoms have completely disappeared.

To some extent, with the best of intentions, medical personnel themselves in the past contributed to the incidence of urinary tract infection. That incidence was markedly reduced as soon as it was realized that in some cases organisms were introduced into the bladder by the catheters used for taking urine samples. Upon substitution of a "clean catch" technique for the catheter, the occurrence of infection was significantly reduced. Other improvements in care, not obviously related to urinary tract conditions, have also reduced the incidence of urinary retention: better anesthesia, early ambulation, less frequent operative delivery, and wider use of antibiotics.

Anemia

We do not treat anemia with blood transfusions nearly as frequently as we did a decade ago. In part this is because we have realized that blood transfusion can be a vehicle to transmit viruses, some deadly, as we became aware in the dramatic revelations relating to acquired immune deficiency syndrome (AIDS). A much less frightening reason is that we know that the expansion of pregnant woman's blood volume is a protection against acute blood loss. Thus, she does not need additional blood unless she has lost enough to cause circulatory difficulty, characterized by a marked increase in the heart rate and a drop in blood pressure. In that case, intravenous fluids are the first step in treatment, followed by transfusion if her bleeding has not come under control.

A woman who is anemic postpartum but who has normal blood pressure and pulse rate may nevertheless find that she fatigues easy. Her anemia is rapidly and safely corrected by oral intake of three iron tablets a day, along with an ample diet. The red blood count will return to normal in three weeks— the fatigue vanishes in less time than that. Iron therapy must be continued for up to six months in order to rebuild iron storage.

Postpartum Examination

Those who have cared for you during pregnancy, labor, and delivery do not consider their job complete until they have seen you through the period of recovery and the return to ordinary activity. We therefore assume that you will return for at least one follow-up examination (and for later maintenance as necessary).

Traditionally this has taken place six weeks after childbirth. There is, however, no medical basis for this particular timing and the postpartum examination can be accomplished at two to three weeks or as late as twelve weeks after delivery. If the patient is completely well and has no complications, an early postpartum visit is ordinarily for the purpose of contraceptive advice for those who are not breast-feeding. The reproductive tract has sufficiently recovered at this point so that a patient who so desires can be fitted or refitted for a diaphragm and instructed as to its use. Insertion of intrauterine devices is probably better postponed until four to six weeks postpartum.

If you have had complications of pregnancy such as an infection or elevated blood pressure, it is urgent for you to appear for a follow-up examination in regard to these items.

Most of us wish to do a pelvic examination at this time to be certain that the internal organs have returned to their normal size and position and to check on any repairs we have made in the vagina. In those who have delivered by section, we inspect the abdominal wound to be certain that it has healed well.

I often find, as do some of my patients, that the follow-up visit is a sentimental occasion. The adults involved have been seeing each other at fairly frequent intervals for seven or eight months and have a sense of accomplishment shared among them. I myself have maintained friendships with women whom I helped in childbirth over the years, in several parts of the United States. I have had the pleasure of following children of my patients into their adult years and watching them achieve success and even prominence; and the joy of sharing the parents' pride in the development of their offspring.

19

Twins and Other Multiple Births

How Many at a Birth?

We read in the works of Ambroise Paré, premier surgeon-physician of sixteenth-century France, that Lady Margaret, Countess of Hagenau, was brought to bed of 365 children at one and the same time in the year 1313. Milady's super-fecundity came about in a miraculous way, through God's displeasure. It happened that, some time the year before, the countess had been walking through the gate of her walled palace when her skirt was plucked by a kneeling beggar woman who said, "My good lady, give me alms."

The countess, haughty and indignant, replied, "Why should I give you alms?"

The beggar woman answered, "Because of all the children I have begot."

The countess looked down upon her in disdain. "Fie upon you, you've had the pleasure of begetting them."

God in heaven overheard, we are told, and he was wroth. The next year the countess was lain in with 365 children, one for each day of the year. There were 182 females, all baptized Elizabeth by the good Bishop of Utrecht, and 182 boys, all baptized John. There was one "scrat" (hermaphrodite), who pathetically remained unnamed and unbaptized. In reporting the same case a hundred years later, Mauriceau said it was either a "miracle or a fable"; we are inclined to the belief that it was a little of both.

Other fabulous cases are recorded, such as "Dorothy, an Italian who had twenty at two births, at the first nine and at the second eleven, and she was so big . . . her belly . . . rested upon her knees."

When we descend to the number seven it becomes impossible to know whether we are dealing with fact or fable. In the German town of Hamelin, which the Pied Piper made famous in 1248, we find the following tablet attached to the front of a house in Emmenstrasse: "Here on this spot dwelt . . . Thiele Romer, and his helpmate Anna Byers. It came about that in the year 1600 . . . at three o'clock in the morning on the ninth day of January, she was delivered of two small boys and five small girls. . . . All peacefully died by twelve o'clock on the twentieth of January and were given the beatitude which is guaranteed to those who believe." That is all we know about the possible, perhaps even probable, Hamelin septuplets.

We come now to undisputed facts outside the realm of the fabulous and the pseudo-fabulous. There are quite a few authentic cases of sextuplets, one reported in 1969, in which all survived.

Quintuplets are reported every few years, but so infrequently that it is impossible to state the mathematical frequency. The first set of quintuplets ever to survive in history were the Dionne sisters of Canada in 1933—not even a single quintuplet had ever survived before.

Natural and Artificial Multiple Births

In 1960, effective hormonal methods of inducing ovulation arrived on the therapeutic scene, bringing with them a noticeably increased incidence of multiple births. The two medicines in use are human pituitary gonadotropin (FSH, follicle-stimulating hormone) and clomiphene citrate, a synthetic steroid that has both estrogenic and antiestrogenic action. Neither of them can be so precisely synchronized with a woman's pituitary and ovaries as are her own hormones. Consequently, with either medication, it is possible that on one occasion no ovulation may result, and on another she may release a great many eggs, all of which can be fertilized.

The most dramatic example I know of the unpredictability of these drugs is a woman whose own pituitary had been removed in the treatment of a pituitary tumor. After this she was treated on two separate occasions with pituitary gonadotropin to induce ovulation; each of these times she had a single normal pregnancy. When she came again for treatment a new, presumably more purified preparation of FSH was available. It was given to her twice, but with no result. Her medical attendants concluded that she had become resistant to the effects of the drug. However, they tried one more time with the same preparation—and this time she became pregnant with, and eventually delivered, quintuplets.

A series of seventy-eight induced-ovulation pregnancies reported from the Tel-Hashomer Hospital in Israel resulted in forty-seven single births, twenty-three pairs of twins, five sets of triplets, two sets of quadruplets, and 1 set of sextuplets. About 16 percent of human pregnancies induced by FSH give rise to more than one baby, and at least 10 percent of clomiphene-induced births do likewise. Since multiple ovulations have occurred, each baby almost always comes from a separate egg; thus, there is not uncommonly a mix of sexes.

In all likelihood the largest multiple pregnancy resulting from this kind of ovarian stimulation has been nonaplets, nine fetuses. Unfortunately, the fetal loss rate among these high numbers is very great. A recent pregnancy with seven fetuses ended with survival of only three. The loss among the pregnancies with four, five, and six fetuses from premature birth or fetal death is sizable despite the use of methods to delay the early onset of labor. There have been no survivors of nonaplet and octuplet (eight fetuses) pregnancies.

In vitro fertilization has also added to the frequency of multiple births. This technique, useful principally among women lacking fallopian tubes, depends for its efficiency on inducing multiple ovulation, in order to provide several eggs for fertilization. It is presently the practice to implant about four early embryos to increase the likelihood that at least one will find a haven in the endometrium. Of course it sometimes happens that all four are successful in doing this.

It has been suggested that these drug-induced and surgically produced multiple births should be termed artificial multiple births and separated out in the statistics. The spontaneous variety can be referred to as natural multiple births; the statistical data given in this chapter refer only to these natural multiple births.

Frequency of Natural Multiple Births

Dionys Hellin, in 1895, stated that twins occurred once in 89 births, triplets once in 89 squared (7,921), and quadruplets once 89 to the third power (704,969). Considering that he used no information concerning the varying incidences of multiple births in different ethnic groups, or the impact of loss of some or all of the babies in quadruple, quintuple, or sextuple births, his estimates were surprisingly accurate. In an analysis of 80 million births in the United States between 1928 and 1955, twins were found to occur once in every 90 pregnancies, triplets once in every 9,300, and quadruplets once in every 490,000.

"What Chance Have I for Twins?"

I cannot answer the question without knowing your ethnic origin, your age, the number of children you have previously given birth to, and whether you or your partner have a family tree featuring a large number of multiple births.

What about your ethnicity? There are marked racial differences in the incidence of multiple births. For example, in Japan twins occur about once in every 154 pregnancies, and triplets once in every 17,200. At the other end of the scale, in Nigeria twins occur about once in every 42 pregnancies; the major studies of multiple births in the Third World are now being carried out in Nigerian hospitals. In the United States twins occur about once in every 73 nonwhite births and once in every 93 white births. These nonwhite statistics are likely to change with the arrival of Oriental populations from Southeast Asia.

What about your age? In the United States white women below the age of twenty have a twinning incidence of 1 in 167 births. As age increases the frequency of twins rises as well. At about forty, the rate is about 1 in 55. Past this age the frequency declines, for reasons we simply do not understand.

What about your parity? Parity is the number of term and premature births you have had, and it exerts an influence on the likelihood of multiple pregnancy independent of age. If you are a white woman in the United States age thirty-five to forty having your first pregnancy, your chance of twins is about 1 in 74; if you are in the same age group having your seventh pregnancy, your chance increases to 1 in 45.

What about your heredity? Multiple births clearly run in some families in which the women tend to produce more than one egg from their ovaries in any particular menstrual cycle. These are fraternal twins. A familial tendency to produce identical twins has been much more difficult to prove. We do not really know how it operates. A tendency to twinning does not skip generations.

There is no evidence that twins are more or less fertile than singletons.

Types of Twins

As I have indicated, there are two types of twins. One variety originates from a single fertilized egg that divides into two very early in its development. In these circumstances, one egg is fertilized by one sperm, and the germ plasm of the two offspring is therefore identical. Consequently they must be of the same sex and exactly alike in skin, hair, and eye color. They also bear a striking resemblance to each other in body build and facial features and possess exactly the same blood factors. Such twins are termed identical, one-egg, or monozygotic.

The other type of twinning results from the fertilization of two different eggs by two separate spermatozoa. The eggs may come from the same ovary or from opposite ovaries. Twins of this variety, known as fraternal, two-egg, or dizygotic, are simply a litter of two and bear no greater resemblance to each other than brothers or sisters at exactly the same age. They may be of the same or opposite sex and may or may not have the same blood types. As we stated, all artificial twins and even all artificial octuplets are of this type.

Monozygotic twins may occasionally, though very rarely, undergo developmental influences *in utero* that cause them to be physically different from each other. For example, one twin at a very early embryonic stage may have lost one of its two sex chromosomes and therefore may develop a female external appearance, a phenomenon known as Turner's syndrome. The co-twin, which is always larger, is clearly male. Unless the problem is suspected and laboratory work is done, the smaller twin will be taken for a small female, and the genetic aberration may not be noted until the child reaches the age of puberty and secondary sexual development fails to take place.

Another possible developmental deviation in one identical twin may be the retention of an extra chromosome 21. This manifests itself as Down's syndrome.

Pairs of twins in which either Turner's syndrome or Down's syndrome has occurred in one twin may nevertheless be identical in all other genetic characteristics. All their other chromosomes, their blood groups, and their HLA tissue types are exactly the same. HLA is a protein material in connective tissue cells; when the HLA types of one individual match that of another, successful organ transplants are possible between them and destructive immune reactions do not occur.

Can You Tell One-egg from Two-egg Twins at Birth?

If the twins are normal and appear to be one male and one female, with the exception noted above, they must necessarily be from two eggs and not identical. If they are of the same sex an answer can be derived from a careful inspection of the placenta. If the two children have a single placenta and examination of the membranes at the point where the two fetal sacs demonstrates only two thin layers (the two amnions), it is overwhelmingly likely that the twins are identical and come from a single egg and a single sperm.

On the other hand, if each twin has a separate placenta, or examination of the wall between the two sets of membranes in a single placenta demonstrates three or four layers instead of just two, nine times out of ten, even though they are of the same sex, they are fraternal and have come from two eggs and two sperm. If the twins have occupied a single amniotic sac, itself a rare event, they are of necessity identical twins.

An absolute decision in some cases must await further testing. One of these tests, readily carried out at birth, is determination of the blood types of the two fetuses. The two bloods of identical twins must be exactly alike in regard to all the early tested blood groups, thirty-one of which are presently identified. HLA typing can be added to this. If the blood types and the HLA types are precisely the same there is only a infinitesimal chance that twins of the same sex are not identical.

The ultimate proof can be accomplished by transplantation of organs from one twin to another. The transplantation of a kidney from one twin to an identical co-twin is always a successful operation. A graft between fraternal twins behaves like the grafts between nontwin brothers and sisters, which have a much lower rate of success.

Frequency of the Two Types

In the United States, in the white population, about one-third of all twins are identical, the other two-thirds fraternal. In the nonwhite population, identical twinning is less common, being only about 29 percent. In direct contrast to this, the twins in Oriental populations are overwhelmingly of the identical type. It is obvious that the difference in the frequency of types of twinning from one ethnic group to another depends upon a difference in the frequency of multiple ovulations in the women in those populations. One-egg identical twinning occurs with the same frequency in all people and is indifferent to ethnicity, age, parity and even—with the few exceptions mentioned above—family history.

Other Multiple Births

Triplets, Quadruplets, and Quintuplets

All the factors just mentioned influence the frequency not only of twins but also of the higher orders of multiple pregnancy; in addition, the rate is clearly affected by the number of artificially induced multiple births.

In six out of every ten instances of triplet pregnancy, two eggs are involved and the fetuses are a pair of identical twins and a singleton; in three out of ten cases all three of the triplets come from a single egg and are identical, and in one case in ten the triplets are fraternal, coming from three different eggs.

Conjoined Twins

In rare instances the splitting of an embryo to form identical twins is incomplete and results in one of the various kinds of conjoined twins. Recent advances in pediatric surgery have improved our success in dividing these twins from one another and allowing them to grow up separately. The birth of surviving conjoined twins is itself a remarkable event, since a high proportion of these unusual infants are lost because of prematurity, and in addition, mechanical difficulties due to their conjunction results in a high rate of unavoidable mortality during labor.

Whether conjoined twins can be separated depends principally on the extent to which they share internal organs. There are instances in which a fetus of nearly normal size has been joined at the chest to an incompletely formed fetus that has failed to develop its own head and is lacking some of the organs normally found in the chest. These twins cannot be separated.

On the other hand, if the twins are joined head to head, and share only the bones of the skull, it can be expected that both will be saved when they are surgically separated. The commonest kind of joining is back-to-back in the pelvic region. Most conjoined twins are female and surgical separation of such twins is apt to be complex, as they often share a rectum, an anus, and a vagina.

The commonly used term for conjoined twins is Siamese twins. The name is derived from a pair of male children born in Siam in 1811, who were united only by a narrow bridge of tissue in the upper abdomen. In 1829 they came to America and were exhibited all over the country by the great showman P. T. Barnum who made them rich and famous. They lived to the age of sixty-three.

Superfetation

Superfetation means conception after an existing pregnancy is already well established in the uterus. This can take place only if a woman has ovulated despite the presence in her body of estrogen, progesterone, and hCG concentrations which are known to inhibit ovulation. It also requires the passage of spermatozoa through the pregnant uterus up into the tube, an event that is out of the question by about the end of the third month, when the pregnancy completely fills the uterine cavity. In the past the evidence for superfetation consisted of a great disparity in weight between newborn twins, or a great delay in the birth of a second twin after the premature birth of a first twin. An interval of as much as sixty days between the births of twins has been observed. For the most part, however, this occurs in women with double uteri, and has nothing to do with superfetation.

It should be possible, using sonography as a diagnostic tool, to prove the occurrence of superfetation if in fact it takes place. To my knowledge no such observation has been made and the phenomenon remains only a theoretical possibility.

Superfecundation

This is the fertilization of two ova during a single menstrual cycle by spermatozoa from separate sexual exposures. There is only one circumstance in which this can be proven: if the woman has had coitus, in a single cycle, with two different partners and become pregnant by each. When the babies are born, a wide difference in appearance between them may suggest the diagnosis, and red-blood-cell and HLA typing may conclusively show that one man could not have fathered both offspring. The first authentic case of superfecundation was reported by Dr. John Archer who, by alphabetical accident, was the first person to graduate from an American medical school. He described a delivery in which a woman gave birth to a white child and a co-twin with distinctly African characteristics. She stated that in her fertile cycle she had had intercourse with a white partner and a black partner within a short span of time. A sufficient number of other credible instances have been reported since that report, so that there can be no doubt that superfecundation can in fact take place. In this case of course the co-twins are within a few days of one another in gestational age.

Pregnancy and Delivery

The Diagnosis of Twins

Twins are identified prior to labor in about seven out of every ten cases. This is most likely to be accomplished when something calls attention to the probability of twins. The larger the infants grow and the closer they get to term the less likely it is that the diagnosis will be missed. If either twin weighs 5½ pounds (2.5 kilos) or more the chances are about eight out of ten that the diagnosis will be made prior to labor. I recall a patient, herself a doctor, who unexpectedly delivered healthy term twin girls. She commented that the previous evening, in view of what she had observed about the size of her uterus and the general constant commotion going on within it, she had said to her husband that if she didn't know better she would strongly suspect that she was having twins. They came as a great surprise in the delivery room the next day.

The following phenomena should raise our suspicion of a twin pregnancy:

1. Extraordinary weight gain, particularly when the uterus is substantially larger than would be expected for the duration of pregnancy. However, twins are not the sole possible explanation for an unusually large uterus. Other things that cause this are hydramnios, fibroids, and hydatidiform mole, any of which may coexist with the pregnancy.

2. A strong family history of twinning.

3. More than the expected amount of fetal movement. This is not the strongest of clues, since fetuses vary considerably from one to the other in their intrauterine activity patterns.

4. A relatively small presenting part in the pelvis, with the cervix starting to prepare for labor four to six weeks prior to term.

The availability of sonography has greatly simplified the diagnosis of twins early in pregnancy. Sonograms can demonstrate two fetal sacs as early as six or seven weeks of pregnancy. Not long after that the two embryos can be separately identified. In an instance of artificial multiple pregnancy in London, five fetal sacs were identified by ultrasound in the ninth week of pregnancy and a clear image of the fetal heads obtained not long thereafter.

When the fetuses are close to term it may be possible by abdominal examination in a slender patient to identify two heads and two fetal trunks. Counting arms and legs is at best confusing. If the fetal heartbeat can be distinctly heard, two separate observers can identify them and count them. To be certain that there are two fetuses present the heartbeats must be counted simultaneously and there must be a difference of 15 to 20 beats per minute between the two. There is considerable error in counting 150 or 160 beats per minute.

Length of Pregnancy

Many studies on the duration of twin pregnancy indicate that the average is about twenty-one days less than that for singletons, apparently slightly shorter when both twins are boys than when both twins are girls.

Most twins are born within a very short time of one another. However, there has been a report of a gap of fifty-four days between the first and second twin from a single uterus, and even longer intervals if one twin is in each horn of a double uterus. In such cases, even at term, the two horns of the uterus may go into labor at separate times. A recent report of the delivery of twins from such a uterus describes the uneventful labor and delivery of one twin. The second twin was not born until labor had been induced in the other half of the uterus, after which the second baby was also uneventfully delivered.

Discomforts of Pregnancy

There is no question that the mechanical discomforts with a twin pregnancy are considerably greater than they are with a singleton. Shortness of breath, severe pressure on varicose veins, hemorrhoids, inability to sleep because of fetal movement, swelling of the legs, and just plain difficulty in getting around are all substantially more common.

Certain complications of pregnancy are more frequent in the presence of multiple pregnancy. Pregnancy-induced hypertension is distinctly more common; this may be due simply to the presence of a larger volume of placental tissue and higher hormone levels in the mother. Since there is a double drain on the iron supply to meet the needs of two fetuses, maternal anemia is more common in the mothers of twins; the diagnosis of twins calls for an increase in maternal iron intake. Hydramnios, the condition in which there is excessive fluid in the uterus, has an increased incidence in twin pregnancies. The excessive fluid usually involves one of the two fetal sacs and is seen more often with one-egg twins than with two-egg twins. The treatment consists of increased bed rest, and if the condition becomes physically intolerable to the mother, amniocentesis with the slow release of the excessive fluid can be done. As the pregnancy goes on, the fluid tends to return and amniocentesis may have to be repeated. However, under these circumstances the uterus may solve the problem by going into premature labor.

Care during Multiple Pregnancy

Because of the mechanical problems attaching to multiple pregnancy, when twins are diagnosed the mother probably should be advised to increase her rest substantially as early as twenty-four weeks of pregnancy. If possible the patient should stop work quite early so that she can take periods of rest, lying down during the day as well as at night. Her caloric needs are increased and the patient should go on a high-calorie diet. Because of the increased likelihood of pregnancy toxemia the patient should come more often for prenatal visits and the red-blood-cell count should be checked at each visit, to be certain that the patient is not becoming anemic.

There has been great interest in the possibility of prolonging pregnancy with twins by maximizing bed rest. In some countries this has been done by hospitalizing the patients starting as early as the twenty-eighth week. It has been difficult, because of the large number of factors involved, to prove that hospitalization is actually of any benefit. Essentially the same thing can be said about the use of drugs to inhibit premature labor in women with twins.

Labor

Most twin labors proceed uneventfully because of the small size of the fetuses and the fact the cervix is often shortened and partially dilated before labor begins. Most plural labors are shorter than single labors. On the other hand, there is a greater incidence of unsatisfactory, sluggish labors among plural births than among single births. This is because the uterus becomes overdistended by the great volume of its contents, and its contractions are then inadequate to move the labor along. If all else is normal, one need only to wait for the labor to complete itself, but if necessary it can be stimulated by the careful use of intravenous oxytocin.

False labor is commoner than in a single pregnancy.

The membranes are more likely to rupture before the onset of labor in multiple pregnancy (29 percent) than in single pregnancy (12 percent).

In regard to fetal position in twins, one finds all the possible combinations and permutations for two fetuses, either of which may assume any of three positions—head, breech, or transverse. One presenting head first, the other breech, is the most frequent combination; although both presenting as cephalic is almost as common.

Conduct of Delivery

In multiple births, the best fetal and maternal results are obtained with the least operative interference.

The delivery of the first infant is managed in precisely the same way that it would be if it were a singleton. If there is an indication for delivery of the first baby by section then both babies are delivered abdominally. It has been suggested that if abdominal delivery of the second baby is anticipated, for example because it is lying in transverse lie, the delivery of both babies be carried out by section. It is certainly more conservative, however, to deliver the first baby normally and then address the birth of the second child as a separate entity.

There has also been considerable discussion about the interval between the first and second baby. Under ideal circumstances observation of the mother who has already delivered one baby but is still pregnant with the second child should be no less vigilant than observations of the mother with a single fetus. Fetal monitoring should be continued, to be certain that the condition of the second fetus is unimpaired. If the second fetus is not in a longitudinal lie, the medical attendant should make prompt efforts at external version (turning the long axis of the baby 90 degrees by manipulations through the abdominal wall). When the first infant has just delivered and the uterus has not yet accommodated to the decrease in its volume, its wall is relaxed and version may be quite easy.

If the second twin is in fact in longitudinal lie, stimulation of the uterus with oxytocin can be begun to hasten the birth of the second child. This ordinarily proceeds quite uneventfully.

A recent study of 115 women thirty-four or more weeks pregnant with twins described intervals between the births of the two babies varying from 1 to 134 minutes. Thirty-nine percent of the births of second twins took place after a interval of 15 minutes or more. It was observed that the greater the delay between the two fetuses the greater the incidence of abdominal delivery for the second fetus. It is known that the condition of the second fetus at birth is frequently not as good as that of the first fetus; this may be due at least in part to maneuvers undertaken to hasten its birth. In the past it was common practice to carry out an internal podalic version and breech extraction for all second fetuses who were not about to be born by the vertex. For such a delivery the patient is ordinarily given a general anesthetic. The operator then introduces a hand into the uterus, grasps the feet of the infant, and turns it into a breech presentation before it is delivered. Internal podalic version has largely fallen out of favor, except in serious emergencies when there is not enough time to deliver the baby abdominally.

Delivery of twins calls for the presence of at least two and preferably three attendants, one of whom should be experienced in some of the procedures necessary to make certain that both babies are born uneventfully in longitudinal lie. Perhaps the most important of these is making sure that the clamp on the severed end of the cord of the first fetus is secure, since identical fetuses have a common circulation and the fetus still in the uterus can bleed from the cord of its co-twin.

Pain Relief for Labor and Delivery

The methods of pain relief during labor with twins do not substantially differ from those with single births. In the event of inadequate contractions the attendants may be inclined to limit anesthetic drugs.

For delivery, local and pudendal block are quite adequate, or epidural and saddle block can also be employed. Because it is necessary to anticipate that general anesthesia may be required for a version, preparations for this should be begun during the first stage of labor. The mother should have an ample intravenous in place, especially in view of the enhanced possibility of postpartum hemorrhage from the enlarged, stretched uterus and from the large placental site.

Postdelivery Care

Except for extra vigilance in regard to postpartum hemorrhage, care is the same as for a single birth. All natural processes go on as scheduled. Breast-feeding presents only the difficulty that there is more of it. The babies can be fed one after the other or simultaneously, and the milk supply will respond to the demand. Each baby may develop a favorite nipple or a preferred way to be held.

The Babies

One twin pregnancy in twenty terminates so prematurely that the fetuses each weigh from 14 ounces to 2 pounds 3 ounces. This compares with the fact that only one single fetus in two hundred has a birth weight in this range (400–1,000 grams). In nine twin pregnancies out of twenty the larger of the twin babies weighs between 2 pounds 3 ounces, and 5 pounds 8 ounces (1,000–2,500 grams); in single pregnancies the chance of such an occurrence is one in twenty. In one-half of all twin pregnancies at least one child has a birth weight of 5½ pounds or more. In 93.7 percent of single pregnancies the newborn weighs at least 5½ pounds.

The average birth weight of single babies is 7½ pounds; the average birth weight of twins, 5 pounds 5 ounces. The disparity in size is due to two factors: the usual earlier termination of multiple gestations, and the relatively unfavorable nutritional environment twins suffer while in the uterus. Twins grow more slowly *in utero*. When a single baby and a twin baby are carried the full nine months, there is an average difference in birth weight of 1½ pounds. The difference in body length is less marked, being about three-quarters of an inch. Not all twins are small at birth. In our series of 1,000 twin infants, 3 percent weighed 8 pounds, in contrast to approximately 20 percent of single births; 0.4 percent weighed over 9 pounds, in contrast to 6 percent of singletons. The largest twin of our series was 9 pounds 2 ounces; the heaviest pair totaled 17 pounds. This hardly competes with a pair reported by Holzapfel in 1935; the twins together weighed 20 pounds 4 ounces.

Difference in Birth Weight between Twins

There may be a great difference in the birth weight between twins, one or two pounds not being extraordinary. In one study the intrapair difference of identical twins was 14 ounces, while in fraternal twins the difference was 6 ounces. It is rare for one of a pair of twins to be as much as twice the weight of the other. In twin births as in single births, male fetuses tend to weigh more than female.

Sex Ratio

Of a series of 126,328 pairs of twins born in the United States, 49,923 were both male, 42,557 male and female, and 40,848 both female. The total of 128,403 male twins and 124,253 female twins produces a sex ratio of 101.6 males per 100 females, instead of the usual 106–to–100 ratio in singletons. Very likely, relatively fewer female than male twins die between conception and birth.

Special Fetal Problems in Multiple Pregnancy

Twin pregnancies experience an increased mortality risk in the first trimester of pregnancy when a heterotopic pregnancy occurs. This term describes the situation in which there are two pregnancies in different locations in the reproductive tract. There may be two ectopic pregnancies, one in each tube or, more commonly, a normal intrauterine pregnancy combined with an ectopic pregnancy.

We have now learned by sonography that the death of one of a set of twins or triplets is more common than has been supposed. When this occurs duing the second trimester it ordinarily has little or no effect on the surviving co-twin. We have known that sometimes, at the birth of a singleton baby, a tiny, long-dead co-twin may be uneventfully passed by the mother before the birth of the placenta. A recent report of the death of one twin, which occurred after the twenty-sixth week, suggests that loss of only that one twin may be associated with the development of the clotting abnormality DIC. In this case the patient was given intense medical therapy during the period in which her clotting was abnormal and after a number of weeks she reverted to normal. Some ten weeks after the death of the co-twin induction of labor was undertaken, with the birth of an infant close to five pounds in very good condition.

Even in the third trimester, there is a greater mortality among babies in multiple pregnancies than among single infants, the largest factor being premature labor and the problems attendant on severe prematurity.

Ordinarily, when both twins are born alive there is no consistent difference in survival between the first twin and the second twin, unless one or the other of them has been subject to an unusual amount of birth trauma. Since as indicated twins are light in weight for their physiological maturity, which is largely determined by how long they spend in the uterus, the prognosis for a twin at any given weight is better than for a singleton. In other words, a twin born alive weighing three pounds has a greater chance for survival than a single baby weighing three pounds. This effectively demonstrates that the chance of survival of a live-born baby is dependent more on its maturity than on its weight.

The death of one identical twin *in utero* has been thought to have adverse effects on the surviving co-twin, but this has not been proved.

The identical twin transfusion syndrome referred to earlier is also the source of some problems. It apparently comes about because of an unusual arrangement of the two circulations in the placenta such that the blood pumped out by one baby actually returns to the other. One fetus then becomes the donor of blood and the other the recipient. The recipient fetus then develops a very high blood count and grows substantially larger than the donor co-twin. In addition to this, hydramnios, the accumulation of excessive amounts of fluid in the amniotic sac, may complicate the situation by bringing on the premature onset of labor. If this happens either twin may experience difficulties in the newborn state, the donor because it is very small in size and anemic, the recipient because it is overloaded with blood to such an extent that the blood may become almost too thick for normal circulation. Accordingly, when hydramnios occurs in the presence of twins, the medical attendant should suspect that this situation may exist and provide for emergency pediatric care at the time of delivery.

Congenital malformations are slightly more common among twins. Two-egg or fraternal twins never show the same malformation except through sheer coincidence. On the other hand, it is rare for an identical twin to suffer from a defect not shared by its fellow. Such identity of abnormalities may appear on the same side of the body of each twin or, through the biological mechanism of mirror-imaging, common in one-egg twins, may occur on the opposite side. This same process of mirror-imaging is responsible for high frequency of opposite-handedness found in adult pairs of identical twins. In 30 to 45 percent of identical twin pairs, one twin is right-handed, the other left-handed.

With the use of sonography it is now possible to do early genetic studies on each of a pair of twins. When one of the two has been proven to have a major abnormality the question of selective abortion inevitably arises. This has in fact been successfully carried out a few times without injury to the co-twin.

20

Early Fetal Diagnosis

Thirty years ago we were pleased to be able to see the beginnings of a fetal skeleton by X-ray at about the fourteenth week of pregnancy. At twenty weeks we were able to hear the fetal heart with a stethoscope. We were just beginning to be able to make some estimate of the severity of Rh disease (erythroblastosis). The ensuing years have been revolutionary. We now have routine screening procedures for a number of fetal abnormalities, and we can visualize the early fetus and scrutinize it for anatomical and functional disorders. We also can obtain samples of placenta, amniotic fluid, fetal blood, and fetal skin to make precise diagnoses.

The need for the diagnosis of fetal disease well before the onset of labor and the moment of delivery has arisen from some of the social changes discussed in Chapter 7. Suffice it to say that, in an epoch when we almost take the safety of the pregnant woman for granted, our attention has been turned to the prenatal diagnosis and treatment of fetal disorders.

Fetal Defects

Chromosomal Abnormalities

The normal number of chromosomes in human beings is forty-six, made up of twenty-three pairs. Twenty-two pairs, the autosomes, carry the genes that encode the information necessary to develop a person from a single-celled ovum. The autosomes are numbered in order of size, the largest being number 1 and the smallest, number 22. The chromosomes consist of short arms and long arms, with relatively inactive material at the point where the arms cross each other, the acrocenter. The short arms of the pair of arms are always on the same side of the acrocenter. The one additional pair of chromosomes, the sex chromosomes, determine the individual's genetic sex and are designated X and Y. A female is XX and a male is XY. The sex chromosomes also carry genes. Each gene occupies a specific position on a specific chromosome; a number of these gene locations have been identified.

During the ordinary life of a cell when it is working and not in the process of division, the material of the chromosomes is mixed up in a diffuse and random manner in the nucleus of the cell. At the time of cell division the chromosomes take form and divide into two equal sets of twenty-three pairs. This process gives rise to two new cells with genetic makeup identical to that of the parent cell. In the formation of spermatozoa and ova, however, the process of division produces individual reproductive cells—eggs or sperm—equipped with only half of the forty-six chromosomes, one of each pair. In fertilization, egg and sperm merge to form a new individual, consisting of twenty-three chromosomes from one parent and twenty-three from the other.

Some genetic defects are the result of abnormal chromosome numbers. A fetus can form and develop lacking one chromosome, if the missing chromosome is one of the two sex chromosomes. Apparently only a limited amount of genetic information is encoded on these chromosomes, and the X and Y do not seem to be equal in this respect. A fetus may develop and survive with only an X but no Y; however, not even an embryo will form if there is a Y but no X. Embryos with one X, designated as 45X, have a high rate of abortion in the first trimester and of fetal death in the second. The 45X individuals who go to full term ordinarily look like females, since there is no development of external genitalia. They have rudimentary sex organs and are commonly short in stature. Some of these deficiencies are now remediable by substitutive hormone therapy, but 45X individuals are infertile.

Occasionally when sperm or ova form they acquire excess numbers of sex chromosomes so that there may be as many as forty-eight or forty-nine chromosomes. In these individuals chromosomes number 1 through 22 have the usual diploid (double) number and the extra chromosomes are all in the sex chromosome group. This can be responsible for a number of abnormalities. Individuals who are 47XXY tend to be tall, gangly males with small genitalia and even smaller testes and are likely to be infertile. The individuals who are 47XXX are externally normal females with normal fertility; a small proportion of these are mentally retarded. The even rarer individuals with 48 and 49 chromosomes all manifest minor degrees of mental retardation and infertility. They may be externally male or female.

The condition known as trisomy occurs because of incomplete separation of chromosome pairs (nondisjunction) during the formation of a sperm or ovum, which may happen in any of the twenty-two non-sex chromosomes. Trisomy of the larger chromosomes and those with ample upper and lower arms ordinarily results in an ovum that cannot survive embryonic life. When trisomy of the chromosomes having very short arms occurs, a live birth is possible, although these fetuses and infants tend to be smaller than normal. The maternal AFP is likely to be low in such pregnancies. The commonest trisomy involves chromosome number 21 and is responsible for Down's syndrome.

Most forms of nondisjunction become more frequent as the mother's age increases. The accompanying table will give you some idea of the frequency of these defects related to maternal age. Although older mothers are more likely than younger ones to produce trisomic infants, the actual number of trisomic babies is greater in women under thirty, because the younger group of women produces a much larger number of babies than the over-thirty group.

Incidence of Trisomy at Birth per 1,000 Live Births,
Estimated for the Midpoint of the Age Groups of Mother

Maternal Age	Down's (21)†	Other Trisomies (13 + 18)†	XXY	Total of All Trisomies*
20–24	0.7	0.1	0.4	2.0
25–29	0.9	0.1	0.4	2.2
30–34	1.5	0.2	0.6	3.2
35–39	6.2	0.6	1.2	8.5
40–44	19.8	3.6	2.8	27.2

*XYY is constant at 0.5/1000. Turner (45x) is constant at less than 0.1/1000. "All others" increase past age thirty from 0.2 to 0.3/1000.

†Number of the involved chromosome

Amniocentesis, the withdrawal of amniotic fluid from the pregnant uterus, is the investigative technique used to verify the presence or absence of trisomy or other chromosomal abnormality. The nuclei of fetal cells can be studied by microscopic techniques: The investigator takes a micro-photograph of a dividing cell, from which the individual chromosomes are identified and arranged in order. In skilled hands this forms a reliable map of the chromosome and a firm diagnosis of chromosomal abnormality can be made.

Defects of Genes

Genes are combinations of amino acids, arranged in sequences as part of a large molecule, deoxyribonucleic acid (DNA), located on the chromosome. Chromosomes are visible under the microscope, but the DNA molecule is far too small to be seen by this technique and therefore cannot be mapped in the same way that chromosomes are. We have nevertheless developed exquisite biochemical techniques for identifying a large number of specific genes and, even more significantly, verifying their absence. It is also possible to find abnormal biochemical products of abnormal genes. For example, the gene that instructs the bone marrow to form sickle hemoglobin can be identified biochemically. As another example, the biochemist can demonstrate the absence of the enzyme the lack of which is responsible for Tay-Sachs disease. These techniques are elaborate, time consuming, and expensive and it is important to know specifically what abnormality to look for in the laboratory in each individual case. We therefore apply the techniques principally to individuals whose pedigrees have already demonstrated the presence of a genetic defect.

Not all defects have been conclusively traced to genes; thus biochemical testing will not necessarily bring to light all genetic disorders. However the list of inherited abnormalities is already sufficiently long to occupy many pages in books on the subject.

Access to the Fetus: Noninvasive Techniques

The steady improvement in the quality of the images produced by ultrasound has made possible the correct prenatal identification of a wide range of anatomical defects. Ultrasound has also made it easier accurately to place a needle in the amniotic sac to withdraw fluid, or a catheter into a body cavity of the fetus. In the same way it aids in placing viewing fetoscopes through which the fetus can be seen.

Another valuable noninvasive screening procedure, useful in detecting neural tube developmental defects and sometimes Down's syndrome or other trisomies, has been the identification of elevated and depressed levels of alpha fetoprotein (AFP) in small samples of maternal blood.

The neural tube forms in the embryo from a flat structure, longer than it is wide. It curls up along its longer edges. These then fuse to form a tube which in turn grows into the brain and spinal cord. Normally the tube closes along its entire length and at its ends, but it may remain unfused at any point, most often at its head end and near its tail end. In either event the skin fails to close over it, leaving nervous tissue on the outside of the body. Cerebrospinal fluid, which contains AFP, can then be secreted directly into the amniotic fluid and the concentration of AFP in amniotic fluid is then far above normal.

Some of the AFP is transferred from the uterus to the mother's blood, so that, with neural tube defects, maternal blood AFP is elevated. Finding this on screening is an indication for sonographic study of the fetus's central nervous system to look for a tube defect. Other causes of elevated AFP are mentioned below.

At the other end of this spectrum, an unusually low concentration of AFP in maternal blood at the sixteenth week is often associated with trisomy, the tripling of a chromosome, which is responsible for such anomalies as Down's syndrome.

Access to the Fetus: Invasive Techniques

Chorionic Villus Sampling (CVS)

At the tenth week of pregnancy the products of conception do not yet quite fill the uterine cavity. The embryo itself is developing inside the sac of membranes, which also contains the amniotic fluid. The outer membrane, the chorion, has already formed a very large number of placental villi. These branch in a treelike fashion, reaching out into the maternal endometrium at the point where the definitive placenta will be located. Elsewhere they simply lie loosely free in the endometrial cavity. These villi, which are entirely of embryonic origin, later shrink down and disappear, but at ten weeks they are growing rapidly.

Under sonographic guidance, a polyethylene catheter can be directed through the cervix to the location of the free villi. By creating a vacuum with a suction pump, a small amount of villus material is sucked into the catheter. These villi can then be used both for immediate study of their nuclei and for cell culture for subsequent chromosome analysis. Since the villi are dividing rapidly it may be possible to find nuclei in which the chromosomes are separate. It is at this time that they can be photographed and mapped. When this is possible an immediate diagnosis of abnormal chromosome number is feasible. Fetal sex and fetal trisomies have been clearly identified by these methods. We can also study cultured villi for chemical evidence of metabolic disorders. The chromosomes of such villi can be readily mapped.

Since CVS can be carried out under moderate sedation and local anesthesia, the maternal risk is trivial. The incidence of intrauterine infection is greater than that experienced with amniocentesis, but infections occur in less than 1 percent of the patients. These usually respond promptly to antibiotic therapy. The risk of fetal loss is expressed as the additional risk of the procedure over the expected rate of spontaneous abortion at this duration of pregnancy; it has been estimated at about 1 percent.

The accuracy of the method is excellent. In one study, among some 500 CVS procedures, usable material was obtained in 489 patients. In 3 of these patients the sex of the embryo was incorrectly diagnosed, but none of these errors had any impact on the outcome of the pregnancy.

Among patients studied in early pregnancy because of advanced maternal age, the incidence of abnormal embryos is substantially greater than when the fetuses are studied at full term. This is believed to result from a selective early loss of abnormal fetuses.

It is accepted that in some cases, the diagnosis made by this still-new procedure must be verified by a subsequent amniocentesis.

Among women studied at about 8 weeks by sonography some 4 percent do not have a live embryo, although they appear still to be pregnant.

Among women studied by ultrasound between the seventh and twelfth week and found to have normal fetuses, approximately 1.5 percent of those less than thirty years of age subsequently abort spontaneously. Among women thirty to thirty-four years of age, 2.5 percent abort, and between thirty-five and thirty-nine years, 4.5 percent abort.

Amniocentesis

Amniocentesis is a procedure in which the amniotic sac is punctured to collect amniotic fluid and the cells or vernix shed into it by the fetus. It can be done after the fifteenth week of pregnancy. Earlier the puncture is technically difficult and carries a significant risk of miscarriage.

When amniocentesis is done for fetal diagnosis and therapy,

it is preceded by sonography to localize the placenta and to find a pool of amniotic fluid. The mother is mildly sedated. She lies on her back, her abdomen is prepared, and a needle is inserted into the fluid pool, usually under local anesthesia. The needle is of the same diameter as those used to draw blood from an arm vein, but is longer, since it must traverse the mother's skin, abdominal wall, and uterine wall to reach the fluid. The uterus is against the mother's abdominal wall so that there is no risk of injuring her other abdominal organs. The chance of complications is the same whether the placenta is anterior or posterior.

Once a suitable fluid sample is obtained, the needle is withdrawn and a small adhesive bandage is placed over the puncture site. Shortly thereafter the mother can get up and go about her business. There may be soreness at the needle stick for a day or two.

Occasionally the fetal skin is stuck with the needle but this does no lasting damage and rarely leaves a trace.

Immediately following collection, the information that can be obtained from studying the cells is limited to determining the genetic sex of the baby. This is done by counting the proportion of the cell nuclei that have Barr bodies (see pages 87–88).

The next step is to put the cells into culture media. After the cells have grown for a few weeks, their cell nuclei can be studied for the distribution of the chromosomes. Fresh amniotic fluid and the liquid culture media can be examined for the presence of abnormal compounds or for the absence of normal substances.

Early in the third timester amniocentesis may be done every few weeks in mothers known to be Rh sensitized. The amount of pigment present, resulting from the destruction of fetal red blood cells by the mother's anti-Rh antibodies, gives evidence of the severity of the fetal anemia.

Amniocentesis has been employed on rare occasions to administer medication to the fetus; it is a part of the process of *in utero* fetal blood transfusion.

Study of amniotic fluid in pregnancies closer to term, to measure the amount of lipid (fatty) chemical substances present, can be used to estimate fetal lung maturity. These amniocenteses are being replaced by noninvasive sonographic study of such items as the amount of fetal fat and the rate of fetal breathing, combined with fetal heart rate observations.

Amniocentesis has also been employed to search for bacteria in the fluid in doubtful cases of amniotic infection.

Fetoscopy

A viewing instrument called a fetoscope, tiny enough to pass through a needle, can be introduced into the amniotic cavity, making it possible to view the fetus under illumination by cold light. The method of inserting the fetoscopy needle is the same as for the amniocentesis, though for this purpose the diameter of the needle is greater.

Unfortunately, the view is not always clear, since the amniotic fluid may be cloudy, due in part to the fetal cells floating in it. The field of view is also limited, so that only very small parts of the fetus can be seen at any one moment. By maneuvering the fetoscope around it is possible to see fetal blood vessels, especially on the surface of the placenta when it is on the posterior wall of the uterus. Employing specially developed miniaturized instruments one can obtain samples of fetal blood and tiny bits of fetal skin, which can then be used for further cytologic and biochemical study.

In at least seven hereditary disorders there are fetal defects that can be seen through a fetoscope. These include: the presence of more than five fingers on a hand; the fusion of fingers together where they should be free of one another, and major defects of the limbs. Even where genes for these defects are present in a family, not every fetus will have the defect and it is therefore important to identify those fetuses in which the defect is present. If sonography reaches a level of precision in which it is possible reliably to count the number of fingers on a fetus's hand, fetoscopy will be obsolete, but we are not even close to that kind of accuracy in sonography at the present time.

Risks of Amniocentesis and Fetoscopy

These procedures are carried out under aseptic precautions with light sedation and local anesthesia in the abdominal wall. Despite care, infection can occur, but this usually responds to antibiotics. The hole made in the membranes may be delayed in healing, or may not heal at all. In either case, the amniotic fluid drains past the membranes and out through the cervix. Fetal death may ensue or, if the pregnancy is prolonged, the fetus may be born prematurely with incompletely developed lungs. The puncture itself may damage fetal blood vessels; such an accident can result in fetal death due to hemorrhage.

Overall the fetal loss rate from amniocentesis is perhaps double the expected loss of about 4 per 1,000 among normally pregnant women with a live fetus at sixteen weeks. As indicated, the loss rate from fetoscopy is probably ten times this. Fetoscopy has a risk of abortion in the vicinity of 5 percent. Its use is presently limited to the very few hereditary diseases that cannot be diagnosed in any other way.

With the continuing improvement in the images possible with sonography, a method of inserting a long needle into the umbilical vein as early as the seventeenth week of pregnancy has been developed. Fetal blood can then be collected directly, greatly simplifying the diagnosis of some fetal abnormalities. The risk is estimated at about 1.5 percent, less than that of fetoscopy but greater than amniocentesis.

There does not seem to be justification for the use of invasive diagnostic procedures on women who do not intend to choose abortion if the study proves an unfavorable diagnosis.

Abortion for Genetic Defect

Since the presence of a defective fetus only rarely affects the mothers medically, the reasons for abortion of such a fetus are psychosocial. The mother should therefore be carefully informed prior to any invasive procedure of the risks to her and to the fetus, including the possibility of error in diagnosis. The decision whether to abort must be entirely hers.

The advantage of CVS is that in some cases the diagnosis can be established early enough so that abortion can be carried out by suction evacuation or by early D & E; by all odds the safest methods. Because a diagnosis of fetal defect cannot be made by amniocentesis earlier than the eighteenth or nineteenth week, except in rare instances, abortion, if elected by the mother, must then be by amnioinfusion or late D&E, both of which methods entail an appreciably greater risk to the mother than do the methods available at the earlier stage.

A few instances of selective abortion, where one fetus in a multiple pregnancy has a defect, have been reported. It is necessary to employ a technique that will abort one fetus without risk to a normal twin or triplet. At present, this can only be done in the second trimester and presents formidable moral and technical problems.

Treatment of the Fetus *In Utero*

Administration of blood transfusion to the anemic fetus *in utero* was the first treatment ever given directly to the unborn child. This was introduced more than a quarter of a century ago by Sir Albert W. Liley when he gave the blood through a needle placed *in utero* into the fetus's peritoneal cavity, the potential space which contains the abdominal organs such as the stomach, liver, intestines and spleen. He did this as early as the twenty-eighth week of pregnancy. It was of course first necessary to develop methods of *in utero* diagnosis of the severity of fetal anemia. If it is certain that the anemia will be fatal *in utero* before the fetus is mature enough to survive birth and subsequent transfusion, then *in utero* transfusion can be done.

Other *In Utero* Treatment

As we have seen, improvement in sonography has now made possible not only highly accurate diagnoses of fetal diseases but also the accurate placement of the devices necessary to treat them. As a result, surgical therapy *in utero* has been expanding steadily in the last decade. Thus far actual operations such as removal of tumors and repair of defects have eluded our skills. What has been accomplished, however, has been the drainage of excessive fluid accumulations in the nervous system and the urinary tract, thus preventing prenatal damage to these essential organs from stretching of the normal structures.

In the urinary tract, obstruction can occur at the point where the bladder connects with the urethra, the short tube through which the baby urinates. Obstruction can also occur at the place where the renal pelvis, the small reservoir for urine in the kidney, connects with the ureter, the conduit that carries urine down to the bladder. If such obstructions are present, urine continues to form and blows up the drainage system to astounding size. This in turn, by back pressure, damages the kidney substance itself. Treatment of this has now been accomplished in carefully selected cases by placing fine catheters into the stretched organs and allowing the fluid to drain into the fetus's peritoneal cavity or the amniotic sac.

The same principle can be applied in instances of obstruction to the proper flow of cerebrospinal fluid: the fluid found within the brain substance itself and also surrounding it and the spinal cord as a shock-absorbing cushion. Obstruction to the flow of this fluid through the proper passages results in hydrocephalus (Greek: *hydro*, "water"; *cephalos*, "head"). By draining the fluid it may be possible to protect the integrity of the brain substance from damage by stretching and pressure.

Not every fetus is a candidate for this kind of intervention. For one thing it has been learned that hydrocephalus is very often associated with a number of other serious anomalies, so that although it may be possible to relieve the back pressure the outcome for the fetus still is not good. If the obstruction is diagnosed late in pregnancy we can deliver the fetus and treat it after birth. How to handle this anomaly must be decided on an individual basis; as our diagnostic techniques improve our decisions will be on steadily sounder ground.

Medical Treatment Prior to Birth

Medicine given to the mother has to be considered as possible medical treatment of the fetus. Most drugs cross the placenta, but in this discussion I wish to consider only those drugs administered to the mother whose intent is not to treat her but rather an abnormal condition in the fetus.

At present the commonest of these are the conditions that cause tachycardia: an unusually rapid heart rate in the fetus. The normal rate for a fetal heart is 120 to 160 beats per minute. When the rate exceeds 220, some fetuses actually go into heart failure. This may be the explanation for some of the "silent" deaths of the fetus, as the fetal tachycardia does not produce maternal symptoms. A number of fetuses with severe tachycardia have now been treated by giving the mother drugs that slow down the heart. These are called cardioactive drugs; the principal ones are digitalis and propranolol. It is possible to achieve the necessary concentrations of these drugs in the fetus without adversely affecting the mother. On occasion the babies may need further treatment after birth, but they are protected from serious damage until they can be born.

When premature delivery between the twenty-eighth and thirty-fourth week is planned because of a complication of pregnancy that may be injurious to the fetus, corticoid medication has been given to the mother with the purpose of accelerating fetal lung maturation. The term "corticoid" refers to the fact that these drugs—actually betamethasone and dexamethasone—have the same effects as hormones secreted by the adrenal cortex. Corticoids are known to be present in increasing amounts in amniotic fluid as term approaches. We do not have complete proof that the treatment works, however.

In one unusual instance a woman who was given radioactive iodine to treat her thyroid disease was found to have been pregnant at the time. It was assumed that the thyroid of the fetus had been damaged by the radiation and therefore later in pregnancy thyroid medication was injected into the amniotic fluid. A normal infant was delivered. We can expect that we will see more of this type of treatment in the future.

In Utero Treatment of Metabolic Defects

What follows is an attempt to look into the future.

A number of uncommon diseases are the result of genetic defects in which a particular enzyme essential to body chemistry is absent. Without the enzyme certain biochemical processes cannot be completed, and abnormal products accumulate, eventually doing damage to the individual. These have been called inborn errors of metabolism.

The commonest of all inherited disorders, cystic fibrosis, is due to the lack of the enzyme that prevents mucus from being sticky. Tay-Sachs disease results from the lack of an enzyme called neuraminidase, which is necessary for the complete normal development of the central nervous system. There are many other such defects.

Laboratory scientists are now able to introduce into animals genes that are otherwise absent. This is done by sophisticated biochemistry, which first synthesizes a gene and attaches it to a virus known not to cause disease in that animal. The virus, when injected, is able to insert the gene into such cells as the bone marrow of the recipient animal. The newly introduced gene can then direct the formation of its enzyme.

Thus far nobody has introduced a functioning gene into a human being, but there is every reason to believe that it will be done. The theory and the laboratory experience are already in place. The gene for neuraminidase could thus be inserted into victims of Tay-Sachs disease and render them normal. Once this has been done successfully with children there is no reason to think that it cannot be done with fetuses.

Conditions That Can Be Diagnosed in the Fetus

Neural Tube Defects

When the neural tube fails to close (see pages 438–39) the alpha fetoprotein in the mother's blood is elevated. This is confirmed by amniocentesis and the diagnosis is proven by sonographic examination of the fetus.

Maternal alpha fetoprotein levels may also be elevated in such conditions as congenital nephrosis (a degenerative condition of the substance of the kidney), fetal death, defects in the formation of the fetal abdominal wall and umbilical cord, and twin pregnancy.

It has been urged that alpha fetoprotein in maternal blood be routinely measured for the early detection of central nervous system abnormalities in the fetus. In Scotland and Ireland, the countries of the world with the highest incidence of neural tube defects (and also in Appalachia in the United States, an enclave of descendants of Scotch and Irish immigrants since the eighteenth and nineteenth centuries), there is no question that this screening is justified, but there is no agreement as to whether it should be applied to all patients.

Interestingly, women who have previously had infants with neural tube defects have only a slightly increased likelihood of having another such fetus. They are nevertheless candidates for alpha fetoprotein screening. All pregnant women should be informed of the availability of such a study.

Metabolic Disorders

This group includes the abnormalities of storage of such substances of lipids and glycogen (the material which is the storage form for ordinary sugar) in the body cells. These are now all detectable by amniocentesis. Women with a family history of such diseases are obviously eligible for such study.

Enzyme Deficiencies

A large number of inherited diseases are characterized by the absence of a particular enzyme needed for an essential body process. Tay-Sachs disease and cystic fibrosis are examples. Combined immune deficiency in children results from the absence of an enzyme essential to the formation of antibodies.

Another member of this group is phenylketonuria (PKU). The blood of newborns can be tested for evidence of this defect, so that if it is present, dietary treatment can be promptly commenced before the baby suffers the brain damage that otherwise results.

PKU, Tay-Sachs, cystic fibrosis, combined immune deficiency, and other less common diseases traceable to the absence of a specific gene or enzyme can now almost all be diagnosed by amniocentesis in the fetus prior to birth. Whenever such a disease exists in the children, both parents must either be carriers or have the disease themselves.

Other Inherited Developmental Defects

There should be mentioned here two other inherited conditions, both rare and of obscure causation, both diagnosable by sonography. One is "brittle bone disease" (osteogenesis imperfecta). This stems from a defect in the laying down of calcium in the bones, which are therefore extremely fragile and may break simply as a consequence of movement of the fetus in utero. The other defect is called spodylothroracic dysplasia; in this the formation of the chest is markedly distorted.

Chromosomal Abnormalities

An abnormal chromosome number may occur simply by accident, as an inherited characteristic, or as an incident of advanced maternal age. Extra chromosomes can occur either among the twenty-two autosomes or in the sex chromosomes. A fetus can survive to term lacking a chromosome only if it is a Y chromosome missing from an XY pair. The absence of any autosome, or of the X from the XY pair, is lethal in fetal life.

The table on page 437 shows the incidence of trisomies at birth per thousand live births, organized by groups according to the ages of the mothers. These figures do not correspond with the higher incidence of trisomies as measured by chorionic villus sampling because, as we now know, some of the afflicted fetuses do not survive to be born alive. Trisomies 13 and 18 are compatible with live birth, but the children are seriously abnormal and do not survive early childhood. Trisomy 47XXY, on the other hand, results in men who are tall, slender, and have deficient male external genitalia. As adults they have poor sperm formation, as a consequence of which they are ordinarily infertile. The steady increase of these trisomies as the mother becomes older is obvious from the table.

The likelihood of Down's syndrome reaches approximately 1 in 100 at about age thirty-nine and a half and the likelihood of all trisomies reaches 1 in 100 slightly earlier than this.

The 47XYY anomaly is apparently accidental and has a constant incidence at 0.5 per 1,000. Most of these individuals are normal males. The 45X Turner syndrome, which produces externally female infertile individuals who are short in stature, occurs at a rate of about 1 for every 10,000 live births regardless of maternal age. All other abnormalities are estimated to increase from approximately 2 per 10,000 to 3 per 10,000 when the mothers pass the age of thirty.

Trisomies should be suspected if screening of maternal serum reveals diminished alpha fetoprotein levels. However, low levels have also been found among diabetic mothers, so that the diagnosis cannot be made from the alpha fetoprotein value alone but requires further investigation of the fetus, by amniocentesis for chromosome pattern and by sonography for its physical development.

Some family trees have an unusual number of instances of Down's syndrome. This may be due to a phenomenon known as translocation, in which two chromosomes with very short arms, one of which is number 21, become stuck together. If one parent is a translocation carrier, one-third of all the newborns will have Down's syndrome, one-third will be carriers of the abnormal chromosome, and one-third will be normal. These diagnoses can be made by amniocentesis or CVS study of fetal cells.

Women with Down's syndrome, since they have an excess chromosome 21, can be expected to have many more children with the chromosome abnormality than normal women, and indeed that is the case. Among 30 pregnancies observed in such women, 10 newborns also had Down's syndrome; eighteen children were normal.

Anemias

Sickle-cell disease, an inherited defect of red blood cells that results in anemia that begins in childhood, can be detected prior to birth by biochemical studies of amniotic fluid. The same is true of thalasemia major, another abnormality of hemoglobin in the red blood cells, which also causes severe anemia.

Rh Isoimmunization

Hemoglobin, the complex red chemical that carries oxygen and carbon dioxide, is in a thick solution in the blood. This solution is contained in tiny disc-shaped bags with characteristics much like those of the bags used to store frozen food. These are the red blood cells (RBC) that give blood its color. A teaspoon will hold twenty million such cells.

On the surface of the plasticlike skin of each red blood cell are the proteins that determine the individual's blood groups. These follow the strict rules of heredity.

The Rh factor is one of these groups. Some 85 percent of Caucasians are Rh-positive, and the rest are negative. African and Oriental peoples are all Rh-positive. Persons who are Rh-negative do not normally have antibodies to the Rh factor. However, if an Rh-negative person is exposed to Rh blood by pregnancy or transfusion, antibodies can form. This process is called sensitization. Since the antibodies are anti-Rh and the person is Rh-negative, no harm results unless and until another Rh-positive transfusion is given, in which event a transfusion reaction occurs. Similarly, an Rh-negative sensitized woman may be carrying an Rh-positive baby. In that case the anti-Rh antibodies can cross the placenta and damage the Rh-positive RBC of the fetus.

Since at least 85 percent of men are Rh-positive, most Rh-negative women will have Rh-positive children. During pregnancy and at the time of placental separation, Rh-positive RBC can enter the mother's circulation and sensitize her.

If an Rh-negative woman has only Rh-negative fetuses, neither she nor the baby can become sensitized. The only way a woman can assure herself of this is to have all her babies by an Rh-negative partner. However, sensitization fortunately is an infrequent event. It occurs rarely with first babies and is most unlikely with any pregnancy if the partner is heterozygous, that is, has the gene for Rh-positive and also the gene for Rh-negative. Even when the partner is homozygous Rh-positive, and all the fetuses are Rh-positive, the incidence of sensitization is low.

Fetal Damage Due to Sensitization

Infrequent though it is, sensitization can be troublesome. When a sensitized woman carries an Rh-positive fetus, the transfer of anti-Rh antibodies across the placenta relentlessly causes injury to fetal red blood cells. The fetus becomes more and more anemic. The hemoglobin is released from damaged RBC faster than the fetus's bone marrow can form new RBC. There is chemical change of the free hemoglobin into bilirubin, a yellow pigment that stains the tissues. *In utero*, the bilirubin can cross the placenta into the mother, who excretes it in her urine.

The fetus then is born very anemic. The blood-forming organs like the liver and spleen are enlarged; the baby turns yellow very rapidly since its immature liver is not equal to the task of disposing of such large amounts of bilirubin. The name of this condition is erythroblastosis fetalis. The treatment is exchange transfusion, in which small fractions of the anemic Rh-positive baby blood are taken out and replaced by equal amounts of Rh-negative donor blood, step by step, until about 94 percent replacement is achieved. This process corrects the anemia and removes excess bilirubin.

The effects of sensitization on the fetuses tend to become worse with each successive Rh-positive pregnancy. Some fetuses die early in the third trimester simply from profound anemia. Others lose liver and cardiac functions and become severely waterlogged. This condition is called hydrops fetalis.

The severity of the RBC destruction during pregnancy can be gauged by studying amniotic fluid obtained by amniocentesis. The yellow color is due to bilirubin and other neuroglobin breakdown products; it reflects the degree of the anemia and can be measured. In severe cases the fetus is given transfusion *in utero* through a needle or a catheter placed through the mother's abdomen in its peritoneal cavity. The goal is to protect the life of the fetus until its lungs are mature enough for it to be delivered. In the most extreme cases, when impending or early hydrops is diagnosed by sonography, transfusion has been accomplished *in utero*, using fetoscopy or sonography. A marvelous technical achievement, exchanges are now successfully done with surprisingly high birth rate of living fetuses.

In Utero Transfusion

In utero transfusion must often be repeated because transfused RBC do not last as long as normal RBC—and in addition, the growth of the fetus necessitates a steadily enlarging supply of RBC. The outcomes with intrauterine transfusions recently reported by the Perinatal Research Group in Winnipeg, for years among the leaders in this field, are truly outstanding. In their most recently treated series they have 100 percent survival of the anemic fetuses and 75 percent survival of those observed to have hydrops *in utero*. The long-term follow-up studies of such infants suggests that despite the injury suffered in the uterus their eventual development is normal.

Treatment to prevent sensitization of the Rh-negative woman has been in use now for a number of years and has resulted in an almost complete disappearance of the problems just described. Human anti-Rh antibodies (Rhogam), precisely the same proteins that cross the placenta and cause trouble in the fetus, are given to women by injection at times when they might experience showers of Rh-positive RBC. The sensitization that would otherwise take place is then effectively prevented. We administer these antibodies whenever an abortion or an amniocentesis is done on an unsensitized Rh-negative woman, unless we can be quite certain that the father of the pregnancy is also Rh-negative.

Rh-negative women who are pregnant by Rh-positive partners and who are not sensitized are given a dose of the Rhogam at the twenty-eighth week of pregnancy. This prevents sensitization from small leaks of Rh-positive blood that may occur during the course of pregnancy.

When an Rh-negative woman delivers it is routine to obtain the Rh blood type on the baby, and if the newborn is Rh-positive, to give the mother a dose of Rhogam immediately. When there has been a difficult operative delivery, when there has been difficulty in the birth of the placenta, or when there have been twins, it is not uncommon for the leakage of Rh-positive RBC into the mother to be greater than in a normal birth. Under those circumstances a double dose of the Rhogam is given. With these techniques Rh isoimmunization has become a rarity and the number of problem cases continues to drop.

Genetic Counseling

As late as the nineteenth century, in the developed world it was common for women to have large number of babies, beginning in their late teens or early twenties. Often, only a few of these children would survive. The others succumbed to infectious diseases of childhood, usually in the first year of life, during which the infant death rate was very high.

Advances in medicine have made spectacular changes in the expectations for babies. The killing infectious diseases of infancy are by now virtually eliminated. We now can expect 99 percent of healthy babies born at term to survive childhood.

This greatly increased rate of survival has been accompanied by a decrease in the number of children born to individual women. The reasons for this are complicated; in recent years, a significant factor has been that an increasing number of women have postponed marriage and childbearing into their thirties. By doing this they obviously decrease their opportunity to replace a child lost for whatever reason, and increase the value of each child that they have. The enhanced importance of the child under these circumstances seems to create pressure on women who are pregnant or contemplating pregnancy to produce a perfect baby at almost any cost. This is almost certainly the explanation for the steadily increasing demand for prenatal diagnosis, even from women who have no reason to expect to conceive an abnormal fetus. Responding to that demand, those of us who give prenatal care to pregnant women are called on to give them information about the techniques available for diagnosing an abnormal child *in utero*, and how they are used.

Candidates for Counseling

The information possessed by individuals or couples who have a family history of an inherited defect usually consists of a mixture of common-sense, fact, old wives' tales, and scientific data. A genetics counselor can sort these out and provide either assurance or warning.

Some defects are sporadic; they appear out of the blue with no prior instances in the family. A complete family tree for several generations is necessary to verify that this has occurred. I recall a couple who produced three children close together; each baby became severely jaundiced after birth and survived, in ill health, for only a few weeks. The couple was advised never to have another baby. Seven years later, following a contraceptive accident, I saw the mother in early pregnancy to counsel in regard to abortion. The couple were Mormon and had a detailed genealogy available. There were no other cases of early infant death anywhere in the family tree. We were able to advise the patient that her chances of having a normal child were about 80 percent. She kept the pregnancy and delivered a normal infant.

On the other hand, some serious conditions are known to result from gene mutation and can therefore be inherited. One of these is retinoblastoma, a malignant tumor of the eye. Either parent with a disease such as this must be advised that he can expect some or all of his children to have it as well, and that because of the genetic origin of the disease a negative family history is of no predictive value.

Autosomal Gene Defects

Gene defects can be autosomal-dominant: That is, the defect is present on one of the twenty-three autosomes and may manifest itself either in the fetus, in childhood, or in maturity, even though the matching autosome of the pair from the other parent is perfectly normal. The severity of the defect cannot be predicted, but that it will appear is a certainty. Huntington's chorea, a severe neurological disorder, follows this pattern. This disease unfortunately does not make itself known until about age forty, by which time the carrier of the gene already has had a family. Recently it has been shown that there may be delicate biochemical tests that can detect carriers of the gene before they develop the disease itself. One half of all the descendants of a man or woman with Hungtington's chorea will eventually develop the disease.

Other gene defects are autosomal-recessive. They become manifest only when both chromosomes of a pair have the defect. This is the homozygous state. If only one chromosome of the pair lacks the gene, the individual appears normal, although sensitive tests may disclose a relative deficiency in, for example, an enzyme produced by the gene. This is called the heterozygous carrier state.

Tay-Sachs disease is an example of this situation. Homozygotes manifest the disease and die in infancy. Heterozygous parents lack the gene on one chromosome. They are normal in all respects except for a slight deficiency of neuroaminidase. The deficiency can be found by laboratory testing, and the carrier of the defect identified. If both parents (or prospective parents) are carriers, one-fourth of their children will be normal, one-half will be carriers like the parents, and one-quarter will have the enzyme defect. The diagnosis can be determined by amniocentesis and probably in the future by CVS.

Other Chromosome Defects

There are familial patterns of defect due to chromosome translocation. Two chromosomes with very small short arms, for example number 18 and number 21, can fuse at their acrocenters to form a new abnormal chromosome. The genetic outcome with this defect in one parent who is a carrier is that one-quarter of all progeny will be normal and one-quarter will have the translocated chromosome only and appear normal. One-quarter will have the translocated chromosome plus a normal chromosome and will have one of the trisomy syndromes. The fourth quarter of the embryos never develops, so that if we consider only fetuses, the proportions are one-third, one-third, and one-third. The diagnosis of translocation can be made by mapping the chromosomes of the parents and the fetuses.

Sex Chromosome Gene Defects

In females, the two X chromosomes match each other and gene defects, with rare exceptions, are heterozygous and recessive. They therefore do not find expression in the fetus or adult. However, if the embryo is a male, the upper short arms of the X are not matched by the Y (which is actually shaped like a V), which effectively has no short arms. Gene defects located on the short arms of the X can then express themselves in the individual. Instances of this kind of defect are hemophilia and most of the muscular dystrophies. The gene is carried by the mother on one of her X chromosomes and the disease is seen only in her male children. The mother herself is necessarily a heterozygous carrier.

When parents are apprehensive that their child may have one of these sex-linked diseases, the sex of the embryo can be identified by CVS, and if it is female, the parents can be reassured that it will not have the problem. If the embryo is a male, it is still possible that it may not be afflicted, and the mother can await the culture of the cells from CVS or later from amniocentesis before committing herself on whether to abort.

Counseling for Advanced Maternal Age

CVS and amniocentesis will reliably identify the instances of the trisomies related to advanced maternal age. The likelihood of these is shown in the table on page 437. It is the role of the genetic counselor and the obstetrical attendant to explain the genetic, pediatric, developmental, and social implications of the particular trisomy involved. For some mothers there is no alternative to abortion if the presence of a defect is verified. For others the decision is more complicated. These mothers may wish to share their problem with a spouse, a counselor, a parent, or a friend, to help them deal with it.

Is the Defect Detectable?

The genetic counselor will have to advise concerned parents of the likelihood of repetition of an abnormal fetus and also whether, if it repeats, the defect can be detected in early pregnancy. We are not yet able to detect every abnormality. In some instances the mother will simply have to await the birth of the baby to know whether it is normal. This inevitable uncertainty may influence her decision about carrying such a pregnancy.

It is also important to know whether the defect is treatable in the event that it does occur. It is now theoretically possible to transfer enzymes into individuals who are lacking them. If the means are found to make such transfer practical, it may be that some of the inherited errors of metabolism, presently uniformly fatal, may yield to treatment in the future, and make possible the survival of an infant that might otherwise have been aborted on genetic grounds.

Availability of Abortion

When a woman has given birth to abnormal children and has had to experience the anguish of watching them sicken and die of untreatable conditions or to see them survive with serious handicaps, she is understandably loath to undertake further pregnancies that might have the same outcome. Prenatal diagnosis and the possibility of aborting abnormal fetuses have gone far to eliminate this anguish.

Some years ago, I was consulted by a woman whose first child had a rare metabolic disorder characterized by chronic severe anemia and extreme sensitivity of his skin to damage on exposure to daylight. She became pregnant again, and it was at least theoretically possible, by amniocentesis, to diagnose the metabolic disorder, although such fetal diagnosis had never actually been done previously. Accordingly, it was tried, and indeed it was discovered that this second fetus was similarly afflicted; it was aborted at the mother's request. Reassured by the knowledge that diagnosis was readily available, she went on through two more pregnancies, each diagnosed as normal by amniocentesis and each resulting in a normal baby. As of this writing, she is pregnant again, and known once more to have a normal infant. Had genetic counseling and diagnostic amniocentesis not been available, this woman might well have terminated her childbearing career after the disaster of her first child, and never had the pleasure of bringing up normal children.

Availability of Genetic Counseling

Competent genetic counseling is now available at every medical school in the United States, and, as I have indicated above, the individual practitioner delivering obstetrical services is required to take the first step to provide such counseling. By now, this field has become very complicated.

The first lessons in genetics were derived from the red and white sweet peas that Abbé Mendel bred to discover the laws of inheritance of physical characteristics. He learned that crossbreeding the pure red variety with the pure white variety produced a pink generation. Breeding the pink sweet peas together yielded a crop that was 50 percent pink, 25 percent white, and 25 percent red. This is the basic pattern of all genetic inheritance if the trait in question is produced by one gene. As you have read above, the inheritance of autosomal recessive genes from heterozygous parents is a process that exactly follows the Mendelian pattern.

Not all genetic traits, however, are so simply derived as to conform to the Mendelian rules. Neural tube defects are an example of apparent deviation from the sweet pea pattern. This may be because several genes, possibly on more than one chromosome, are involved in producing the defect. We know, also, that eye color shows a complex pattern of inheritance involving several genes. A competent genetic counselor will be able to teach parents, or prospective parents about the genetic aspects of the particular features with which they are most concerned, as well as the influences of environment and other relevant factors on genetic inheritance.

Certainly any patient who has had an abnormal child or who comes from a family with a history of genetic defects is well advised to consult a genetics counseling clinic. In most cases the advice available there will be reassuring as to the outcome of the pregnancy, but if that is not possible, it will point the couple in the direction of competent diagnosis and care.

21

Family Planning

Throughout history, when faced with overcrowding and scarcity of food, human beings have attempted to control their numbers. If the natural limitation by starvation, disease, and accident failed, they resorted to infanticide, often selectively eliminating females, since they were economically less productive. In the hostile environment found in parts of the Arctic, female infanticide was common into the first quarter of the twentieth century. Existence of the practice is demonstrated by some statistics compiled in 1932. Among the Netsilik Eskimos the sex ratio in the age group up to eighteen years was 48 females to every 100 males in the population; in the Barren Grounds area the ratio was 46 to 100. This contrasts with the expected sex ratio at birth of about 100 females to 106 males.

It is uncertain at what stage of our history our precivilized forebears came to the realization that sexual intercourse was what brought babies into being. We suppose that it must have happened relatively recently, as measured by the approximately two-million-year history of our species. There are three major reasons why we presume that early humankind did not associate intercourse with the birth of offspring. First, they had no systematic method for recording the passage of time, and therefore were unable to associate the birth of a baby with an event far in the past—an event, moreover, that would probably have been repeated many times over in the meanwhile. Second, sexual intercourse was commonplace between children, and such intercourse necessarily did not result in babies. There was nothing momentous about the sex act, any more than there was about sleeping or eating, and therefore there was no reason to associate it with so dramatic a happening as the birth of a child. It was easier to credit a thunderstorm or the foam from the sea with the performance of a miracle. Finally, among primitive peoples as among their descendants some men and women engaged in intercourse throughout their lives without ever generating a pregnancy. There is no reason to identify the causal quality of the sex act, if it has no observable consequences.

Early References to Contraception and Abortion

When the Babylonian Code of Hammurabi was drawn up in about 1800 B.C., abortion was important enough to be discouraged through the penalty of death by crucifixion. Among the medical treatises written on papyrus by the priest-physicians of the ancient Pharaohs four thousand years ago, seven of which survive in part or in whole, three are gynecological works which contain contraceptive and abortifacient recipes for ladies of the court. By the time that the first book of the Old Testament, Genesis, was written about 1500 B.C., contraception by coitus interruptus was sufficiently widespread among the early Hebrews that four verses (Genesis xxxviii: 7–10) were devoted to its interdiction through the parable of Onan.

Which Is Older, Abortion or Contraception?

We do not know with any certainty whether abortion or contraception is the older form of family limitation.

The early hunters slew pregnant animals and saw the uterus and the fetus within. No doubt some of their pregnant females had their bellies ripped in accidents and they must have witnessed the residence of the unborn fetus. Did they attempt to deliver it forthwith? Did they recognize it as a living creature? When did they realize that externalized semen is infertile? It may be stated categorically that few if any people throughout history have bred or breed to their full capacity. Some method of family limitation—continence, often through taboos; abortion; or simple means of contraception—has always been employed. The average woman who commences her reproductive life at seventeen and makes no effort at family limitation will produce thirteen living children. Today and in recent years this degree of unrestrained fertility is met only occasionally. At present it is seen largely in unusual religious sects such as the Hutterites in this country.

Contraception versus Abortion

Soranus, the famous gynecologist of antiquity, in Chapter XIX of his *Gynecology*, written in about A.D. 130, discusses the question: Which is the better method to limit child birth, abortion or contraception? He concludes that it is safer to prevent conception than to destroy its product. However, this decision was made on the basis of the substantial physical and psychological trauma that resulted from the inept and dangerous methods of abortion that were the only recourse at that time.

In the centuries that followed the pronouncement of Soranus, abortion continued to present extreme hazard to the life or health of a pregnant woman. This was true until the twentieth century, when practitioners began to invest their ingenuity in developing methods of abortion that would be both safe and effective. One of the most successful of these methods is the use of suction evacuation. The late Christopher Tietze pointed out the almost incredible safety of abortion by suction evacuation at the seventh week of pregnancy. The use of this technique as a backup in case of a failure of a barrier method (such as the condom or the diaphragm) results in the lowest risk so far achieved for women practicing contraception. It is recognized therefore that abortion has become a form of family planning. This of course assumes conscientious use of the barrier methods and, if they fail, timely resort to abortions. Otherwise it is probably correct, on safety grounds, that contraceptives are to be preferred.

These considerations must be dealt with if we are to reduce the present exceedingly high rate of adolescent pregnancies in the United States. Not until we establish the educational means to teach early adolescents how to avoid pregnancy, as part of their education in the family, in schools, and in religious institutions are we likely to make any headway. Very few adolescents are motivated to have either an abortion or a pregnancy. If we recognize that they fall under serious peer pressure to be sexually active we must then accept the responsibility of providing them with a means of preventing pregnancy and the knowledge of how to use those means.

Prohibition of Birth Control in the United States

Before 1873 there were no laws in the United States concerning contraception. However, in that year, Anthony Comstock, secretary of the New York Society for the Suppression of Vice, persuaded the Congress to pass a federal anti–birth control law. He then persuaded many state legislatures to pass their own statutes. The acts of Congress were enforced nationwide by a prohibition on mailing contraceptive devices and information. As has always been the case, these laws principally penalized the poor.

Margaret Sanger

The first full-time American evangelist to fight for the liberalization of birth control was a trained nurse, the mother of three children, Margaret Sanger. She had had good training in fighting for causes on the picket lines of the I.W.W. and in the struggle for woman's suffrage. Her focus of interest was concentrated on birth control through her experiences while nursing among Jewish and Italian immigrants in the slums of lower Manhattan. There she saw at first hand the misery resulting from unplanned and unwanted pregnancies, which led to either life-threatening abortions or a plethora of ill-provided-for children.

In 1912, at age thirty-three, she defied the United States Postal Department regulations by writing articles on birth control for the *Call*, a socialist paper widely distributed by mail. When indicted she fled abroad, where she used her self-imposed exile to study birth control in England, France, and Holland. When she returned to the United States she brought with her the knowledge and appreciation of the usefulness of the diaphragm. Mrs. Sanger's motivation in the espousal of birth control, a term she coined, was singleminded—prevention of unwanted conceptions among the married poor. This ideal was not influenced by efforts to limit population growth, for then there was no problem in the United States or elsewhere of excessively rapid population growth.

Mrs. Sanger opened the first birth-control clinic in the Western world in the slums of Brooklyn in October 1916, which immediately led to her arrest—the first of eight. Under her leadership federal and state anti-birth-control statutes were eroded by public and judicial opinion. In November 1921 the dispersal by the police on the order of Cardinal Hayes of a public meeting which she was to address in New York's Town Hall brought the American press to her side.

Legal Emancipation of Birth Control

In 1936 there was a landmark decision by the New York Circuit Court of Appeals in the case of *The U.S.* v. *One Package*, the package being three diaphragms imported from Japan. The favorable opinion of the three-judge court legalized prescription of contraceptives by the medical profession for health indications. The final blow against the statutory ban on birth control was the United States Supreme Court's decision in 1965 declaring the prohibitory law of Connecticut unconstitutional, largely as an invasion of privacy.

Reasons for Effective Contraception

There is no longer any reason (if one ever existed) to deny women the right to be sexually active without the threat of unwanted pregnancy. Pregnancy and childbirth do carry a health risk for the woman, however safe they have become. Furthermore, responsibility for child-rearing ordinarily falls upon the mother, and this has a major impact on the way in which she spends the rest of her life.

The availability and use of effective contraceptives is essential to accomplish family limitation. Each couple should be given the means to tailor the size of the family to suit personal desires and plans. Since 97 of 100 babies born alive in the United States reach adulthood, women should be offered the opportunity to plan with reasonable assurance the number of children they want to rear.

As I noted earlier, until fairly recent times a couple had to have a large number of children in order to be certain of having a few who might look after them in their old age. Now, however, the number of children is a personal decision. There is no over-all ideal family size because the ideal varies from person to person and couple to couple, affected by age, health, income, social and religious mores, and emotional needs for parenthood.

Many countries in the world are now suffering from hunger and related health problems because their populations have outgrown their land's ability to feed them an adequate diet. In the United States we are an affluent society, and we can afford to allow the decisions on family size to be made, unregulated, by the parents and prospective parents themselves. The kind of rigorous restriction of family size that has become a matter of public policy in China has not yet become a necessity in our country. There is no biological reason why people should not have their children as close together or as far apart as they wish. We have no scientific data at present to show that the health of a normal woman on an adequate diet is adversely affected by having her children as close together as she pleases and nature will allow. With lengthy intervals the situation is different because the woman has become substantially older with each birth and, as has been shown, her fertility normally will decrease with advancing age.

Demographers have uniformly observed that as a society becomes more affluent its birth rate steadily falls. In the United States at the present time the overall birth rate is below the level which provides for replacement, and the death rate continues to fall, so that the population is slowly expanding. However, on a global scale, we are still experiencing a population explosion. This has come to public attention in such areas as Bangladesh and sub-Saharan Africa, where mass starvation has brought about immense mortality rates. As we bend our efforts to feed the hungry, to prevent epidemic disease, and to achieve a peaceful world we may be courting disaster from over-population.

The alternative is population control. In the United States it is clearly preferred that this be accomplished on a voluntary basis. To do so requires widespread diffusion of contraception knowledge and materials. Birth control must be taught at the schools with the practical goal of promoting responsible sexual behavior. This means that we must cease to use age (or youth), marital status, or financial ability as reasons to restrict the distribution of contraceptives and contraceptive information. In addition, we must continue to expend money and scientific talent to improve birth control methods through basic research.

Medical Factors Associated with Planning a Family

There are several considerations worth mentioning, if for no other reason than to give emphasis. First, youth is a respected ally of successful pregnancy and delivery. Second, no physical harm has been proved to result from having children close together. Third, having borne many children and being relatively advanced in reproductive age are both factors that prejudice the efficiency and safety of childbirth. Fourth, if one is unfortunate enough to have a child born with a serious congenital abnormality it is imperative to seek highly competent genetic counseling before another pregnancy is undertaken to get expert opinion on the risk of repetition. After the degree of risk is spelled out a couple can then make a knowledgeable decision about future childbearing.

Special factors may place a woman in an individual category, so that a doctor may feel it necessary to offer specific advice rather than generalities. These are some of the commoner conditions that make advisable a short interval between the termination of one pregnancy and the beginning of the next:

1. A woman starts her family at the age of thirty-five or more and wants several children.

2. Fibroid tumors of the uterus are present and their removal is not contemplated. Since the speed of their growth is unpredictable, one had better make hay while the sun shines.

3. The couple for whom it required several years to achieve a pregnancy cannot afford to wait, as it is impossible to know whether relative infertility will thwart them again. Usually it does not, but nobody can be sure.

When pregnancy has resulted in a spontaneous abortion, a stillbirth, or a newborn death, it is better that the couple complete the often painful task of grieving before embarking on a new pregnancy.

There are a few conditions that argue in favor of a postponement of a new pregnancy:

1. Malignancy, particularly cancer of the breast. Until the status of a breast malignancy has become quite clear, pregnancy should not be undertaken.

2. Major psychiatric illness, particularly depression. Especially when the woman is dependent on the use of lithium, it is best to postpone pregnancy.

3. Chronic debilitating disease, which given sufficient time, can be expected to improve. An example of this is a serious bout with ulcerative colitis, which may necessitate extensive bowel surgery.

Neither of these lists is intended to be complete. If you are in doubt about decisions regarding your health you should consult your own doctor. However, it is reassuring that recent cesarean section, diabetes, chronic renal injury, recent abortion, chronic high blood pressure, or recent experience with toxemia of pregnancy and eclampsia need have no direct impact on your decision either to have or to postpone any pregnancy.

Methods of Contraception: An Overview

There are many methods of contraception, some relatively new, some antedating written records. Even the two newest, the pill and the intrauterine device (IUD), had their progenitors in the deep past. The Talmud, more than fifteen hundred years ago, recommended a "cup of roots" to prevent pregnancy. One such prescription was to dissolve in beer Alexandrian gum, alum, and the bulb of the crocus and "to drink thereof." All folk people have a particular plant reported to diminish fertility. The American Indians made tea from *Lithospermum ruderale*, which grew on the western slopes of the Rockies, and each spring the squaws and braves who sought no pregnancy drank it. Temporary lodgement of a foreign body in the uterine cavity, an IUD, was first used by sixteenth-century Arabs to prevent their camels from becoming pregnant. A long, hollow reed loaded with a small stone was introduced through the vagina and cervix and a stone blown into the uterine cavity. When pregnancy was desired, it is said, the stone was milked out.

I propose to list the presently available contraceptive methods roughly in order of their effectiveness and provide some numerical estimate of their success. I shall then list them under three general headings: those that depend upon the woman; those that depend primarily on the man; and finally the rhythm method, which requires the cooperation of both partners.

The estimates of effectiveness are best stated by indicating the average number of pregnancies that would occur among 100 fertile women using the method for one year. We know that in the absence of contraceptive methods and without suppression of ovulation by breast feeding, 80 out of every 100 fertile women who are sexually active will be pregnant within the year. There is, of course, a difference between method effectiveness and use effectiveness. A couple must choose a method that has a high degree of acceptability for both of them. There is therefore no best method of contraception in use, but there is a best method for an individual partnership. The very large psychological component in sexual satisfaction makes it unwise for partners to choose a contraceptive method in which they lack confidence or which they fear because of side effects or which is unesthetic or objectionable to either partner.

The following listing of contraceptive techniques is in order of their method effectiveness: that is, the measure of the results attained when the method is used correctly and consistently:

1. The greatest method effectiveness is achieved with the hormonal contraceptives. At the present time this involves the use of female sex steroids, administered in a number of ways. The commonest is by mouth. Steroids can also be given by injection, implanted in silastic tubes, or included in intrauterine and intravaginal devices. The overall effectiveness of these

hormonal preparations is approximately 99.8 percent or about 2 pregnancies in every 1,000 woman years.

2. This category includes intrauterine devices. Overall they are about 98.5 percent effective. The latest ones, which consist of inert plastic partly encased in copper or loaded with progestins, when used by properly selected patients are among the safest contraceptives. Unfortunately, for reasons of legal liability, the major manufacturers have stopped marketing IUDs in the United States. They continue to be approved by the FDA, so there is no reason why, if available, they cannot be used, nor is there any medical reason to remove them from those women presently wearing them.

3. The next category includes the most commonly used barrier methods, the condom and the diaphragm. These techniques are also associated with an effectiveness of about 98.5 percent or about 1.5 pregnancies per 100 woman years, but only, it must be emphasized, when they are used consistently and correctly.

4. Much less effective is a group of methods that have in common with the condom that they do not require a doctor's prescription. The intravaginal foams and sponges, which depend on chemicals to destroy sperm but also provide some mechanical barrier to semen, attain a rate of effectiveness of about 96 percent. Intravaginal creams, jellies, and tablets are associated with between 8 and 10 pregnancies per 100 woman years.

5. Our information about withdrawal (coitus interruptus) as a method is woefully incomplete but a pregnancy rate of 10 to 20 seems a reasonable estimate.

6. Methods that rely on timing a woman's menstrual cycle and abstinence from intercourse during the supposed fertile period result in 15 pregnancies per 100 woman years, even with careful recording and computation. When they are supplemented by study of the woman's basal body temperature and of the moisture and sugar content of her cervical mucus, both methods that reflect ovulation, the pregnancy rate may be reduced to about 8.

7. The so-called morning-after pill is a hormonal method in which large doses of sex steroids are used for a short period. This is most appropriately employed as part of preventive med-

ical care of rape victims. It appears to be very effective, but may have unpleasant side effects, and so should be advised only for emergency situations and not as a regular reliance.

8. We have no statistics on the efficacy of postcoital douching. It may be better than no method at all, but, since sperm ascend into the uterus within minutes of their deposition in the cervix, it cannot be very effective.

Methods for the Woman

The Birth-Control Pill

The pill, if taken as directed, is the most effective contraceptive known. Its active ingredients are two hormones, estrogen and progestogen, both synthetically produced. These manufactured hormones are similar to, but more potent than, naturally occurring hormones and they exert their contraceptive effect by four physiological actions. The primary action is inhibition (prevention) of ovulation; absence of an ovum makes impregnation impossible. The way it works is that when the two hormones are present in sufficient concentration they prevent the hypothalamus (a specialized area on the underside of the brain) from sending a signal to the pituitary gland to mobilize the two gonadotropic hormones, FSH (follicle-stimulating hormone) and LH (luteinizing hormone), which trigger ovulation.

A secondary action of the pill prevents the cervical mucus from entering its mid-cycle profuse, watery phase, a phase that creates a perfect fluid medium for penetration by sperm cells. Instead, under the influence of the pill, the cervical mucus remains scant, viscid, and relatively impenetrable to sperm.

Another action affects the lining of the uterus, the endometrium. For a fertilized egg to implant successfully the endometrium must present a very specific pattern of cells, glands, and blood vessels. The pill alters the endometrial pattern materially. Then too it may affect the transport of the egg down the tubes. These four antifertility actions combine to prevent pregnancy, and if one is lacking the action of the others will suffice—accounting for the pill's unparalleled contraceptive effectiveness. If the pills are taken precisely as prescribed, without omitting a single dose, theoretically there should be no more than 0.1 unplanned pregnancy per year per 100 women using the pill (1 per 1,000). However, the practical pregnancy rate (use effectiveness) is 0.7 unplanned pregnancies per 100, the higher rate stemming from departures from the strict regime.

Administration

The pill (in reality a tablet) is begun on the fifth day of the menstrual cycle, counting the first day of menses as day 1, or on the Sunday following the onset of menses, and taken once daily, preferably at the same hour, for twenty-one days. Then no medication is taken for one week, or, if easier for the patient to monitor, she takes a different-colored, inert, placebo pill daily for seven days before recommencing the twenty-one-day (birth-control pill) regimen. Many women find it easier to take a daily pill rather than go through the mathematical routine of twenty-one days yes and seven days no.

There are a large number of brands of orals available at the present moment, and introduction of minor variations continues. Virtually all pills now combine estrogen and progestogen; the makers can vary the relative and absolute potencies of each and still maintain almost complete contraceptive effectiveness. The side effects do vary, and this makes it possible to find an optimum pill for each patient. A few combinations, such as Ortho-Novum 7/7/7, include smaller amounts of progestogen early in the twenty-one-day period. Triphasil varies the proportions of estrogen to progestogen throughout each cycle. Others, such as Micronor, consist of progestogen only taken daily, and are slightly less effective.

About seventy-two hours after taking the last birth-control pill vaginal bleeding, which can be considered a menstrual period, commences. In actuality it differs physiologically, since pill bleeding is from a different type of uterine lining than normal menses. A pill menses is usually briefer and scantier than a true menses and is almost always free of menstrual cramps. In approximately 3 percent of pill cycles no bleeding episode occurs after the last pill. This makes no difference, and despite absence of bleeding the woman starts her new twenty-one-day cycle precisely one week after the conclusion of the previous pill cycle. If there is no bleeding for two successive cycles, it is wise to consult a physician to rule out the unlikely possibility of pregnancy.

If for some reason you wish to postpone bleeding for a trip or participation in an athletic contest, there is no harm in taking the pill continuously for thirty or forty days instead of twenty-one. However, it is deemed unwise to take the pill continually for an indefinite period, since the creation of cyclic bleeding mimics nature's normal pattern and probably maintains the reproductive tract in better condition.

Extreme youth is no bar to use of the pill, nor is an approaching menopause.

Contraceptive protection is given in the first cycle if the pill is started on day 5, but if it is started later than day 5, additional means of contraception should be used through the first cycle.

You can adjust yourself to a Sunday start of orals by continuing your first cycle on them until a Saturday, using an extra package of pills for the purpose. Thereafter, starting on Sunday and stopping on Saturday, you are likely to find yourself bleeding in the middle of the usual work week. This adjustment may be complicated if you are on a triphasic pill such as Ortho 777 or Triphasil. In that case you should consult your doctor for advice.

There is no time limit on how long the pill can be used. There is no need to discontinue it after two or three years and substitute another contraceptive method for a few months before resuming its use. Such a pill "vacation" is not medically indicated.

If you are on an oral containing fifty micrograms or more of estrogen (the strength is listed on the label under the name of either mestranol or ethynyl estradiol) and miss two daily doses in a cycle, your ovaries may release an egg and pregnancy becomes possible. Either sexual abstinence or the use of another method for the remainder of the cycle is advised. With the thirty- and thirty-five microgram pills, missing even one day may require a backup method.

If pregnancy should occur because of either use or method failure in a patient taking ordinary doses of oral contraceptives, there does not seem to be any likelihood of abnormality in the fetus. For a while it was thought that anomalies occurred among babies exposed to orals. However, later studies have failed to confirm this.

Effect on Subsequent Fertility

In most individuals there is no effect on subsequent fertility. At first it was thought that the pill increased fertility by granting physiological rest to the ovaries and pituitary, but there are no hard data to confirm this theory. Ordinarily, true menses—not the immediate withdrawal bleeding—resume four to six weeks after abandoning the pill. About 30 percent of women report initiation of pregnancy within three months after stopping the pill. A small percentage (0.75 percent) have amenorrhea (absence of menses) associated with sterility for six months or longer after terminating the pill. If the menses are not reestablished after nine months, Clomid, one of the two ovulatory drugs, is ordinarily given and usually, though not always, triggers normal ovulatory cycles. If Clomid fails, treatment with human pituitary gonadotropins (Pergonal) is likely to succeed. Spontaneous return of menstruation has been delayed as long as seventy-two months after stopping the pill.

Side Effects

Oral contraceptives are potent drugs with effects on a wide range of body systems in addition to the reproductive tract. For that reason, prior to starting on orals, a patient should have a physical examination, which should include a breast and pelvic examination and a Papanicoloau (Pap) smear. Blood pressure should be taken and the urine should be examined for sugar.

There are a few contraindications to the pill. One is breast-feeding, unless this is well established and copious. Others are: previous breast carcinoma; a history of prior problems with phlebitis or pulmonary embolism from deep vein thrombosis; a history of recurrent jaundice during pregnancy (since this jaundice tends to recur with orals); high blood pressure and diabetes are not mandatory contraindications but the drug must be used with great care in patients with these conditions, since it is possible that the conditions may be aggravated.

The commonest side effects of orals are mostly minor and mostly nuisances. They include nausea, vomiting, a sense of fullness in the breast and pelvis, and breakthrough irregular vaginal bleeding while taking the pill. Weight gain is commonly attributed to oral contraceptives, but when this has been studied carefully it is clear that this is a psychological and not a hormonal effect.

Some other side effects, observed in the first ten years when we were using oral contraceptives in much larger doses, are no longer seen.

A proven serious side effect of the pill is an increased tendency to form blood clots in the veins. It is estimated that this occurs among women using orals five to ten times more frequently than among women of similar age and parity who are not doing so. The difficulty with this statistic is that it is based on studies of British women who took orals at a dose of one hundred micrograms, in contrast to the presently employed dose which is half that or less. There is reason to think that the reduction in dose will substantially reduce this effect, but there is no way of saying that it will be reduced to zero. The danger is that the clots that form in these veins can break off and go to the lungs; in severe cases this can obstruct the flow of blood through the lungs, with possibly fatal consequences. The incidence of this complication does not seem to be greater in long term users of oral contraceptives than in short term users. Once oral contraceptives are stopped the incidence appears to drop to the same as that of people who have never used the pill. There is a minor correlation of the incidence of this with increasing age.

Orals and Heart Disease

Investigators have given considerable attention to the relationship, if any, of oral contraceptive use to heart disease. These studies also come largely from Great Britain and were also done while the estrogen dose was substantially larger than it is now. In these reports, the orals relate to an increased occurrence of coronary artery disease among women past the age of thirty-five. We cannot ascribe this increase solely to the pill, however, as a substantial number of pill users are also cigarette smokers, who are thus subjecting themselves to an added risk of coronary artery disease over any that may result from using orals. In fact the risk of coronary artery disease associated with smoking alone is more than the risk associated with orals. But because the danger, though small, is real, and is enhanced by the increasing age of the woman, serious consideration should be given, before prescribing the pill, to the medical and family history of any patient over the age of forty who wishes to use it.

Gall bladder disease appears as a complication of orals, usually in the first year of use. It may be that the effect of the pill is to call attention to already existing but still silent disease. The risk of hospitalization is about 74 per 100,000 users per year. There is no relationship between use of orals and cancer of the gall bladder, nor indeed to cancer in other organs such as the stomach or the intestines.

Women on oral contraceptives experience symptomless alterations in body chemistry, such as changes in the blood lipids (triglycerides and cholesterol), increased blood copper levels, abnormal tests of sugar tolerance, and even shifts of body water. These effects are all transitory and we have no evidence that they do any permanent damage.

An occasional woman notes a leakage of breast milk after discontinuing orals, usually in the first year off medication. No harm comes of this.

If you wear contact lenses, you may notice a change in their fit when you start or stop taking orals. It may also be that orals and some antibiotics compete for transport substances in the blood, and so the contraceptive effect is diminished. To be cautious, you can add a barrier method while taking the antibiotics.

Orals and Cancer

Oral contraceptives have been in use long enough so that we have convincing information about their relationship with human cancer, particularly in the reproductive tract. Women who have used orals for any substantial periods of time subsequently have a significantly decreased incidence of cancer of the lining of the uterus (endometrial carcinoma) and of the ovaries. It has been estimated in an excellent study by the Centers for

Disease Control that, among these former users of orals something like seventeen hundred cases of ovarian cancer and two thousand cases of endometrial cancer are prevented every year. We believe that this is probably because these organs are put at relative rest during the period when the patient is using orals.

It has been stated that women who use orals have an increased risk of developing cancer of the cervix. On further study of the data, it emerges that the women using orals were more likely than the women using barrier methods to have changes in the cervix before starting the use of orals. These changes had been shown on their Pap smears done prior to use. Further study has also shown that users of orals are more likely to be smokers and also to have multiple sex partners. Both these factors are in some way limited with cervical cancer. The final verdict is not in, but it seems probable that a continent nonsmoker with a normal Pap smear is exceedingly unlikely to increase her cervical cancer risk by taking orals. Indeed, she may even reduce it, by having fewer pregnancies.

There is an increase among long-term users of orals over thirty in the frequency of hepatoma, a nonmalignant tumor of the liver. The incidence seems to be about 3 cases per 100,000 users per year.

There is evidence that infection of the internal female genitalia, especially the tubes and ovaries, is less common among women exposed to venereal disease if they are taking orals. This is believed to be due to the thickening of the cervical mucus, which prevents bacteria as well as sperm from ascending the cervical canal to the uterus and tubes.

Several other conditions appear to be less common among women who use oral contraceptives. The diagnosis of benign breast disease is made infrequently among such women and consequently the rate at which biopsies of the breast are indicated is reduced. Ovarian cysts are less likely to form. The reduction in uterine bleeding is such that pill users have decreased likelihood of having iron-deficiency anemia. Finally, of course, there is a reduction in ectopic pregnancy.

Should You Take the Pill?
Both the United States Food and Drug Administration and the British Committee on the Safety of Drugs feel that the advan-

tages of the birth control pill, its almost complete protection against an undesired conception and its greater acceptability because it permits spontaneous intercourse without preliminary contraceptive preparations, outweigh the infrequent hazard to health. This is also the verdict of the American public.

Among American women under the age of thirty, the most popular method of birth control is orals, and it is estimated that among women of all ages, there are about ten million users. From time to time there have been flurries of concern about side effects, which have brought about a drop in the rate of use but this phenomenon has been counter balanced by a subsequent rise in the rate as reassuring information has been published. The continuation rate for orals after two years is about 80 percent. Reasons for discontinuance vary, and include perceptions of unpleasant side effects; preference for other methods more suited to the woman's sexual activity, or simply a decision to become pregnant.

The Alan Guttmacher Institute has gathered figures for the year 1982, showing the relative prevalence in use of the different methods of contraception among American women aged fifteen to forty-four.

Of a total of 33,425,000 women using some kind of contraceptive technique, 35 percent were relying on sterilization of either themselves (24 percent of the total) or their partners (11 percent of the total). Next most popular as a method was oral hormonal contraceptives, 29 percent; after this came condoms (13 percent); intrauterine devices (7 percent); diaphragms (6 percent); and spermicides (4 percent). Methods not depending on surgery, devices, or chemicals accounted for the small remaining percentage.

From my point of view as a practitioner, orals are the method of choice in early marriage. Properly used, they pretty well guarantee postponement of pregnancy until the couple are ready to start a family, and in addition, because they are not directly associated in use with the sex act, they permit safe and wholly spontaneous sexual behavior, thus enhancing the pleasure of both partners.

The method least to be recommended in early marriage, or before a woman has ever had a baby, is the IUD, because of its potential to cause pelvic infection, which may lead to infertility. Apart from this, there is no reason why a woman or a couple should not use any available method of contraception that appeals to them, if they know its failure rate and that rate is acceptable.

Other Hormonal Contraceptives for Women

Combined orals—those with both estrogen and progestogen—tend to suppress lactation at least briefly; thus nursing women may prefer to use pills containing only a progestogen. The method effectiveness of this minipill is about 97.5 percent in contrast to the 99+ percent with the combined orals.

Hormonal contraceptives can be given by injection, with long intervals between consecutive doses. The hormone most used in this way is medroxyprogesterone (Depoprovera). This preparation has been widely used in the Third World. An injection is given every four to six months and the method effectiveness is at least as high as that of orals. It has the great advantage that it does not call for the patient to do more than remember to return for the next dose. In cultures where male partners restrict women's access to contraception, the male need not even know that the hormone has been injected. The side effects are similar to those of combined orals. The significant undesirable effect is irregular and unpredictable uterine bleeding, in contrast with the regularity that most women enjoy on orals.

The administration of very high doses of Depoprovera to laboratory monkeys has resulted in a small number of cases of cancer of the uterus. There is simply no way of repeating this experiment in human beings. We only know that in large human populations in such countries as Thailand there is no evidence of such a result from the much smaller doses used for contraception. However, the consulting committee for the Food and Drug Administration recommended that since there was doubt, based on the monkey experiment, of the safety of the injected drug, and since in the United States other methods of birth control are readily available, Depoprovera should not be approved for contraceptive use in this country.

Another long-acting method of administering hormonal contraceptive is to implant capsules containing levonorgestrel, a potent progestogen, immediately under the skin. The capsules are made of silastic, a synthetic material permeable to drugs. Small amounts of the steroid leak out of the capsules into the woman's circulation and suppress ovulation. The method is in its infancy. It is not known how long these implants can be left in place. Studies are being done with various doses. It is, however, easy to insert the implants with needles of proper size, and equally easy to retrieve them, through small incisions in the skin, with tweezers, almost like removing a splinter. Continuation rates with implants are in the vicinity of 90 percent and the pregnancy rate even after five years is no more than 2 per 100 woman years of use.

The combination of estrogen and progestogen can also be incorporated in a silastic ring which is placed in the vagina in the same way as a contraceptive diaphragm. The hormones are slowly released over the three or more weeks in which the ring is present. The woman herself can readily remove the ring when she wishes to experience bleeding. The clinical trials of this device are in their earliest days.

The final form of administration of hormones has been to include them in intrauterine devices, again in silastic tubing from which the steroids leak out slowly over a period of time. It appears that a levonorgestrel-releasing IUD can be allowed to remain in place for seven years without losing its hormonal effectiveness.

The Morning-After Pill

Women who have had unprotected intercourse can substantially reduce the risk of pregnancy from a single exposure by taking combined orals on the following two days. This calls for using pills containing at least 50 micrograms of estradiol and at least 0.5 milligrams of a progestogen per pill and taking four pills on each day. The best information we have on efficacy has been obtained on the basis of the use of Ovral.

The likelihood of pregnancy resulting from one unprotected exposure is something like 5 percent, taking into consideration that the odds are well against the woman's being in her fertile period at the time. Using the morning-after pill reduces the pregnancy rate by about 85 percent of the unprotected level.

As the morning-after dose greatly exceeds the daily dose used in routine administration of hormonal contraceptives, it obviously cannot be used as a substitute. It is, however, very useful and should be offered to any patient directly following rape unless she is known to be pregnant.

The mechanism of this protection against pregnancy is not fully understood. In view of the disastrous experience with DES it is probably wise to offer a patient abortion should the contraceptive fail to work.

Intrauterine Devices (IUDs)

Contemporary intrauterine devices are all based on plastic, which can be deformed for insertion into the uterus and which will resume its original shape once in place. All are impregnated with material to make them visible by X-ray and they are readily seen by sonography. Some are covered by copper wire (the Tatum T and the Cu7), some have sections that release hormones (the Progestasert), and others simply consist of inert plastic (the Lippes Loop).

For insertion, they are drawn into a hollow tube, the introducer, which is much like a thin drinking straw. The introducer is passed through the cervix into the uterine cavity; anesthesia is not necessary for women who have previously been in labor, since their cervical canals are slightly open, particularly at the time of menses. Most women experience some cramping, much like menses, as the introducer is placed, and the IUD then resumes its shape inside the uterus; it is inserted there by pushing a plunger into the introducer or by pulling the introducer off the IUD. Insertions are done with sterile technique.

Almost all IUDs have a nylon thread attached to the lower end, a few inches of thread being allowed to protrude from the mouth of the cervix into the upper vagina. This serves a dual purpose. The protruding thread permits self-examination to make sure the device is still in position and has not been unknowingly expelled. Also, the thread can be easily grasped by the physician and the IUD simply removed by traction.

Millions of IUDs are in use in the developed countries; it is estimated that in China, where a vigorous campaign to limit family size is under way, 70 million women are wearing IUDs.

The way an IUD works is still not entirely understood. A recent study has failed to find hCG late in the menstrual cycle in a group of women wearing IUDs, although if very early unimplanted pregnancies were present, the test should have been positive. Fertilization infrequently occurs. The presence of an IUD causes chemical changes in the uterine fluid which are hostile to both sperm and ova. Microscopic studies show a mobilization of scavenger-type white blood cells in the uterine lining where the IUD rests. Since the frequency of all pregnancies is reduced, that of ectopic pregnancies is also, but not as much as that of intrauterine pregnancies.

It has been demonstrated that the presence of copper increases the concentration of the scavenger cells in the uterine cavity. This added effect of copper is employed with the Tatum T and Cu7 (Cu is the chemist's symbol for copper) so that the IUD can be made smaller. It is therefore easier to insert and causes less irritation to the interior of the uterus. This reduces the likelihood of two of the annoying side effects, cramps and increased uterine bleeding. The T is shaped like a T and the 7 like the numeral. The copper wire is wound around the long arms. The present generation of FDA-approved copper bearing IUDs can be left in place at least three years without losing effectiveness. Copper IUDs wound with more copper have also been approved; it will be possible to leave them in place much longer.

The first IUD to include steroids, the Progestasert, employed progesterone. It was suggested that this device be replaced each year. Presently under study at the Food and Drug Administration is an IUD containing levonorgestrel, which appears to be effective for at least seven years without replacement.

The Lippes Loop is made of solid plastic in a double S shape; despite its name it is open-ended and is readily deformed into a straight shape for insertion into an introducer.

Effectiveness of IUDs

Two unplanned pregnancies can be anticipated each year in 100 women wearing the all-plastic IUD. If pregnancy occurs the presence of the IUD does not interfere except for the risk of abortion, which is somewhat increased.

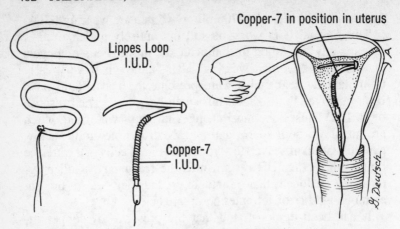

Copper-7 in position in uterus

Lippes Loop
I.U.D.

Copper-7
I.U.D.

H. Deutsch.

IUDs. On the left is a Lippes Loop, in the center a Cu7. The native copper wire is wound around the stem. The strings come out through the cervix into the vagina. On the right, one wall of the uterus is cut away to show how a Cu7 lies in the uterine cavity.

When pregnancy does occur, the IUD lies outside the fetal sac and is pushed aside by the developing fetal membranes. It never makes contact with the fetus. In such pregnancies followed to term there is no increase in fetal malformations.

Insertion

IUDs are best inserted on the waning days of menses. The advantage of this time is that one can be sure that the patient is not pregnant. Also, because the cervical canal is ordinarily more open, insertion is technically easier and less uncomfortable for the patient.

For insertion the cervix is exposed by a vaginal speculum and grasped by a clamp to steady it. Aseptic technique is required. The introducer, having been loaded with the IUD, is threaded through the cervical canal into the uterine cavity and the device deposited in the uterus.

The risk of this procedure is that in the hands of inexperienced operators the IUD can be thrust through the uterine wall.

This is most likely to occur in nursing women. In most instances the IUD should be retrieved if perforation has taken place. The reported incidence of perforations is about once in every twenty-five hundred insertions.

Side Effects

The major side effects of IUDs are chronic pelvic infection and uterine perforation. The latter may occur at the time of the initial insertion. It tends to be somewhat painful and therefore to be recognized promptly. Occasionally even properly placed IUDs work their way out through the uterine wall into the peritoneal cavity or come to rest among the supporting structures of the uterus. If the string disappears from the cervix the IUD can be localized by sonography. If the uterus is perforated it may be wise to remove the device. Inert IUDs can be allowed to remain in some abnormal locations, but copper devices must be removed.

Acute pelvic inflammatory disease in the presence of an IUD can be cured by conventional antibiotic treatment. However, the smoldering infections, ordinarily due to an unusual microorganism named Actinomyces israeli, may not respond rapidly to antibiotics. Should this happen, the IUD should be removed and intense and prolonged antibiotic therapy undertaken. This complication occurs about once in every fifteen hundred cases. If neglected it can require removal of the uterus, tubes and ovaries to protect the woman's life. About two deaths from this cause per hundred thousand users per year are reported. The subtle form of the infection can damage the lining of the tubes and thereby cause infertility. For this reason I am reluctant to provide IUDs to women who have not yet had children. The minor side effects of the IUD are expulsion, pain, and irregular bleeding, or profuse menses. If an IUD is reinserted, about 50 percent retain it the second time. Cramps during the first twenty-four hours are not unusual and can ordinarily be tolerated with the aid of simple analgesics, such as acetaminophen (Tylenol). If pain lasts beyond forty-eight hours the doctor may decide to remove the device. Staining or mild bleeding after insertion is usually transitory. Profuse menses or irregular bleeding during the cycle may be sufficiently worrisome to dictate discontinuance. The cases of pain and of bleeding account for about 11 percent of removals of IUDs during the first year, less frequently thereafter.

Acceptability

Like the hormonal methods, the IUD has the great psychological advantage of being separated from the act of intercourse. Once the IUD is in place no preparations have to be made nor does any medicine have to be remembered.

Because of the cramps and bleeding the rate of discontinuation is higher than it should be if effectiveness were the only consideration. The smaller IUDs, which use either copper or hormones to enhance their effect, produce less by way of side effects and have higher rates of continuance.

Despite the current acceptability, safety, and effectiveness of IUDs, there has been a proliferation of lawsuits in the United States against the manufacturers. These actions have been based on uterine perforations and pelvic infections that have led to disability, operations, and even hysterectomy, with resultant sterility. The stage was set for this by the earlier experience with the Dalkon Shield. The major manufacturers have recently decided to discontinue marketing the devices.

IUDs continue to be approved on medical grounds by the FDA. But the manufacturers assert that the expense of legal defense against the claims of injury exceeds whatever profits they can make from the sale of IUDs, despite the fact that, except in the case of the Dalkon Shield, in most instances they have not been found liable.

Women presently wearing IUDs can continue their use, particularly if they have been properly counseled as to the risks. Dalkon Shields should be removed, however.

The Diaphragm

It has long been known that when semen is ejaculated into the vagina pregnancy cannot result if an obstruction prevents the seed from entering the cervix. In preliterate societies gums, leaves, fruits, and seedpods were used for this purpose. The Hebrew Talmud, compiled in the fifth century, recommends stuffing wool in the upper vagina. None other than Casanova suggests that a half lemon, squeezed of its contents, be inserted over the cervix as an obstructive cup.

One hundred and sixty-five years ago a German physician created a removable, individually molded cap for his patients to insert over the cervix. Over one hundred years ago a Dutch physician published a study on a vulcanized-rubber, domed cap attached to a circular watch spring, which occluded not only the cervix but the upper vagina as well. Known as the vaginal diaphragm, it was prescribed virtually routinely in all birth control clinics in the days before the pill and IUD.

Today the diaphragm is made of latex in the shape of a shallow cup with a metal spring forming its circular rim. It comes in a range of sizes from 55 millimeters to 105 millimeters in diameter. Since the vagina is a distensible structure that will accommodate a sphere the size of a baby's head it is clear that the vagina itself does not hold the diaphragm in position. Instead it is held by the muscles and connective tissue of the pelvic floor against support provided by the bones forming the forward part of the pelvis, the pubic arch. When properly placed in position, the diaphragm covers the cervix.

Like gloves and shoes, a diaphragm must be carefully fitted to the individual woman. The practitioner estimates the necessary size, makes a trial fitting, and prescribes a diaphragm of the appropriate size. When such a diaphragm is in place the wearer should be unaware of its presence.

The mechanical barrier alone is not sufficient for contraceptive effectiveness. About a teaspoon full of a contraceptive cream or jelly designed for use with a diaphragm is smeared around the rim. This acts as a lubricant for insertion and provides a chemical seal against the semen. The contraceptive creams and jellies, in additon to the vehicle and the perfume contain a potent agent that destroys sperm.

I recommend to patients that they experiment with both cream and jelly before deciding on one or the other. Women who produce a great deal of natural lubricant when they are sexually excited will probably prefer the cream, while those women who can use additional lubrication may prefer the jelly.

Because the vagina enlarges in response to sexual stimulus, as was pointed out by Masters and Johnson, the patient should be fitted with the largest size diaphragm she can comfortably wear. Many women can accommodate a larger diaphragm after they have delivered a baby and may therefore need a new fitting at that time. A diaphragm that is either too large or too small may be readily displaced by the penis during intercourse.

When a patient is initially fitted with a diaphragm she should practice inserting it before leaving the office or clinic so that she can be confident that she is inserting it in the right place and that it is not uncomfortable. Some women like to use a specially designed plastic device to insert the diaphragm. It is nevertheless important that the patient learn to feel with her fingers inside the vagina to be certain that the diaphragm covers the cervix.

There is a common opinion that the diaphragm needs to be refitted if the woman has either gained or lost a great deal of weight. This is rarely if ever the case, since external weight gain does not particularly affect these internal measurements.

The vagina is relatively smaller in the early months of breast-feeding. Thus the prechildbirth diaphragm may seem snug the first time it is used. This may or may not signal a need for a new size diaphragm.

Time and Duration of Diaphragm Use
The diaphragm and cream or jelly must be in place in the vagina before there is any penile penetration. Some men have a discharge of fertile semen, capable of impregnating their partner, prior to a recognizable ejaculation. The diaphragm should be left in place for at least six hours after the act of intercourse. In the event that there is a second episode of intercourse it is probably advisable to insert an additional amount of jelly or cream into the vagina without disturbing the position of the diaphragm. The diaphragm once removed can be rinsed off with soap and water and dried with a towel or a tissue. A light dusting with cornstarch may help prolong its life. From time to time you should test the diaphragm's ability to hold water. If it leaks, you should immediately replace it.

A diaphragm can be used during menses; if you do this, you would do well to remove it promptly when the requisite six hours have elapsed.

Side Effects
Use of diaphragms has no known side effects except in those few individuals who may be sensitive to contraceptive jellies

or creams. A diaphragm confers protection against bacterial venereal disease by providing a barrier against the bacteria. Nearly two million women in the United States rely on it.

The Cervical Cap

The cervical cap is a cup made of plastic designed to fit securely over the cervix, much as a thimble fits on a finger. The cervix projects into the upper portion of the vagina and is about an inch in diameter and an inch and a half in length. A cup of the proper size can fit snugly over it, held in place by negative pressure, and undisturbed by intercourse. It acts effectively as a diaphragm. Since cervixes vary considerably in size, the cap, like the diaphragm, must be fitted by an individual experienced in this technique.

Unlike the ease of diaphragm insertion however, self-insertion and placement of the cervical cap are difficult for some women because the cervix is located so deep in the vagina. It is even more difficult to remove a cervical cap than to insert it. This may have played a role in the recommendation by some that the cap, once properly placed, be left over the cervix for long periods of time, even throughout menses. I would not endorse this recommendation. Our experience with toxic shock syndrome indicates that one cause is the presence of a foreign body in the vagina for long enough to allow the toxin-producing Staphylococci to multiply. This would suggest caution against recommending that the cervical cap be left in the vagina for long periods of time, particularly during menses, which provides an especially rich culture medium.

Early studies with the cervical cap suggest that the pregnancy rate is greater than 15 per 100 women years, a rate of approximately ten times that achievable with a diaphragm.

Over-the-Counter Vaginal Preparations

Vaginal foam, jellies, creams, suppositories, and a vaginal sponge are now available without prescription. They all depend on nonoxynol-9 to destroy sperm; only the vehicle to carry the nonoxynol varies among them. These preparations are used without a diaphragm. For ideal effectiveness they must all be placed in the upper vagina against the cervix. The foams and suppositories must be sufficiently viscous and sticky to remain in place in that location.

The trade names of the vaginal foams are Because, Delfen, Emko, and Koromex. The vaginal suppositories are sold under the names of Encare, Intercept, Prevetts, and Semicid. The vaginal sponge is sold under the name of Today.

The reported pregnancy rates of all of these depend upon consistent use and vary widely from one study to the next. I think we must assume in a fertile population that the failures are likely to be more than 5 pregnancies per 100 woman years and may even exceed 10 pregnancies. Some women or their partners are sensitive to the nonoxynol-9. Interestingly, these preparations appear to reduce the risk of contracting gonorrhea by about 50 percent.

These methods are to be recommended to women who have intercourse infrequently and to those who try to reinforce the effectiveness of the condom. They share the great advantage of the condom that they are readily available without a prescription, but they should not be used when maximum effectiveness of the contraceptive is a crucial consideration.

The Contraceptive Douche

This is unquestionably the least effective method. Its pregnancy rate is between 25 and 30 per 100 users per year. The entire responsibility for this method of contraception falls upon the female partner since, to be effective at all, the douche must be taken immediately after ejaculation.

There are two main types of douching apparatus. One is a flexible bag that allows the flow of the fluid to proceed under gravity. This bag should be no more than a few feet above the level of the vagina, since injection of fluid under high pressure can cause it to flow into the peritoneal cavity and thus produce a chemical and a bacterial peritonitis. Bulb syringes are the other type of douche device. They are less desirable than a bag properly used, because they can produce high pressure.

Almost any nonirritating solution can be used. Plain water will work, or a small amount of lemon juice or vinegar can be added to it, to dissolve vaginal mucus. You should put several irrigations of water through the vagina for maximum benefit.

Methods for the Man

Hormonal Methods

A number of methods to reduce male fertility have been tested. All have been significantly successful for that purpose, but all have also had the highly undesirable result of producing an almost complete disappearance of sexual drive and a conspicuous diminution in the man's ability to maintain an erection. Under these circumstances it is irrelevant that the male's sperm count is simultaneously reduced to infertile levels. These apparently inevitable side effects, strikingly different from the effect of hormonal contraceptives for the female, account for the fact that there is at present no practical hormonal method of male contraception.

The Condom

Condoms are presently employed by about 13 percent of all couples practicing contraception, a rate approximately twice that of the diaphragm and about half that of the oral contraceptives. Condoms are harmless, have virtually no side effects, are simple to use, and can be purchased without a prescription. Approximately one billion condoms are manufactured in the United States every year. Condoms have the great advantage of protecting each partner from acquiring venereal disease from the other.

Early History of the Condom

The derivation of the word is uncertain. It is claimed without strong evidence that a certain Dr. Condom was attached to the court of the seventeenth-century English King Charles II, who perhaps holds one of the world records for creating royal bastards. Dr. Condom is said to have invented the sheath for the welfare of his monarch, who had become alarmed by the number of illegitimate offspring he had fathered. For the relief his device supplied, it is said, Dr. Condom was knighted by his grateful sovereign. Doubt is cast on this intriguing story by the evidence that animal bladders were probably used as penile sheaths in the days of imperial Rome and that, as early as 1564, an Italian physician, Guy Fallopius, in his poem on syphilis, mentions the value of a linen penile sheath in the prevention of venereal disease. The less romantic but more likely etymology of the word "condom" is its derivation from the Latin *condo*, meaning "to sheath."

Modern Use

Shaped like the finger of a glove, condoms are placed on the erect penis before intercourse and receive the man's ejaculation during orgasm. They can be purchased without prescription in drugstores and elsewhere. When used properly and regularly, they will provide a very high degree of protection against unwanted pregnancy.

Condoms are relied upon by 7 percent of married couples currently practicing contraception, and are probably used more frequently outside of marriage. Their popularity is explained by the fact that they are harmless, simple to use, and easy to purchase, and do not require medical advice.

The upper, open end of the condom, usually one and three-eighths inches in diameter, is surrounded by a rubber ring; its closed end may be plain-ended or have a pocket or teat, in which the semen can be trapped. The teat-ended variety, which is supposed to be less likely to burst after ejaculation, is more popular in Europe than in the United States. Condoms are about seven and one-half inches in length and are made of such thin material that each weighs only one-twentieth of an ounce. They are packed rolled in aluminum foil, cardboard boxes, or metal containers in quantities of three to a dozen. Some latex condoms that are packed singly in fluid are said to increase enjoyment. Packaged condoms have a shelf life—the period of time during which a packaged product can be kept before it deteriorates—of at least two years.

Improvements in manufacturing permit automated production of condoms, which are virtually free of defects. Testing procedures instituted by the manufacturers themselves now utilize electronic methods which can pick up even minute flaws. A single worker is able to check more than two thousand per hour. A few years ago I (A.F.G.) watched an electrical testing machine at work in the family-planning headquarters in Stockholm, which acts as the national purveyor of contraceptives in Sweden. A technician was check-testing a mixed batch of British and American condoms, which had had their initial tests in the country of manufacture. The lot was so perfect that after several minutes the demonstrator had to stick a pin in a condom to demonstrate how the machine automatically rejects a condom with a flaw.

Condom Accidents

Condoms provide a very high degree of protection against conception, but accidents can happen. The major cause of failure is rupture of the condom during use, which occurs approximately once in 150 to 300 occasions. Two steps may help to forestall this. First, if the condom is the usual plain-ended American variety, it should be unrolled on the erect penis with a half-inch of space or overlap left at the end to accommodate the ejaculate. Second, if the natural moisture in the woman's genital tract is scant, the outside of the condom should be lubricated to prevent tearing on insertion. The best lubricant is one of the many medical contraceptive jellies or creams. Vaseline or other oils should not be used.

Failure may sometimes be caused if the condom slips off when the penis is being withdrawn after orgasm. When this happens, some semen may be spilled into the vagina. This can be avoided if the man does not dally and securely holds the ring at the top of the condom to prevent spillage as he withdraws.

Despite these precautions, however, accidents can occur. If this happens, the woman should immediately insert an applicator full of contraceptive cream or jelly into her vagina. If such equipment is not available, immediate douching is second best. Plain water acts as a spermicide, and, since time is of the essence, it is unwise to delay by preparing a douche solution. It is ill advised to insert the erect penis into the vagina before adjusting the condom, as there may be loss of preejaculatory secretion containing perhaps sufficient sperm to impregnate.

Advantages and Drawbacks of Condoms

Despite the popularity of the condom, some couples do not like to use it for a variety of reasons. One objection is that love play must be interrupted to put the condom on, but imaginative couples have found this presents no difficulty: It becomes a part of the pleasurable preparation for intercourse with the woman undertaking its placement as a signal of her readiness. Some men claim that the condom interferes with normal sexual response by dulling sensation, and others tend to ejaculate prematurely while placement is being made.

On the other hand, there is ample evidence that many couples find condoms perfectly satisfactory and use them in preference to all other methods.

There is one kind of situation in which the condom can play a strong role in controlling a medical problem that may affect a couple who are regular sexual partners. An example is infection with Trichomonas, in which the woman may have a symptomatic vaginitis, while the man harbors the organism in his prostrate or bladder but is symptom-free. The consequence of this may be that they simply pass the infection back and forth between them.

The treatment here is to give both partners metronidazole, an antibiotic, simultaneously, and to reinforce the effect of the drug by having the man use condoms for their barrier effect in preventing transmission of the organism between him and the woman. In this way the ability of the medicine to eradicate the infectious material is enhanced, and the cure is expedited.

Personal Preference

Some couples prefer the condom for essentially esthetic or psychological reasons. If a woman finds it distasteful to use a diaphragm, it is undesirable to prescribe one; and if she also rejects the idea of the pill or IUD, the condom might well be indicated. Likewise, many couples find the condom reassuring because they can see clearly that it works by preventing semen from entering the vaginal canal. This may be particularly true for couples whose knowledge of sexual anatomy and physiology is limited and who therefore feel less security with other contraceptive methods. Certainly for promiscuous sexual encounters a condom has special utility.

Coitus Interruptus (Withdrawal)

Coitus interruptus has many synonyms in the vernacular including withdrawal, "pulling out," and "taking care." It may well be the oldest method of birth control, since it is mentioned in the Old Testament (Genesis 38:9), and worldwide it probably is still the one most extensively used. The decline in birth rates in the developed countries in Europe in the eighteenth and nineteenth centuries is largely attributed to the practice of coitus interruptus. In the United States at the present time, however, fewer than 3 percent of sexually active adults use it as their principal method of birth control, although perhaps five times as many employ it occasionally. This makes it difficult to state the method effectiveness of withdrawal. It is likely to be less than 90 percent.

Withdrawal is a simple method requiring no equipment or preparation before the sex act; it costs nothing and is always available. And though it requires intercourse to be terminated rather abruptly by the male, it permits full contact between the sex organs of the partners. However, withdrawal has had a poor reputation among doctors, and some physicians still attribute many male and female ills to this technique.

The absence of substantial evidence to support these accusations makes it difficult to assess them. Many now believe that the charges stem more from an author's personal dislike of the method than from his professional observation. Perhaps I lean toward this view because of the evident fact that happy, sexually well-adjusted American as well as European couples find this method of conception control satisfactory.

Withdrawal is a legitimate method of contraception and should be considered by couples in deciding which method to employ. If it has been used with complete satisfaction for both partners, there is little reason to change. It is probably more satisfactory in later marriage, when husband and wife have established a consistent pattern of sexual response, and the man is better able to control and anticipate ejaculation. Obviously the cause of failures in this technique is reluctance by the man to withdraw before ejaculation has started. Spilling even the initial drop of semen in the vagina is dangerous, since it has been demonstrated that the first portion of the ejaculate contains the greatest bulk of the spermatozoa, the latter part being mainly a diluent. This method, therefore, places a great responsibility on the male partner.

Gossypol

Gossypol, an orally administered preparation derived from Chinese herbal medicine, has had considerable use in the Far East, particularly in China. It is said to result in marked decrease in sperm count without other undesirable side effects. It has, however, not been studied under rigorous conditions that would allow it to be compared for its effectiveness with other common methods of birth control, nor do we have any clear notion of the full range of its side effects. It is said to be unique in reducing sperm count without diminishing sex drive or potency.

Methods for the Couple

Natural Family Planning—The Rhythm Method

The theory of natural family planning is that it uses the woman's physiological recurring cycle of fertility and sterility to determine when intercourse will not have the consequence of pregnancy, and to restrict intercourse to only those times. It is a "couple" method because it requires the understanding and cooperation of both partners, but nevertheless it is the woman who must do most of the bookkeeping. It is, furthermore, the only method other than total abstinence that has been declared licit by the Pope. In the United States, natural family planning is the method of choice for 1.7 percent of all women using birth control. This technique has a use effectiveness of about 80 percent, though its theoretical method effectiveness is higher than this. It is the cheapest of all techniques, as it requires no equipment and no devices, and it is physically harmless.

Normally a woman ovulates once each menstrual month.

The egg cell survives for about twelve hours, during which it can be fertilized. A man's sperm has a fertile life of forty-eight to seventy-two hours following ejaculation into the female reproductive tract. These facts lead to the conclusion that a woman can become pregnant as a result of intercourse during only about eighty-four hours each menstrual month, three days before ovulation and half a day thereafter. In order to utilize the rhythm method, therefore, it is necessary to determine exactly when ovulation is going to take place, and that is where the difficulty lies.

There are presently four ways now in use to identify a woman's fertile period:

1. The calendar method, which assumes that the woman has regular and predictable menstrual cycles;

2. The temperature method, based on the rise and fall of basal body temperature throughout the menstrual cycle; and

3. Collection of cervical mucus for chemical study.

4. Over-the-counter home urine tests to identify the day of ovulation are now available. They are based on estimation of hLH levels and we do not yet know their precision or reliability. They are expensive as compared to the methods above but should be more accurate in determining fertile days, especially for women with irregular cycles.

The Calendar Method
This was the original rhythm method.

A normal woman usually ovulates twelve to sixteen days *before* her next menstrual period begins. If a woman menstruates every twenty-eight days, she should ovulate halfway through the cycle—on the thirteenth to the seventeenth day after menstruation begins. Similarly, if her cycle were regularly thirty-three days, her ovum would be released between the eighteenth and twenty-second days after the first day of menstruation.

The difficulty, of course, is that few women ovulate or menstruate with clocklike regularity. In most women the cycle can—and does—vary considerably, and then too, ovulation does not always occur precisely fourteen days before the next menses.

To make allowances for irregularities, it is necessary to lengthen the period of abstinence to provide a few days' margin of safety before and after the day on which it is believed ovulation will take place. To figure out the safe period by the calendar technique:

1. Keep a written record of the menstrual cycles for twelve consecutive months. Count the first day of menstruation as the first day of the cycle, and the day before the next period as the last day of the cycle. At the end of twelve months, choose the shortest and longest cycles for that year.

2. Subtract eighteen from the number of days in the shortest cycle. This determines the first fertile, or unsafe, day of the cycle.

3. Subtract eleven from the number of days in the longest of the twelve cycles. This determines the last fertile day of the cycle, or the day on which the safe period begins. For example, Jane Doe's shortest cycle was twenty-seven days and her longest thirty. $27 - 18 = 9$ and $30 - 11 = 19$. No intercourse should take place between 9 and 19, inclusive.

The "eighteen and eleven rule" will help a woman determine with some degree of accuracy which days of the month are "safe" and which are fertile. It is as accurate as any special calendars, slide rules, wheels, and other assorted devices produced as "aids" to calculate the safe period. As each month is ended, substitute its length for the same month last year. This keeps the twelve menstrual intervals current and permits for physiological changes in cycle length caused by age and other factors.

The Temperature (BBT) Method

A far more accurate means of practicing rhythm is the use of the basal body temperature (BBT). This depends on the fact that during the first half of the monthly cycle, the days preceding ovulation, a woman's temperature is relatively low and with the occurrence of ovulation it rises about six-tenths of one degree Fahrenheit, remaining elevated until just before menstruation. If pregnancy ensues, the temperature remains elevated and does not show the premenstrual drop. The reason for the temperature rise is that ovulation causes a wound in the ovary with the rupture of the follicle; the wound is immediately filled in by a rapid growth of cells forming a new gland, the corpus luteum, which promptly manufactures the chemical progesterone, a thermogenic substance causing the temperature to rise. Therefore in the absence of any other cause for temperature elevation in mid-cycle, such as a cold or sore throat, it is safe to assume ovulation has occurred.

To use the BBT rhythm method the woman takes her temperature each morning on awakening, before getting out of bed. After the thermometer is kept in for the necessary three minutes, she can put it aside to read at her leisure. She charts the temperature daily, preferably on widely spaced graph paper, and when she notes that the temperature has risen a half degree or more and that it remains elevated for three consecutive mornings, she can be relatively certain ovulation has occurred and intercourse is very unlikely to result in impregnation. A bad cold or tonsillitis makes the method useless for the time being.

Special thermometers that are calibrated only from 96° to 100°, so that the tenths-of-degree marks are more widely spaced, make the BBT technique easier; also rectal temperatures are more reliable than mouth temperatures, though if care is taken mouth temperature is satisfactory.

Using BBT is far superior to the calendar technique, but it usually restricts the days for intercourse to the last ten or eleven days of the menstrual month, no intercourse being permitted during the entire month before the third day of elevated temperature.

With meticulous use of the temperature method, 90 to 92 percent effectiveness in preventing pregnancy can be accomplished.

The Cervical Mucus Method

Of the four methods of natural family planning, we have the least scientific evidence on the cervical mucus method. It depends on a woman's having a thorough understanding of her own anatomy and physiology, because it requires her to study the amount, consistency, and color of her own cervical mucus. A sample of cervical mucus can be obtained by touching the cervix directly even without seeing it.

Early in the cycle, about the sixth day after bleeding begins, the cervix is dry and the woman can be expected to be infertile. The mucus next becomes sticky and tacky but scant. Up to the fourteenth day, or the day of ovulation, it increases steadily in amount and is clear and liquid, like raw egg white in its consistency. Immediately after ovulation the cervix starts to dry again. The important thing is to identify the peak of mucus: the one or two days when the volume and the liquidity are at their maximum. On these days pregnancy is most likely to take place since the sperm can persist in this hospitable medium for at least forty-eight and sometimes up to seventy-two hours.

Not every woman can use the mucus method. Patients who are nursing, those with vaginitis, and patients who occasionally use contraceptive chemicals in the upper vagina will find it very hard to interpret their cervical mucus. The success rate of the cervical mucus method is approximately 90 percent in patients who meet all the requirements for the effective use of the techniques. Like the BBT method, it requires daily record keeping, but the mucus method does not at all depend on regular cycles for its interpretation. The number of fertile days as determined by the cervical mucus method is ordinarily approximately fifteen as compared with eight by the calendar method and twelve by the temperature method.

As described in the discussion of *in vitro* sterilization, we have precise techniques now for determining ovulation based on daily and sometimes twice-daily assays of pituitary hormones in the patient's blood, combined with sonographic study of her ovaries. The expense and inconvenience of completing such studies takes this out of the realm of natural family planning.

Limitations of Natural Family Planning
The great hope for improving natural family planning lies in development of simple procedures that will enable a woman either to predict when ovulation will take place, or to cause it to occur at a given time. There is evidence that such procedures are scientifically possible.

Approximately 15 percent of women menstruate with such irregularity that they cannot use rhythm at all. Moreover, this method is not recommended during the months immediately after childbirth, since the first several postpartum menstrual periods may be very irregular. It is probably safe to apply the "eighteen and eleven" formula only after the third menstrual cycle following childbirth.

For the 85 percent of women who can use them, however, these methods are far more effective than no contraceptive method at all, although less effective than the pill, IUD, condom, or diaphragm.

It has always puzzled me why some couples fail so consistently in preventing pregnancy even while using rhythm correctly. Perhaps Masters and Johnson have given the clue. Through laboratory observations, they discovered that a very small percentage of women, like the female rabbit, cat, and ferret, ovulates out of cycle, after orgasm.

Research in Contraception

Currently, the most promising direction of research in contraception is the clinical application of gonadotropin-releasing hormone (GnRH) and its antagonists. Early reports encourage the hope that suppression of ovulation can be accomplished without a drug-induced hormonal menopause. In the male, however, it does not seem likely that GnRH or its antagonists will reduce sperm production without producing impotence and loss of libido.

Other current studies attack the problems of eliminating the need for a daily pill for women who use hormonal contraceptives. One promising approach seems to be a long-lasting dose, administered by means of such devices as silastic implants and hormone-impregnated vaginal rings.

New spermicides for vaginal use are constantly under tests, even including gossypol, the drug referred to above as being used in China in men to reduce the sperm count. There are reports, as yet unverified, that gossypol can suppress ovulation.

When prostaglandins first entered the picture as abortifacients, investigators hoped that these drugs would also function as contraceptives by causing disruption of the ovarian corpus luteum. This expectation has not been realized, but active study of other prostaglandin effects continues.

The possibility of developing vaccines that would interfere with the hormones that regulate ovarian and testicular function continues to be an attractive possibility. Genetic engineering may yet make it feasible to alter egg and sperm production even more directly. However, a sober appraisal of what we now know does not encourage us to expect an imminent breakthrough like the one that took place with the introduction of combined oral contraceptive pills.

Permanent Contraception (Sterilization)

Sterilization as a contraceptive measure is any procedure that permanently prevents union of sex cells. Castration by removal or irradiation of ovaries and the testes accomplishes this end, but the attendant hormonal deficits have restricted its use to certain rare medical indications. Hysterectomy should not be performed for the sole purpose of sterilization; procedures interrupting the fallopian tubes have excellent success rates and a far lower risk.

In the vast majority of sterilizations, the operator blocks the pathway of the sex cells without removing the testes in the male or the ovaries or uterus in the female. In men a portion of the *vas deferens*, the conduit for sperm from the testes to the seminal vesicles, is removed and the cut ends tied. In the female a similar procedure is done upon the fallopian tubes, thus preventing the upward passage of sperm and the downward migration of eggs.

I repeat that today sterilization operations are not the equivalent of castration. They leave the sex glands intact and have no effect on the secretion of the hormones that physiologically determine an individual's sexual drives and performance. Modern sterilization is thus not a desexing operation and sexual activity is not affected. In fact, because it eliminates the possibility of pregnancy it may result in a more spontaneous and enjoyable sexual relationship.

Women have been led to feel that tubal sterilization will bring on the menopause prematurely; this is simply not so. Ovarian function is unaffected and menstruation continues unchanged. Sex hormones are secreted without alteration. If there has been a hysterectomy for medical reasons and one or both ovaries have been left in place, the patient experiences no change other than the absence of menstruation.

Legal Status

Sterilization falls under the jurisdiction of the several states. There is no generally applicable federal law on the subject. However, the differences from state to state in legislative prescriptions are not great.

In the 1920's there was a drive to improve the human species by compulsory eugenic sterilization of the "unfit." This received the approval of the United States Supreme Court in 1927, and many states thereafter passed laws mandating sterilization for loosely defined defects such as mental retardation. In the 1950's, with the vastly improved knowledge of genetics and the revulsion against the performance of compulsory sterilization in the Nazi concentration camps in the 1940's, compulsory sterilization fell into disfavor and has been virtually abandoned. Inheritance of intelligence and social behavior is so complex that it cannot be significantly altered by selective sterilization.

In the absence of restraining statutes, voluntary sterilization of competent adults on medical, moral, and social grounds is legal; no state completely prohibits voluntary sterilization.

Consent is required only of the individual to be sterilized. Some hospitals, some doctors, and some local jurisdictions require the consent of the spouse. In the case of a minor or an individual declared incompetent by an appropriate court, permission from a responsible relative or a court is needed. Coercive sterilization ordered by local courts for women who have had children out of wedlock has been held illegal by the federal courts.

Medical Attitudes

Sterilization policies vary from community to community, from hospital to hospital, and from doctor to doctor. Some hospitals have committees that review and validate every case of female sterilization done within the hospital. Other hospitals have simply left the decision to the doctor and patient. Some hospitals and doctors have prescribed a numbers game: To comply with its rules, the product of the number of living children multiplied by the mother's age is required to exceed a certain number, commonly in the neighborhood of 120. If the woman is 30 years old and has had 4 children, this meets the requirement, but if she is only 29, she would have to have 5 children. The absurdity of this is now generally recognized and such numerical standards are for the most part no longer in use. Vasectomy, unlike tubal ligation, is an ambulatory service and not under the jurisdiction of the hospital. The only consent required is that of the individual being sterilized, provided he is of age and competent.

Roman Catholic hospitals do not sanction operations whose purpose is sterilization, but removal of diseased organs where sterilization is a secondary effect is not prohibited.

Medicare recipients and all women in the City of New York are required to wait thirty days after giving consent for sterilization before the operation can be carried out. The sole exception to this is emergency surgery occurring seven days or more after the consent has been given if the surgical procedure is such that the sterilization can be carried out at the same time. Both Medicare and New York City require that the woman be over twenty-one years of age regardless of her medical and child bearing history.

No court has ever judged a doctor guilty of a crime for performing a contraceptive sterilization. No physician has been held responsible for civil damages if, prior to the operation, properly executed consent for the procedure was obtained.

On the other hand there have been substantial judgments for damages when sterilization has failed and the woman subsequently became pregnant. It is therefore imperative that all patients be made to understand that the procedure has limited reversibility but that the possibility of failure always exists.

Who Does Sterilizations?

A recent survey in the United States makes clear that approximately two-fifths of the physicians in the reproductive-health-care field, including general practitioners, general surgeons, and urologists, as well as obstetricians, provide sterilization services. Actually 94 percent of all obstetrician-gynecologists will provide sterilization.

Religious Scruples

No patient should ever be made to feel that she is being coerced into accepting sterilization against her own religious convictions. By the same token, doctors whose religion proscribes doing sterilization operations cannot be forced to do these operations.

I cannot lay down the law in a situation where a patient's life or health would be endangered by another pregnancy, and I conscientiously advise her to have a tubal sterilization. In such a case, if the patient's religious scruples stand as an obstacle, I counsel her to consult a trusted religious advisor and members of her family or friends whose advice she values, and then act as her conscience may dictate. If the decision were against the indicated treatment I would have to honor it, but I would urge her to take the most effective measures available to her to prevent further pregnancies.

When Should Sterilization Be Considered?

The most skilled efforts to reestablish fertility in women after sterilization are successful no more than 50 percent of the time. It is therefore wise to assume that the procedure is irreversible when deciding whether to undergo it. The decision to be sterilized should in any case be made carefully and deliberately, taking into account all relevant social, medical, and economical factors. The precise spectrum of influences varies greatly from one individual to the next.

Among the variables are the preferences for family size and for the desired age intervals between children, the stability of the marriage as perceived by the parties, how many children the parties think they can afford, and their economic prospects in general and the family history of genetically transmitted disease. This is by no means an exhaustive list. What is always of first importance is that the decision be made without coercion, and earnestly desired without major misgivings.

As a physician, I would not ordinarily recommend sterilization when temporary methods of contraception are perfectly adequate. Sometimes, even for ideally healthy people, they are not—as when a patient seems to encounter the failure rate of every method she tries, and turns to sterilization in disgust and desperation. At the other end of the spectrum is the woman suffering from a condition in which her life might be imperiled or her health permanently impaired by pregnancy. For this woman sterilization is a medical necessity. But in such cases it may be safer not to operate but to use more routine forms of contraception, with early abortion as a backup.

Sterilizing the Mentally Retarded

The two pervasive questions that haunt this subject are: how to obtain an informed, voluntary consent, and whose consent should be regarded as sufficient. Mental retardation is not necessarily synonymous with incompetence, so that the first step that needs to be taken is to determine whether the person to be sterilized is competent to make her own decision whether to accept or refuse sterilization. If she is competent—that is, if she is old enough to consent, and can understand the nature and meaning of the operation—then her consent is sufficient, and it is only necessary that it be voluntary and informed, as with any other candidate for sterilization.

The matter becomes more complex if the mentally retarded person is below the legal age to give consent, or is severely enough retarded to be incompetent in the legal sense.

Moderately and even severely retarded individuals are ordinarily not aggressive sexually; promiscuity is not one of the problems they present, either to their therapeutic communities or their parents. But the retarded woman, especially if she is out in the community, is vulnerable to unwanted and perhaps incompletely understood sexual abuse. In addition, many of the retarded are unable to cope with the responsibility of parenthood. It seems therefore not unreasonable to make sterilization available to them, if it is actually in their best interests to do so. What is important is to make sure that the sterilization is for the benefit of the mentally retarded person, and not for the convenience of someone else. If the person is underage and in the care of her parents, consent of the parents for sterilization may be sufficient. If the individual is an adult, has been declared incompetent, and is under the care of a legal guardian the consent of the guardian (who may be the parent) is required, but it may be safer, and may even be required, that application also be made for court approval. If medical opinion and the parents' or guardian's decision are at odds, then the dispute should be submitted to an appropriate court for resolution. In either event, the help of a lawyer familiar with the local law should be sought.

Mildly retarded adults who are clearly able to understand what is being proposed may be considered quite competent to give or withhold consent to the procedure and should in no case be subjected to it against their will.

Incidence of Sterilization

Overwhelmingly the commonest form of birth control among adults over the age of thirty in the United States is one or another form of permanent sterilization. Between 1971 and 1982, almost 13 million people were sterilized by procedures other than hysterectomy. In 1981 alone it is estimated that over 1,100,000 sterilizations were performed in the United States, 700,000 of them among women. In 1982, as a consequence of a flurry of publicity purporting to connect vasectomy with a variety of unwanted consequences, the incidence of vasectomy fell below 300,000. It now appears that the existence of such a connection has never been properly verified. The panic, in any case, was of very short duration. In 1983 there was a dramatic increase in the number of procedures, which rose to

455,000. The number of female sterilizations in 1983 fell to 622,000 but the total of male and female sterilizations was once again in excess of 1 million.

The vast majority of those sterilized are partners in a stable marriage that has already produced the number of children the couple want. About the only decision that such a couple has to make once the partners have decided on sterilization is which one of them should undergo the operation. There are individuals who find it most difficult to contemplate being operated on and others for whom it is a matter of relative indifference.

As will be described below, the sterilization procedures for the male are materially safer and less uncomfortable than those for the female. It is undoubtedly a reflection of attitudes toward sexuality in this country that tubal procedures continue to be done more frequently than vasectomies. The decision as to which partner in the couple will have the operation is entirely personal; there are seldom any genuinely medical grounds for making the choice.

Female Sterilization

For term pregnancy to occur a woman must have at least one functioning ovary, one fallopian tube open throughout the five-inch course, and a uterus. Therefore, if both ovaries are removed, or if both tubes are removed, or if the canals in both tubes are interrupted so the egg cannot pass down and the sperm cannot pass up, or if the uterus is removed, a woman cannot become normally pregnant. All sterilization procedures are based on these basic facts.

Most procedures intended to achieve sterilization are carried out by operations on the fallopian tubes. Tubal operations for sterilization are termed tubectomies or, more technically, salpingectomies. Sterilization may be accomplished by the total and complete removal of both tubes or by a much simpler operation which consists of interrupting the passage through the tube. Today this is usually done either by the Pomeroy operation, or by laparoscopy.

The Pomeroy Technique

A Pomeroy operation consists of raising a knuckle of fallopian tube and placing a tie around the base of the knuckle. The knuckle is then cut off, the tie having been tightly drawn so that, when cut, the two severed ends are squeezed together. This controls immediate bleeding. Catgut suture is used for the tie. Body enzymes dissolve the catgut in four or five days, by which time the blood has clotted but the healing of the tube has just begun. The cut ends of the tube pull away from each other and the peritoneum closes over them. If permanent suture material is used, the tubal ends are held together and repair may reestablish tubal continuity. The patient has no sensations when the tubal ends separate. If a second abdominal procedure is done months or years later the two ends are found an inch or so apart, well sealed and free of adhesions.

The tubes must be exposed by an abdominal incision. In nonpregnant women this is usually made in the lower abdomen across the upper margin of the sexual hair. In slender women it need be no more than two inches long. Indeed, when special instruments are available an even smaller incision can be made. This is called a minilaparotomy, an excellent operation for use on an ambulatory basis.

The tubes can also be approached in nonpregnant women by incision into the peritoneal cavity at the top of the vagina behind the cervix. This involves no skin incision. Because complications from bleeding and infection are more frequent with this operation than with an abdominal incision, this approach is employed infrequently.

At the time of cesarean, when the abdomen is already open, it is a matter of only two minutes to carry out the Pomeroy technique on both tubes.

The operation can also be done shortly after a normal delivery. In this case it is called puerperal sterilization. This is the safest time for a tubal ligation. The abdominal wall is relaxed and the top of the uterus is near the level of the navel. Minimal anesthesia will suffice. A semilunar incision is made just below the umbilicus; the tubes are easily found and tied. The hospital stay is no different from that of a normal birth.

In the nonpregnant patient almost the entire time of the operation is spent making the incision and repairing it. All told it takes twenty to twenty-five minutes.

The recovery from the procedure is almost always uneventful. The incision is uncomfortable for a few days. The patient can leave the hospital in eight to forty-eight hours after the procedure and resume normal activity as soon as she feels up to it. It is possible to do the procedure on an ambulatory basis.

Failure of Pomeroy Sterilization

Failure to achieve sterilization comes to light if the woman becomes pregnant after the operation. This may occur as much as five years or more later. When it does, it is usually traceable entirely to the body's great capacity to heal, and only rarely to surgical error. We do submit the removed knuckles of tube to the pathologist for examination to be certain that we have cut the tube properly. The failure rate of the Pomeroy technique is about 1 in 350 procedures done in the nonpregnant or the puerperal state. Tubal ligation done at cesarean fails more frequently; we do not have a clue to the reason.

The Pomeroy technique is the easiest to reverse of all tubal sterilization methods. This is because there is so little scarring. The location of the removed knuckle is such that the healed ends are close to each other in size and therefore are not too difficult to attach to one another.

Complications of Tubal Ligation

All tubal ligations are subject to the risks that attend other abdominal operations and should be carried out with the same conditions and precautions that surgeons use to minimize complications. There is the occasional flare-up of pelvic infection and, though rarely, a wound infection.

Laparoscopy

Laparoscopy literally means looking into the abdomen. The word is used to describe a means of access to the tubal sterilization in which the tubes can be cauterized or clipped through a very small opening in the abdominal wall. The operation is carried out under general anesthesia or under local anesthesia supplemented with pain-relieving drugs and a tranquilizer. With the patient lying flat on her back the abdomen is prepared for a general surgical procedure and draped with sterile towels. A specially designed needle is then thrust through the abdominal wall into the peritoneal cavity, a potential space. A suitable gas, usually carbon dioxide, is then pumped in through this needle to blow up the peritoneal cavity, much as one blows up a balloon. It generally takes two or three liters of the gas to lift the abdominal wall well away from the internal organs. A small incision is made just below the navel and a metal tube is put through it into the peritoneal cavity. This is done by fitting a sharp pointed tip into the tube. The abdominal wall can then be pierced. Once the tube is in the peritoneal cavity, the sharp tip is pulled back out of it and replaced with the viewing scope, to give visibility of the interior. Alternatively, the abdominal wall may be opened by incision under the direct vision and the tube rapidly inserted before the gas can escape.

In either case, a viewing telescope is passed through the tube. It is fitted with fiber optics that deliver cold light by which the operator can get an excellent view of the abdominal contents.

Laparoscopy can be used to inspect the upper abdomen, including the stomach and the gall bladder, but is usually employed to visualize the pelvic organs. Slender operating instruments can be passed alongside the viewing telescope or through a second tube inserted into the abdominal wall under the direct vision of the already placed laparoscope. With these operating instruments in place the fallopian tubes can be cauterized, preferably in two places. Another method calls for attaching a plastic clip to each tube. The advantage of this latter technique is that it does not introduce any heat into the peritoneal cavity. Tubes occluded in this way are much easier to reconnect surgically later if the patient wishes to have the procedure reversed. The pregnancy rate subsequent to tubal clipping is slightly higher than that following cautery.

Advantage and Complications of Laparoscopy
The advantage of sterilization by laparoscopy is that it can be done as an outpatient procedure. This results in a great saving of time and money even if general anesthesia is used.

The complications of laparoscopy are infrequent but may be serious. With the blind insertion of the metal tube there have been accidental injuries to the major blood vessels on the posterior wall of the peritoneal cavity. This accident necessitates immediate abdominal operation to repair the vessel lacerations. If cautery is inexpertly used, it may burn the bladder or the bowel.

Sterilization by laparoscopy is contraindicated in the presence of multiple previous abdominal operations in the lower abdomen, which may have produced adhesions. The procedure is also more difficult to do in patients with a marked degree of abdominal obesity.

"Tying" the Tubes

On page 507, I gave a description of the sterilization operation known as a tubal ligation. The vernacular name for this operation is "tying the tubes"—a name that has given rise to some misconceptions that I would like to correct.

Fallopian tubes are not tied in a bow like shoelaces, nor in a knot like a string around a package. Both the shoelaces and the package string can be untied, and are then in much the same shape they were in before they were tied. The tubes, however, are tied with suture material, which is like string, before being cut and, as I indicated in my description, the suture material dissolves and disappears after a few days. This leaves separate segments of tube on either side, which do not rejoin if the operation is successful. We therefore cannot untie the tubes that we have tied. If we hope to reverse the operation and reestablish the continuity of the passage through one or both tubes, we must put the open ends of the two segments together, using very delicate and meticulous techniques that are much more difficult than was the initial ligation.

Reversal of Female Sterilization

This is done by removing the scarred portions of the tubes and reconnecting the two freshened ends. The operation requires major abdominal surgery because a large incision is necessary. The best results have been obtained by experienced surgeons working under magnification with very fine suture material. It requires skill and experience to sew the muscle and the lining of each cut end of the fallopian tube to the other with precision. About 25 percent of the patients thus operated on subsequently have a normal full-term pregnancy. In about twice as many patients as this the continuity and patency of the tubes is actually restored, but the women do not achieve uterine pregnancies. There is an increased incidence of ectopic pregnancy following this operation.

Hysterectomy for Sterilization

Hysterectomy should not be done when its sole purpose is sterilization, because it is accompanied by an unacceptable degree of risk compared to the other available choices. It is the case that in the United States the operation is performed on large numbers of still-fertile women and is the second commonest operative procedure resulting in female sterilization. The commonest reason for a hysterectomy on a woman in her childbearing years is to treat fibroid tumors of the uterus. When the fibroid tumors are symptomatic or disabling, they are substantial reasons for removal of the uterus. However, if the tumors are small and do not cause discomfort or disability, the conservative approach is to leave them in place and do a tubal sterilization procedure, rather than incur the greater morbidity from hysterectomy.

The same principles apply to hysterectomy combined with cesarean section. The removal of the uterus increases the risks of complications at the time of section, and therefore, if the only purpose is sterilization, the tubal method is the procedure of choice.

In some parts of the United States, vaginal hysterectomy is done on young women with a frequency disproportionate to that of the same operation in the same age group elsewhere in the country. The reasons usually given have seemed to me insufficient to justify the operation when, if the real purpose is sterilization, a less formidable tubal procedure would be sufficient and safer.

Hysterectomy, of, course cannot be reversed.

Unproven Methods of Female Sterilization

Efforts have been made for years to produce blockage of the tubes where they enter the uterus. This point can be seen by passing a hysteroscope through the cervix into the uterine cavity. Like the laparoscope, the hysteroscope consists of a slender viewing telescope equipped with fiber optic cold light. In the past, various corrosive materials have been injected into the fallopian tubes by this route with some degree of success in achieving closure. Attention has now turned to the injection of fast setting polymers which are injected as liquids but very rapidly solidify to form a plug. The best results with this technique so far have achieved about an 85 percent rate of bilateral tubal blockage.

In the People's Republic of China, investigators are currently working on a technique of tubal injection in which the catheters used are put through the vagina and cervix and into the opening of the tube inside the uterus by touch and feel rather than under direct vision. Until we know more about the long-term follow-up of this method, it has to be watched with interest but considered experimental. The advantage of these injection methods is that they do not involve abdominal surgery and can readily be done on an ambulatory basis.

Male Sterilization

Vasectomy

Sterilization of the male for permanent contraception is carried out by vasectomy, which is a simple operation. Since there are two testicles the operation must be done on both sides. Vasectomy consists of blocking the duct which leads from the testicle, where sperm are manufactured, to their point of exit, the penis. Blocking is accomplished by cutting out an inch or an inch and a half from the passageway, the *vas deferens*.

Vasectomy is simple surgery since no body cavity is entered. The procedure is done either in a doctor's office or in a clinic or hospital. It is ordinarily performed by either a genitourinary surgeon, who specializes in male reproductive and urinary problems, or by a general surgeon. Occasionally general practitioners perform vasectomy.

A local anesthetic, a cocaine derivative, is injected into the operative site to eliminate pain. Some physicians and some patients prefer a general anesthetic.

A small incision, about an inch in length, is made in the upper and lateral region of the scrotum, directly over the large tube called the spermatic cord. The cord carries within it not only the much smaller duct, the *vas deferens*, but also blood vessels and nerves. The incision is extended about a quarter-inch downward from the skin until the cord is reached; then the cord itself is incised and the *vas deferens* isolated from other structures within the cord, much like isolating the largest wire in a coaxial cable. Two sutures of a relatively nonabsorbable material are tied around the *vas deferens* an inch and a half apart and the intervening portion cut out.

The skin incision is closed with one or two sutures and a dressing is applied. The man is advised to wear a suspensory to support the testicles so they don't make traction on the wound, which might be painful. The operation requires fifteen or twenty minutes, most of the time occupied in injecting the local anesthetic. If the operation is performed in the hospital, the patient is discharged twenty-four hours later. If done in the doctor's office, or in an outpatient clinic, the man is kept under observation for an hour and then is allowed to go home and advised to refrain from strenuous activity for forty-eight hours. The skin suture is usually removed five or six days after operation.

In 99 cases out of 100 vasectomy is completely successful. The 1 percent failure rate is attributed to the fact that the two severed ends of the *vas* are able to find each other and grow together again to form a new canal.

However, since there is storage of the sperm in the ampulla of the *vas deferens*, spermatozoa do not disappear immediately after vasectomy. It may take as many as six or more ejaculations before all fertile spermatozoa are washed out of the system. It is therefore advisable that contraceptive methods be continued until the man has ejaculated at least six times. Even then it is probably advisable to have a semen specimen examined under the microscope to be certain that the operation has not failed. Once this proof is obtained, sexual contact without contraceptives will not result in pregnancy. Some surgeons feel since reunion of the *vas* may occur within the first six months after the operation, that for complete safety it is advisable to examine a semen specimen every six or eight weeks during that period.

The vasectomy does not change either libido or sexual performance. The spermatozoa constitute a negligible proportion of the semen and the volume of the ejaculate is not appreciably diminished. About 60 percent of men who have had a vasectomy are subsequently found to have circulating sperm antibodies. This, however, so far as we know does no harm except that it may possibly interfere with the success of subsequent efforts to reestablish fertility. Sperm continue to be produced after the procedure, but with their passage blocked they disintegrate and are reabsorbed by the body.

Complications of Vasectomy

Leakage from the artery that runs alongside the *vas* can introduce a mass of blood into the scrotum, producing a hematoma (from the Greek roots for "blood" and "mass") that is quite painful. This heals itself slowly and completely unless it becomes infected, in which event it must be drained.

Reversal of Vasectomy

Like fallopian tubes, the *vasa* can be reunited. This also calls for meticulous surgery, often carried out under magnification and employing very fine sutures. About 75 percent of these reanastomoses result in the presence of sperm in the ejaculate and approximately 50 percent of the men subsequently successfully impregnate their partners. As is the case with the original vasectomy, this second operation has almost no risk.

Expense of Sterilization

According to a survey carried out on a large national sample, the total fee for a female sterilization done on an inpatient hospital basis in 1982 was $1,335. The same procedure on an ambulatory hospital basis was $1,275. The average fee for the small numbers of female sterilizations done in a doctor's office is reported as $614.

The total fee for in-hospital vasectomy, on the other hand, was $511, or $240 for a procedure carried out in the physician's office.

The total expense of female sterilization should also be calculated to include time lost from the work place, which will be substantially greater than time lost for vasectomy.

22

Infertility

A discussion of infertility follows naturally after consideration of family planning. Moreover, I know that the previous editions of this book have been read by many people before they married or had contemplated pregnancy. The book has also been recommended in many college courses on family formation. Therefore I cannot assume that all the readers of this book have already tested their fertility.

Many questions arise about the ability to become pregnant. What are the prospects of an infertile marriage? How long should a couple be thwarted in their attempt to initiate pregnancy before being concerned, and how long before being seriously worried? What type of specialist should be consulted and how does one locate a competent doctor in the field of infertility? What tests are performed to diagnose the cause, or causes, of an infertile mating? If such and such an abnormality is found, what treatment should be tried? I hope that this discussion will answer these and other questions.

The Chances of an Infertile Marriage

It has been estimated that about one in seven married couples in the United States are unable to have a child. There seem to be no inherent social, economic, or racial group differences affecting the ability or inability to create a baby. Existing group differences in family size are probably dependent upon the employment or lack of employment of contraception.

Years ago the theory was that the explanation for the smaller size of professional and white-collar families, by comparison with blue-collar and laboring families, was related to their occupations. The difference does exist, but research seems to show that couples with above-average income or education resort more frequently than do those who are less well off to measures to limit family size and to defer the first pregnancy. The prolonged use of contraception may postpone attempts at conception beyond the age of highest fertility.

Effect of Age and Coital Frequency on Conception

The effect of age on fertility has been studied in two samples, one from the Canadian province of Quebec and the other from England and Wales, to determine the percentage of childless unions for couples who use no birth control but marry at different ages. When the women married before age twenty, 4 percent remained childless; between twenty and twenty-four, 6 percent; between twenty-five and twenty-nine, 10 percent; and between thirty and thirty-four, 16 percent. Other studies differently constructed show little decline in the fertility of the woman before age thirty, but declining fertility thereafter.

Recent studies based on observations made in France have given rise to controversy about the effect of a woman's age on fertility. The consensus is that as women become older their fertility declines until it ceases at the menopause.

Little attention has been paid to the relationship of a man's age to his fertility. However, MacLeod has reported on the relationship of the husband's age and his ability to cause his wife to conceive in six months or less. Of men less than twenty-five years old, 75 percent impregnated their wives in six months or less; twenty-five to twenty-nine, 48 percent; thirty to thirty-five, 38 percent; thirty-five to thirty-nine, 26 percent; and forty and over, 23 percent.

The only other general factor in addition to age which seems to influence fertility is frequency of intercourse. As a rule, couples having sexual intercourse four times and over per week are far more likely to achieve pregnancy in less than six months than couples practicing coitus once or less often per week. Since coital frequency is correlated to age, perhaps these two modifying factors of fertility are in large part one and the same.

Usual Time Required to Initiate Pregnancy

Of 5,574 couples whom we studied who achieved pregnancy, one-third succeeded the first month, and more than half within the first three months. Fifteen percent required four to six months; 13 percent, seven to twelve months; and 8 percent, one to two years. More than 6 percent of those who eventually had a baby took more than two years to initiate pregnancy. The median time, or most usual time required, was about two and one-half months.

When to Seek Medical Help

If both partners are less than thirty-five years of age, there is no urgency about seeking medical advice until they have been trying for at least a year and no pregnancy has ensued. On the other hand, if either is above thirty-five, they should see a doctor after six months of unsuccessful attempts.

Whom Should One Consult?

The choice of the doctor is important. Treatment of infertility is a complicated field, and many family doctors have not had the training to manage it. However, the family doctor can refer the problem to a specialist or to a clinic. Most infertility specialists are members of The American Fertility Society; names of members in a specific geographic area can be obtained by writing to the Office of the Director, 1608 Thirteenth Avenue South, Birmingham, AL 35256, telephone 205-933-7222. Then too, a first-rate local hospital, especially a teaching hospital, can refer an inquiring couple to qualified members of its staff. Furthermore, there are fertility clinics in many cities of the United States. If you are unable to locate such a clinic in your community, write for help to the Planned Parenthood Federation of America, 810 Seventh Avenue, New York City, NY 10019. In the New York area, the world-famous Margaret

Sanger Center, 380 Second Avenue, New York, NY 10010, telephone 212-541-7800 or 212-677-6474, is available for consultation.

The Medical Consultation

It goes without saying that both partners of an infertile marriage must participate in the study. A medical history is essential to look for such chronic disorders as diabetes, hypertension, thyroid abnormalities, anemia, severe psychological trauma, or any large weight change. The medical history of either partner may include episodes of venereal disease. A history of birth control practices in the past is relevant, since we know that young women who have used IUDs prior to pregnancy have an approximately double likelihood of being infertile subsequently, due to chronic inflammatory processes in the tubes. The occupation and hobbies of the partners should be recorded to screen for the possibility of exposure to environmental toxins or a history of intense physical activity such as marathon running and ballet training in the woman. Both are associated with disturbance of ovulation and menstruation.

It is important to obtain a sexual history from each partner in separate interviews. Such matters as frequency of intercourse and the timing of intercourse in relationship to the woman's cycle should be recorded. Does the woman find intercourse repellent in any way? Is she in the habit of douching, washing, and voiding immediately after sexual relations? Some couples occasionally use lubricants such as vaseline, which can damage sperm cells and reduce the likelihood of conception. I have seen one couple who limited their sexual activity almost entirely to the time of menses. The problem in another couple was the fact that the husband was unable to have an ejaculation during coitus. With this kind of information from both partners, the physician may ultimately be able to solve the problem, in some cases by making a few simple suggestions for changes in the couple's sexual practices.

Both partners should then be put through a physical examination sufficient to confirm general good health and to be certain of the normality of the external genitalia. One husband whom I examined under these circumstances had virtually no testicular tissue to be found in his scrotum; on further questioning it turned out that in childhood he had had a severe attack of mumps, a disease that can involve the testicle and cause testicle shrinkage without interfering with the production of testosterone, the male sex hormone.

It is essential to complete the usual screening laboratory procedures such as a complete blood count and a urinalysis before proceeding to specialized and expensive hormonal determinations.

Tests for the Man

After getting the pertinent historical data, the specialist proceeds with a series of tests. It usually starts by examining the sperm content of the man's semen. The specimen is collected directly into a wide-necked, dry, clean bottle or jar, and the man must be very careful none is lost, as the first few drops of the ejaculation contain the bulk of the sperm cells. If the first few drops are lost, normal semen may test as defective. The specimen can be collected at home either by masturbation or withdrawal, and taken within a few hours to the doctor's office, where it is tested to determine whether it meets certain requirements. To be normal it must be about a teaspoon in quantity and have a sticky, but not a ropy, consistency, and under the microscope there must be twenty or more million sperm cells per cubic centimeter, of which 80 percent must show a progressive type of swimming movement in the seminal fluid. Then, too, at least three-fourths of the cells must appear normal in form when stained and studied.

If repeated examination of the semen demonstrates a subfertile specimen, it may be because of chronic infection in the male system that transports sperm. A common cause of this is chronic chlamydia infection, manifested by the presence of pus cells in the ejaculate. This infection has proven to be amenable to antibiotic therapy, although it is unreasonable to expect spectacular increases in fertility after the infection is conquered. A wide range of hormonal therapies has been undertaken for the subfertile sperm, none of which seems to have been particularly effective. Some efforts have been made to ameliorate this condition by harvesting as large a proportion as possible of the normal active sperm from the first portion of the ejaculate and using these for artificial insemination.

If sperm cells are completely absent from the semen specimen, two possibilities present themselves. Either no spermatozoa are being produced in the two testicles, or they are being produced but their egress through the penis is blocked so that they cannot appear in the ejaculation. Such blockage usually occurs in the tiny tubules of the epididymis, where the testicle joins the *vas deferens*, the conducting tube that conveys the sperm cells upward. A biopsy, the removal of a fragment of tissue from the testicle for microscopic study, will determine whether the absence of spermatozoa is due to failure of their formation or to blockage. If sperm cells are being formed, a bypass operation around the point of blockage is successful in about one-third of the cases.

Occasionally, surgical elimination of a hydrocele, a cystlike collection of fluid outside the testicles, improves poor semen, as may ligation of large varicose veins of the scrotal sac. Close-fitting jockey shorts, which may raise the intrascrotal temperature, should be abandoned in infertility cases.

Tests for the Woman

There are several requirements for fertility in a woman: normal ovulation (egg production); proper functioning of the tube for picking up the egg; unobstructed passage through the tube for the ascent of spermatozoa and descent into the uterus of the fertilized egg cell; and implantation of the early conception into the lining of the uterus, specifically prepared by naturally occurring hormones.

The simplest way of identifying ovulation is to record your body temperature daily under standard basal conditions. You take your temperature each morning immediately upon awakening before activity and, if possible, at the same time every day. This is the basal body temperature, or BBT. It should be written down immediately. The BBT is low during menstruation and for a week or so thereafter. It then begins to rise gently or rapidly at mid-cycle and remains at an elevated level until about twenty-four hours before the next period. All these temperatures are within normal limits. The maintained temperature rise in the second half of the menstrual cycle is strong evidence of ovulation, but its absence does not prove anything one way or another.

Another test for ovulation involves an endometrial biopsy in which minute pieces of the uterine lining are removed, with little discomfort, just prior to menstruation or during the first twelve hours of the flow. These fragments are studied microscopically. If ovulation has occurred that month, the resulting corpus luteum will cause the tissue to show a so-called "secretory pattern," which is the body's preparation for the reception and implantation of an egg. If ovulation does not occur and therefore no corpus luteum is formed, the uterus omits this chapter of its story and characteristic secretory changes are absent.

Other tests less often used to detect ovulation are frequent examinations of the mucus of the cervix to determine whether during mid-cycle it goes through a "watery" phase, and observation of daily vaginal smears to seek for "cornified" or mature cells, which are found only during a month in which ovulation takes place.

Still another way is to identify, by a blood assay, the mid-cycle surge of lutenizing hormone (LH) from the pituitary gland. The surge immediately precedes a release of eggs from the ovary. LH is the hormone that also guides the formation of a corpus luteum at the place in the ovary which produced an egg.

If the endometrial biopsy shows evidence of poor quality response to ovulation, some authorities believe that taking progestins in the latter half of the cycle in subsequent cycles will increase the secretory state of the endometrium sufficiently to support implantation of a fertilized egg.

If ovulation is persistently absent the examinations should go further to study the patient's hormonal balance and particularly to determine the blood level of prolactin, a hormone that can seriously interfere with normal ovulation. Elevated prolactin levels are often associated with adenomas (benign epithelial tumors) of the pituitary gland. Such levels of prolactin can be reduced by the administration of bromocriptine (Parlodel) with the consequent establishment of normal ovulation and menstruation.

Persistent failure to ovulate is associated in some circumstances with polycystic ovarian syndrome, a complex hormonal situation that probably is due to several different factors. It is a condition with multiple small cysts, which derive from the failure of graafian follicles to rupture normally through the surface of the ovary.

Most patients who are simply anovulatory are treated by the administration of clomiphene (Clomid), a drug which is principally an antiestrogen. It may work by suppressing the pituitary briefly. When the drug is discontinued, the pituitary resumes function. Clomiphene is given initially in daily doses of 50 milligrams for five days. This course may be repeated and the subsequent doses increased up to a level of about 150 milligrams a day for five days. About 70 percent of nonovulators will ovulate with clomiphene therapy, and approximately half of them become pregnant.

Patients who do not respond to clomiphene therapy can then be treated with injections of human pituitary gonadotropin (hFSH) supplemented with human chorionic gonadotropin (hCG). These drugs are expensive and must be given by injection, in contrast to Clomid, which is given by mouth. The combined therapy with these two hormones produces a pregnancy rate of about 50 percent.

About 15 percent of the pregnancies resulting from induction of ovulations are multiple. As these drugs cause the release of two or more ova in any given cycle, the fetuses are fraternally related and not identical.

The most recent development in this field has been the injection of gonadotropin releasing hormone (hGnRH) at 90- to 120-minute intervals by electric pumps. This apparently reasonably accurately mimics the normal functioning of the hypothalamus, the structure in the base of the brain which produces this hormone. It is too early to know what the expectation will be of multiple pregnancies with this technique and of its success, but this is a very promising development.

Blockage of the Fallopian Tubes

When it has been demonstrated that an infertile woman is ovulating regularly, attention turns to the fallopian tubes. They must be open so that the eggs can proceed down and the sperm travel up to impregnate the ova. The common cause of tubal obstruction is infection, although in some instances the obstruction is due to endometriosis. The common causes of infection are gonorrhea and chlamydia. Infections following childbirth or abortion, unless they are extraordinarily severe, are very unlikely to have this effect. Because of the danger of blockage of the tubes from severe tubal infection, we have learned that early intensive therapy of acute pelvic inflammatory disease is mandatory if fertility is to be preserved.

Accurate identification of the location of tubal blockage involves two procedures. One is an X-ray of the pelvis while a radiopaque fluid is injected through the uterus into the tubes. The material that is used is quickly absorbed by the body. When the tubes are open and the fluid passes rapidly through them, it spills into the peritoneal cavity behind the uterus and produces a readily recognized picture. If the radiopaque material cannot pass through the tubes it can be seen up to the point of obstruction. This X-ray procedure is called hysterosalpingography (from the Greek and Latin roots meaning uterus, tube, and picture). This procedure may have some curative value in itself. Occasionally a patient will become pregnant with no further diagnostic or therapeutic undertaking. With modern X-ray equipment the amount of irradiation delivered to the pelvis is minimal and without measurable genetic hazard. The best time for the test is a few days after the cessation of menses, in order to avoid unnecessary radiation of a new pregnancy.

If the tubes appear to be nonpatent, the next step is direct visualization of the pelvic structures by laparoscopy, described on page 508. The laparoscopist can usually tell whether the tubal obstruction is due to pressure from the outside or whether the tube itself is damaged. This information greatly helps the doctor to estimate the possibilities of surgery and therefore the wisdom of advising a major operation whose chance of success is unfortunately limited. Among patients who have had previous tubal surgery, not uncommonly a previous sterilization operation, laparoscopy gives an accurate picture to the surgeon of what needs to be accomplished. Diagnostic laparoscopy can be done as an ambulatory procedure under general or regional anesthesia.

If the outer end of the tube is scarred closed but the remainder of the tube is normal, delicate surgery, usually done under an operating microscope, can be done to open this up. The microscope facilitates identification of the layers of the tube, so that they can be accurately sewn to one another; the suture material used is of a delicacy unimagined a decade ago. Areas of obstruction along the length of the tube can also be excised and the tube brought together again. The most difficult problems are encountered when the obstruction is in the very narrow portion of the tube as it passes through the uterine wall. Occasionally the outer end is also obstructed, blocking the tube, so that it fills with fluid (hydrosalpinx). The chance of correcting this or a thickened tube is quite small.

The Postcoital Test

Even if normal ovulation is occurring and the tubes are patent, pregnancy will not result unless the husband's sperm cells can make the four- or five-inch journey to the site in the midportion of the tube where fertilization takes place. It is important to know that there are live sperm present at the starting line in the cervix following sexual intercourse. To prepare for the test, the patients must be sure not to use a barrier method of contraception out of habit. The woman then comes to the doctor's office shortly after intercourse. Samples of fluid from the vagina and from the mucus of the cervix are aspirated separately and placed under the microscope. Live, motile sperm cells should be present in the vaginal sample and certainly must be present and actively moving in the cervical mucus. These postcoital tests should be carried out at about mid-cycle, when the mucus is at its best for sperm penetration.

If only dead sperm are found in the cervical mucus on repeated tests this may be due to antibody reactions, which are as yet poorly understood. It is known that antisperm antibodies in the woman are a reasonably common cause of infertility. It is possible to detect their presence in the laboratory by tests which will also demonstrate that the woman's body fluids have an adverse effect on sperm survival and motility. Treatment for this condition has been undertaken by having the male partner use a condom until the laboratory evidence of sensitivity disappears. The process may be hastened by suppressing the woman's immune response with cortical steroids. The sensitivity may be to the seminal fluid rather than to the sperm themselves. Studies have therefore been done in which the sperm are concentrated, washed twice and then used for artificial insemination. The success rate is about 15 to 20 percent. Sperm antibodies are found in 20 to 30 percent of infertile couples, a rate substantially higher than that among normally fertile people.

Surgery to Treat Infertility

In the Male

1. Very infrequently the urethra, the excretory tube leading through the penis, has an opening at the base of the penis instead of its tip (hypospadias) and therefore the semen is delivered externally. A plastic-surgical procedure will close the defect, allowing the semen to exit from the tip of the penis.

2. Bypassing an obstructed epididymis is sometimes surgically feasible, a procedure termed epididymovasostomy.

3. If the testicles are retained in the abdomen, either hormonal or surgical correction must be carried out before puberty, as described on page 559.

4. If a male with a poor semen specimen has a varicocele (large scrotal varicose vein), this condition is usually eliminated surgically.

5. If the man has been sterilized by vasectomy (a tie or ligature placed around the *vas deferens* on each side and a small segment removed) 50 percent of these men are able to initiate a pregnancy. The procedure can be undone surgically in about 75 percent of the cases.

In the Female

1. Efforts to reestablish patency of the fallopian tubes have a success rate well above 50 percent in instances where adhesions around the tube are responsible for the obstruction and the lining of the tube is normal. However, where the tubes are

scarred and closed from disease the success rate with the very best of surgery is much lower than this. Patency is reestablished in no more than 25 percent of the patients upon whom it is tried, and the pregnancy rate is lower still. Unfortunately in such reconstructed tubes the rate of ectopic pregnancy is distinctly increased.

2. Surgical removal of fibroid tumors of the uterus that have distorted the endometrial cavity and have been associated with either infertility or repeated miscarriage results in a high success rate in patients who are otherwise normal.

3. If the woman has been sterilized by laparoscopy or laparotomy it is possible to reestablish tubal patency and in many cases to reestablish fertility. The great majority of these are women who have been sterilized solely because they have been pregnant several times. They are quite normal from a hormonal standpoint. If the sterilization has been done by applying clips to the tubes through a laparoscope, the success rate of tubal reanastomosis is higher than if the tubes have been burned through the laparoscope. The best success rates are achieved with patients who have had the Pomeroy type of sterilization by laparotomy. In this last group approximately 60 percent of the patients can expect to have future pregnancies after operation to rejoin the tubes.

Artificial Insemination

If the woman appears to be fertile and her partner irremediably sterile or if he is unable to ejaculate into her vagina, conception may still occur through artificial insemination. In this procedure semen is simply placed in the upper vagina. Insemination can be done either with the husband's semen or with a fertile semen donated by a third party. Donor insemination may be undertaken for genetic reasons when both husband and wife are carriers of a recessive genetic defect. Substitution of semen from an unrelated donor eliminates the possibility that the defect will be inherited from both parents and will express itself in the fetus. Donor insemination has the advantages, as compared to adoption, that the woman and her partner go through the experiences of pregnancy and delivery.

Donor insemination was condemned by Pope Pius XII in

1951. In 1962 the Presbyterian Church bestowed its approval on the technique, but few other Protestant groups have taken any public position. Orthodox Judaism forbids donor insemination, but a child resulting from this transgression has been ruled legitimate.

The legal status of a child conceived by donor insemination is somewhat clouded and has tended to vary from one jurisdiction to another in the United States. Several states have legislation on the subject and the courts have interpreted the rights of the biological father in several different ways. For this reason donor insemination probably should not be undertaken casually and surely not without consultation with an attorney experienced in this field. There is very wide disagreement within the medical profession as to what documents should be completed by the couple to make a record of their consent to the proceeding, and besides, it is most important to see to it that the personal and property rights of the child conceived by donor insemination are maximally protected.

The Procedure of Artificial Insemination

The few days on which the woman is maximally fertile can be selected on the basis of the menstrual history, BBT chart, inspection of cervical mucus, and measurement of LH in the urine.

When the semen is obtained from a third party, the donor and recipient should never know each other's identity. There have been some painful court battles in instances of surrogate motherhood, which involves many of the same problems, where this kind of anonymity has not been appropriately protected.

From one to three inseminations can be carried out during one menstrual cycle depending upon the convenience of all concerned. The greater number of inseminations the higher the likelihood for pregnancy. In a large series of 690 cases of donor inseminations gathered by six different physicians, the rate of success has varied from 55 to 78 percent, the average being 69 percent. In one small series, using three inseminations per month, 80 percent of the successful inseminations occurred in the first two months, and with an additional two months the rate reached 90 percent.

The fetal outcomes from artificially inseminated pregnancies do not differ from those of normal pregnancies. Patients have been known to seek donor insemination repeatedly. Donor insemination has also been used by single women and lesbian couples who wish to have a baby.

In any event the procedure should not be undertaken unless the women and their partners have seriously considered the possible emotional pitfalls and are nevertheless enthusiastic for it.

In Vitro Fertilization (IVF)

Until recently a woman who had lost both her tubes due to infection, tumors, or ectopic pregnancies had no possibility of becoming pregnant. Now, making use of exquisite hormonal studies and elegant ultrasound combined with laparoscopy, it is possible to time ovulation quite accurately and to harvest fertilized eggs from the ovary.

The woman's spontaneous ovulation is often controlled by the use of gonadotropin-releasing hormone (hGnRH). The woman is then given hFSH, which produces ovulation in a carefully timed manner. The eggs are then harvested by laparoscopy or aspiration under sonographic guidance. The goal is to harvest as many eggs as is possible, sometimes as many as six to eight. These eggs are then fertilized in the laboratory (hence *in vitro*, meaning in glass) with fertile sperm and allowed to develop for a few days. At the present time three or four of those embryos which have exhibited evidence of fertilization are injected into the mother's uterus, using a syringe and a fine catheter. If implantation takes place they grow there for the remaining 263 days. Multiple pregnancies have occurred in cases of this sort.

The most experienced clinics, which select their patients very carefully, have a success rate of about 25 percent. IVF can be repeated, and with six attempts the rate of success rises to a remarkable 65 percent. Combining blood hormone studies with detailed sonographic examination of the ovaries to determine when follicles are ripe and then with the surgical skills to harvest the eggs by laparoscopy calls for a large and experienced team of specialists and a battery of expensive laboratory procedures.

The method is certainly in its infancy. Consideration has been given to freezing unfertilized eggs for subsequent use, in order to reduce the number of times laparoscopy is necessary, but we have little information as to the safety of this procedure. Our colleagues in Australia, who are in the forefront of the use of freezing, have done this with early embryos. After two months of storage the embryos were used to implant in a woman who was not the donor of the eggs with the outcome of a normal live birth. On at least one occasion a fertilized ovum has been implanted in the uterus of a woman with no ovaries of her own and the fetus carried to term.

Eggs have been collected from a woman whose uterus had been removed because it ruptured during labor. After IVF, the ova were transferred to the uterus of her sister, who had previously delivered healthy children. The baby thus produced was of course genetically the child of the donor of the eggs and her husband.

Ethicists and moralists have started to discuss the implications of these new kinds of relationships, and public bodies have begun to issue regulations controlling medical practice. The law and legislatures characteristically move slowly in dealing with these complex issues.

Ovum Transfer

Another new approach for the woman who is infertile because she lacks fallopian tubes or functioning ovaries is ovum transfer. In this circumstance a normal fertile woman arranges to establish an early pregnancy, which is then irrigated out of her uterus, identified under the microscope, and transferred to a recipient by injecting it into the uterine cavity as with *in vitro* fertilization. The recipient woman then goes through a pregnancy with a fetus with whom she has no genetic relationship. A few such pregnancies and even two in women with no ovarian function of their own have implanted successfully and gone on to term. Not enough instances of ovum transfer have been reported to give us any inkling of its likelihood of success.

Surrogate Motherhood

Some normally fertile women have agreed to be inseminated by fertile husbands whose wives for one reason or another are unable to conceive: because for example, they have had a hysterectomy, or have an anatomical anomaly such as a congenital absence of the uterus and vagina. These women cannot have an *in vitro* fertilization or an ovum transfer. The recipient mother agrees to go through pregnancy and then to turn the baby over for adoption by the couple. There is already a foundation established in the Midwest that advertises its services in arranging for surrogate motherhood to frustrated infertile people.

The legal status of this is very unclear. For example, who is responsible for the care of a defective child born from such an arrangement, however unlikely such an event might be? And how can an agreement of the sort described above be enforced if the woman carrying the baby, or the one whom she is carrying it for, changes her mind?

Organ Transfer

We have now had a report of a transplant of an ovary and a fallopian tube from one woman to another. In this case the women involved were identical twins, one of whom had lost her own ovaries and tubes through disease. Early studies have indicated that this particular transplantation has succeeded, but it is as yet not known whether this can result in a pregnancy, which is after all the ultimate criterion of success.

Genetic Implications

There are limits to the utility of genetic counseling in connection with the procedures described above, since either or both of the biological parents of the children produced in these ways may be unknown.

A Message to the Infertile

If you are one of the couples who have unsuccessfully been trying to establish a pregnancy for a year or two, what are your chances? Two decades ago the likelihood of your having a baby was perhaps in the neighborhood of 25 percent. Now it is much more likely to be in the neighborhood of 50 percent. Some of the astonishing methods described briefly above are so new that we do not know how much of a help they will turn out to be. But in any case you do not have to greet infertility with inaction and guilt. It is probably wiser for you to seek skilled medical assistance to help you exhaust all possible avenues of having a baby. If these all fail, you may wish to adopt one or more children or simply continue in a strong and loving relationship with one another, if you are so blessed.

23

The Newborn Baby

All of us are programmed from childhood to consider newborn babies as attractive, cute, cuddly, darling, and angelic. Indeed most of them are, but some of the babies have their appearance temporarily altered by the processes of labor and delivery and this may give some concern to the unprepared. It is, therefore, appropriate in the final chapter of this book to direct attention to the newborn baby, its needs and its care and, of course, its appearance. The Professor of Obstetrics at Harvard of a previous generation once stated emphatically that a woman does not go to a doctor to have a case of obstetrics, she goes to have a baby. This, after all, is the appropriate climax of these events.

First off, what is the immediate care of the newborn? In a completely normal birth, it has become my practice to hand the baby to the mother so that she can place it on her chest, or else to put it there myself. Studies have demonstrated that when the baby is placed on the mother's bare skin, particularly on her chest, that the baby's temperature loss after birth is much less than if the baby is wrapped or put under an infrared warmer. I generally toss a towel over the baby to reduce its heat loss but do little more than that. This procedure does not quite conform to usual middle-class standards of neatness, since the baby is always wet, frequently covered with vernix caseosa (the cheeselike material found on the skin of term newborns), and, not infrequently, somewhat bloody.

Babies placed in this warm, comfortable environment ordinarily initiate breathing quite promptly but do not cry vigorously, probably because they are right back near the mother's heartbeat where they have been for the previous eight months. I like to think that they find this reassuring. Babies handled in this way continue to look blue for a substantially longer period of time than babies rubbed and dried off with towels and, as was frequently done in the past, spanked to get them to cry. They are nevertheless vigorous and alert and in no difficulty. With a normal birth there is no hurry about clamping and cutting the umbilical cord. There have been debates in the medical literature in the last twenty-five years as to whether the cord should be clamped early or clamped late and whether the baby should be above or below the placenta during the time before cord clamping. Over the long run this does not seem to be of any material importance to the healthy newborn. My practice is to clamp and cut the cord several minutes after birth, when the pulsations of the umbilical arteries have ceased. However, with a healthy newborn there is no hurry to do this, except for the fact that while the baby is still attached to the placenta, handling it may be a little clumsy. The ordinary length of the umbilical cord is sufficient to permit the baby to be placed on the mother's chest but not much more.

Cutting the Cord

To cut the cord, I put a clamp on it a short distance away from the navel. A second clamp is also attached nearer the baby about a half inch from the first one, and the cord cut between the two. Each clamp prevents the cord from bleeding; the critical one is the clamp closer to the baby. The exact device for clamping varies from hospital to hospital. Some hospitals use a metal clip, some use a plastic device that clamps the cord off. The clips or plastic clamps can be removed in thirty-six to forty-eight hours, and the stump of the umbilical cord ordinarily falls off in five to seven days. The place where it has been will sometimes look a little bit unclean and may have a minor amount of exudate, which gets on the diaper. All that needs to be done with this is to wash and dry the area and otherwise disregard it, unless it continues to exude pus and the skin around it reddens.

When the mother delivers by cesarean, her chest is completely covered with sterile drapes, and this defeats the purpose of laying the newborn down upon it. Furthermore, because the edges of the uterine incision tend to bleed and need prompt attention, the obstetrical team is likely to pass the baby over to other hands as soon as is practical. Accordingly, at an abdominal delivery, the cord is clamped and cut promptly, and the baby passed over to the waiting pediatrician. The baby usually reacts to these events with vigorous cries of annoyance while the pediatrician is making certain that it is in good condition. It can then be suitably wrapped in warm blankets and handed over to the mother's partner. If the mother has delivered under conduction anesthesia and is awake there is no reason why she cannot see, touch, and feel the baby with her free hand, and she can therefore certainly share the baby's first few moments with her partner.

We have recently begun putting small knitted caps on the babies because we have become aware of the fact that heat loss from the baby's scalp is substantial. It is easier to maintain the baby's body temperature at a more normal level if this heat loss is prevented.

A Distressed Baby

When a distressed baby is born it is promptly turned over to pediatric care. If there is meconium-stained fluid in the nose and respiratory passages, the pediatricians will apply suction to remove it, and will look at the baby's vocal cords to see how far down the passages the meconium has gone. As contact with meconium irritates the trachea and bronchi, it is advisable to suction it out of these passages as promptly as possible.

A baby who is depressed may need positive-pressure ventilation with oxygen mixtures. This can be facilitated in the delivery room by passing a tube down into the baby's trachea. Such babies as this, babies who do not breathe well on their own, and those born to diabetic mothers, are usually taken to special-care units for further observation.

The other step taken in the delivery room immediately after birth is some form of identification. How and sometimes when this is done may be mandated by local health agencies and by hospital practice. In most of the hospitals where I have worked, this includes fingerprinting and footprinting and attaching identifying bands to the mother and to the baby. Identification can be carried out while the baby is on the mother's chest or while it is being held by the mother's partner.

The procedures I have described above are used in the hospitals where I have worked, but newborns in other hospitals may be handled differently. Most commonly, the parents are shown the baby, who is then placed in a newborn baby warmer and, while there, is inspected by the nurse in the delivery room or by the pediatrician, if one is present. There may be an overhead warmer to reduce the newborn's inevitable heat loss, and it is common for someone to dry the baby off and clean it up a bit. The identification procedures may then be completed.

Once all this housekeeping has been done the baby may be wrapped and returned to the mother or placed in a closed baby warmer preparatory to being transported to the nursery. Alternatively the baby may be placed in the warmer and kept alongside the mother until she is transferred to a nearby recovery room. Some hospitals keep the baby with the mother in the recovery room for varying periods of time, while others transport the baby directly from the delivery room to the newborn nursery.

As we have become increasingly aware of the benefits of early bonding of the baby to its parents, the trend has been to keep the baby in close contact with them in the immediate newborn period. Competent studies show that an alert infant kept in proximity to an alert mother establishes bonds between them that makes newborn care in the subsequent days and weeks notably smoother. You may find it helpful to inquire at the hospital where you intend to deliver what its practices are in the immediate care of the newborn.

Appearance of the Newborn

The skull of a newborn baby consists principally of seven separate skull bones, which are connected with one another by relatively pliable connective tissue. This allows molding to take place to accommodate the shape of the baby's head to the shape of the mother's pelvis and thereby to facilitate birth. This may result in a head that at birth looks more like a loaf of French bread than like the classical image of a Gerber baby, but this process is very rapidly reversed. The baby's head resumes its almost spherical shape within twenty-four to forty-eight hours after delivery.

The scalp of the baby's head where it presents into the dilating cervical opening sometimes becomes edematous— swollen into what is called the caput succedaneum. This often looks like a somewhat distorted skull cap on the top of the baby's head, at the point where the caput has been leading the head through the birth canal. When scalp electrodes have been used in monitoring or blood samples taken from the scalp for studies during labor, the puncture marks made thereby will be found somewhere on the skin of the caput.

More conspicuous distortion of the shape of the baby's head can occur when there is bleeding under the periosteum, the connective tissue covering of each of the bones of the scalp. The distribution of this mass of clotted blood (known as a cephalhematoma) is limited by the attachments of the periosteum to the margins of the bones so that it does not cross the midline of the skull and does not extend all the way from the back of head to the front. It is therefore necessarily asymmetrical and may give the baby's head a lopsided appearance. It also has a fluctuant feel much like that of a plastic bag full of liquid. Cephalhematomas do not clear up immediately and indeed may last for several weeks. The baby's body, however, is very efficient in eventually removing the clot of blood and making use of the material in it in the formation of new blood.

Breeches

The baby born by the breech may have swelling and bruising on its buttocks from the same factors that produce these effects on the scalp of the baby born head first. Occasionally, the structures look purplish and the external genitalia may be somewhat swollen. This is much more noticeable in the scrotum of boy babies than on the labia of girls but is present in both. The head of a baby born by the breech does not undergo molding and is therefore nice and round like the idealized picture of the classic newborn. Breech babies very often lie in the uterus with their legs extended and their feet right in front of their faces; they may continue to occupy this position in the first several hours of life. This position is strikingly different from that of the baby born by the vertex, who usually has its legs flexed.

The heads of babies born by cesarean section, except for those delivered late in labor, exhibit none of the changes associated with labor. Like breech babies, therefore, they present the appearance of the idealized newborn.

Vernix

This is a fatty material, which looks for all the world like very soft cream cheese, spread over the surface of many newborns. Vernix caseosa is just about the best skin cream ever. I wish the standard of neatness in hospitals did not make it necessary to wash the vernix off. Left alone, it disappears over the course of a few days. Meanwhile, it is an excellent moisturizer for the baby's skin, which otherwise has a tendency to dry out in the newborn period.

When the baby is first born, before it has established much gas exchange through its lungs, its skin tends to be of a somewhat dusky purplish color, particularly in the hands and feet. This is succeeded by a bright red when the blood vessels of the skin open up widely in response to its sudden exposure to the air and to a change in temperature. As the baby becomes accustomed to being out at room temperature the deep red color that is characteristic of the first day or two of life gradually fades off to the more familiar ordinary skin color, although the hands and the feet often remain rather blue or turn blue from time to time, mostly when the baby's hands and feet are cold. These changes are entirely natural and require no treatment.

Newborn skin is also subject to a wide variety of rashes and irritations, most of which clear up entirely on their own with exposure to the air. The very common newborn rash is called erythema toxicum, a frightening name for a totally benign condition in which there are red blotches in the skin with little tiny pustules in their middle. Extensive rashes, particularly with raised edges and large pustules which tend to drain, can represent a true infection that requires some medical attention. These rashes are ordinarily due to infections with Staphylococcus, commonly referred to as staph. Treatment may consist of bathing with hexachlorophene, an antibacterial chemical, or antibiotic ointments, or even antibiotics by mouth. Something like 30 percent of all newborns have these staph organisms on their skin and on occasion some do become infected. The best way to limit the likelihood of this is careful hand washing by all who have contact with the baby. Fortunately these infections are seldom serious.

Another common skin infection of the newborn is caused by a common fungus, monilia (Candida). It is manifested in the diaper area by small red raised patches. When it occurs in the mouth it is called thrush, and it appears as a white coating on the palate and the tongue. The treatment consists of nystatin, an antifungal agent.

Other markings on the skin are occasional dark brown to blue-black pigmented areas, located on the low back or over the buttocks and of no particular significance in the normal newborn. There are also patches of dilated blood vessels (hemangiomas) of a variety of shapes and sizes. These can be identified because they are usually slightly raised and bright red and fade out with pressure on the skin. The vast majority of these hemangiomas is quite benign. Even if they appear on the face, they constitute a cosmetic rather than a medical problem.

Fingernails

A newborn baby has very fine fingernails and the babies that are born well past term are generally have rather long ones. Thus, in its unguided random activity the baby may scratch itself rather badly and make itself unsightly and uncomfortable. Rather than allow this to occur, you should keep the baby's fingernails trimmed, using fine nail scissors. You may find this a little daunting the first few times you try, but you really cannot inflict any harm in doing it, even though the baby is tiny and wiggly and you may cut a little bit too deep at first.

Body Hair

Newborn babies ordinarily have hair on their heads, eyebrows, and eyelids. Over the trunk there may be some fine blond hairs, which are called lanugo hairs; these ordinarily vanish quite soon after birth and normally do not reappear.

There are babies that come from families with a strong tendency toward hairiness and these babies may have dark hairs over their shoulders and on their foreheads. These hairs disappear fairly early in the newborn period. Indeed the hair on the head is not absolutely clear evidence of the hair color the baby will eventually have. I myself was born blond and in later childhood became a very unmistakable brunet.

Breast Engorgement

All babies in the uterus are exposed to the mother's increased concentration of female sex hormone and as a consequence newborns usually show some enlargement of breast tissue. This, of course, is not conspicuous, but on occasion the breast may become engorged for a brief period in the newborn state. Left entirely alone, this clears up without event. There may even be a small amount of secretion, picturesquely called witch's milk, the appearance of which gives no cause for concern.

Eyes

Eye color is almost a uniform dusky gray in the newborn, with the sole exception of albinos, whose irises have no pigment and are therefore bright pink from the blood circulating in them. The newborn gray color does not give any solid ground for prediction of the eventual eye color of the baby, as the definitive pigment in the iris appears somewhat later on. Newborn babies, no matter how hard they cry, do not form tears until they are about a month old.

With all newborns we are concerned about the possibility of infection in the conjunctival sac, the space just under the eyelids, and in the cornea, the clear transparent structure through which we see. If a mother is a carrier of gonorrhea in her vagina at the time of the baby's birth, the conjunctival sac and cornea can readily become colonized with gonococci. This can cause a disastrous infection which, given a foothold, scars the cornea so badly as to produce blindness. Every health department in the country has a regulation requiring that some sort of medication be put in the baby's eyes to prevent this condition, which is known as gonococcal ophthalmia. Most hospitals now instill an antibiotic ointment in the baby's eyes. This is effective and free of the undesirable irritating effect of the silver nitrate drops that were formerly used. The silver nitrate caused a transitory inflammation of the eyes, with pus in the conjunctival sac that inevitably interfered with the baby's vision.

Recently, we have observed a different sort of eye infection in newborns, caused by chlamydia. This generally does not appear until the baby is a week or ten days old. It is characterized by the formation of a purulent discharge from the eyes. It responds to antibiotics. Fortunately, mandatory gonorrhea prophylaxis reduces the incidence of this chlamydia infection as well. Should your baby develop a discharge from the eyes, however, you should promptly report it to the pediatrician.

Do not become alarmed if you see your baby's eyes moving independently of each other. Many newborns can do this, so that they look cross-eyed some of the time. This often occurs when the baby is half asleep and not paying attention to what it is doing. When the baby actually looks at something its eyes work together.

The Face

The baby's nose at birth does not have fully formed cartilage and therefore may appear temporarily to be smashed out of shape. Furthermore, the chin of a normal newborn is small by adult standards and this may sometimes give the baby an odd appearance. These features will duly straighten themselves out before long, and better proportions will appear.

There may be small hemorrhages in the skin of the face and neck, particularly in a baby who has had the umbilical cord wrapped around its neck in such a way as to tighten as the head descends through the birth canal. Hemorrhages also occur in the retina, at the back of the eye, and can be seen with an ophthalmoscope. They occur with surprising frequency at the time of normal birth, but evidently have no late consequences. Unless the baby's eyes are examined by a skilled ophthalmologist we are likely to be blissfully unaware that anything of the kind has happened.

Behavior of the Newborn

Most babies cry for a brief while after they are born. This serves to expand the babies' lungs and provides for an adequate exchange of gases. Once this is accomplished, the babies tend to doze off and sleep a great deal in the first eight to twelve hours. They are more likely to sleep if the mother initiates breast-feeding as soon as the baby is born; this seems to be reassuring to the baby.

Each baby has its own sleep-and-wake cycle, which is manifested fairly early and may actually be a continuation of prenatal behavior. On the evidence that we have from fetal monitor recordings, this cycle appears to be on about a ninety-minute basis. It takes a long time before this is completely entrained to the social cycles of older children and adults, which are related to the periods of light and dark. The ordinarily rolling and wiggling movements that the newborn baby manifests are probably in no way different from their acrobatics *in utero*.

Newborn babies have episodes of sneezing, and particularly those who have hiccoughed in the uterus will continue to do so after birth. Occasional babies go through periods of snorting. All these phenomena are perfectly normal, and do not, in any event, persist past the newborn phase.

As I have said earlier, it was for a long time believed that newborns were born like blank slates, not capable of anything more than eating and sleeping, and having no personality traits of their own. It was also thought that they did not see or hear for several weeks. But we now know that not only is it possible for a baby to learn *in utero*, but also that it is probably born with familiarity with its mother's voice, gained prior to its birth. Once born, the full-term baby can hear, see, mimic facial expressions, cry, suck, swallow, grasp things with its hands, move its hands, turn its head from side to side, and, placed on a flat surface, will move around, unless it is restrained.

Newborns respond to loud noises with a startle response much like that of an adult. In a more subtle way, newborns show a preference for slightly high-pitched voices. Many adults are subconsciously aware of this and talk to newborn babies in such a high-pitched squeaky voice. The baby will turn its head toward a voice and follow it for 180 degrees. It will follow a light. Since we know now that a baby exposed to a light *in utero* will blink, it is not surprising that a baby does this very soon after birth as well. It has been demonstrated that the baby has a preference for looking at concentric circles and for grids. Bright colors like red and orange are preferred over subtle ones even though there is some evidence that color vision is not established until later. The baby also has a preference for human faces, and the combination of a face and a familiar voice is particularly alluring. Not only this: A baby will mimic the expressions of the face of a person the baby is looking at. Most of these accomplishments are expressed best when the infant is in a quiet, alert state, neither asleep nor fully awake and crying, but with the eyes open and searching. Newborns do more of this than used to be believed.

Newborn Temperament

It became clear that newborn babies have a specific temperament that is characteristic of them; it has been described on a scale ranging from very easy to very difficult. Such items as the fraction of the day spent crying, the amount of motor activity, the sleep patterns, and the feeding difficulties may describe a baby's temperament. It is important for both you and the baby that you should understand your own baby's temperament and adapt to it rather than suffer unnecessary guilt feelings because you are thinking of the baby as a blank slate on which you may have written all your shortcomings as a parent.

The infant's instinct to suckle is very strong. Most babies are able to nurse shortly after delivery, making use of what has been called a rooting reflex. When a newborn baby's cheek is stroked, the baby will turn its head in the direction of the stroke, open its mouth, and suck on almost anything that will go into it. There is protective gag reflex which prevents babies from choking and if by any chance they happen to get any material into the trachea, which is the "wrong tube," they cough it up promptly.

Most babies urinate very shortly after birth with no embarrassment whatever. The stressed baby, as has been pointed out, may pass meconium even before it is born. The unstressed newborn usually pushes out meconium sometime in the first twelve or twenty-four hours. This initial meconium, which is gluey and dark green in color, is followed by transitional stools, when bacteria get down into the lower intestinal tract from the initial feedings. The pigments change and so does the consistency of the material coming out. Babies who are on artificial feedings with cow's milk have stools that are larger, more formed, and a chalky yellow in color. The stools of breast-milk-fed babies are smaller in volume, usually wetter, and the greenish color of the meconium tends to persist a little longer. This kind of stool should not be confused with the diarrhea stool.

Almost all babies experience weight loss in the first few

days of life. They are disposing of the extra water with which
they are loaded at birth, as a resource against any delay in the
start of lactation in their mothers. This is an entirely healthy
mechanism. There is no rush to deliver calories to a healthy
newborn. The newborn has reserves that will last a surprisingly
long time. Babies are programmed to survive nicely on a limited caloric intake for as much as several weeks should the
occasion arise.

Feeding the Newborn

Human milk provides perfect nutrition for the full-term infant
and for most premature infants. In addition to its nutritional
elements it contains antibodies to viruses and bacteria and also
white blood cells that help to prevent many diseases. These
immunizing mechanisms are very important, because they assist in the prevention of the diarrheas that are the major cause
of disease and death of infants throughout the world. Intolerance of mother's milk is a great rarity.

The most difficult part of breast-feeding is to get it started.
A hospital is not the ideal place to accomplish this. If the
hospital staff is motivated and knowledgeable, however, they
can assist in the initiation of the process. One of the positive
aspects of the trend toward an abbreviated stay following delivery is that the mother returns to the relatively tranquil environment of her own home, where she can give her attention
to nursing free of hospital routines and interruptions by strangers.

At home it is helpful to have the support of people who will
encourage you in breast-feeding. You ought to be in touch with
someone able to answer any questions you might have. This
role in bygone days was filled by other women in the extended
family. Now it is played by the occasional friend or grand-
mother and in some cases by the La Leche League.

A decision to abandon breast-feeding because it does not
seem to be going well should never be made on the basis of
experience in the hospital but deferred until breast-feeding has
been continued in a quiet environment where a more natural

rhythm can be established. It is obviously important to prepare in pregnancy for breast-feeding as well as for childbirth, if you intend to nurse your baby.

The concept that babies should be fed every four hours by the clock derived from earlier investigations of the emptying time of the stomachs of babies on artificial feeding. It also relates to the work schedule of personnel in hospital nurseries and to housekeeping needs at home, rather than to physiological processes in the baby. But in breast-feeding, the baby should be free to establish its own schedule on demand if the process is to be successful.

More About Breast-feeding

The more a baby is put to the breast and sucks at it the sooner the milk comes in. Most breast fed babies are ideally fed at first every two to three hours even though the duration of the feeds themselves may be short. There is great variation however in how often the babies feed. Some have periods when they feed very frequently and then have longer stretches between feedings. Others are more regular in their pattern. In the first two or three days many are sleepy and do not demand many feedings at all. Do not be discouraged if this occurs, for very shortly your baby's appetite and interest in feeding will increase. You need to learn to sense your baby's own rhythm and not pay attention to your wrist watch.

Newborns feed best when they are awake and hungry and indicating their hunger by moving around, sucking on their fists or just sucking on the air and crying. Over a twenty-four-hour period a normal newborn will take enough milk but each individual feeding may not be the same in amount as the previous one, nor will the timing be on any rigid schedule. If the mother can trust herself to respond to a baby's cues and trust what her own breasts tell her, she can breast-feed successfully. Frequent sucking will bring the milk in best and can also help to reassure the mother that she is in fact accomplishing something. Frequent feedings may also help you avoid engorgement, a condition in which your breasts become very full of milk, feel hard, and may even be painful. For babies, frequent feedings help them to have reflex bowel movements, to urinate often, and to assure that they are receiving lots of fluids. Additional water or supplementary formula are usually unnecessary since there is really no hurry to provide extra water or calories to a normal newborn.

In the beginning you may not think your baby is getting much because you usually do not see milk dripping out from the breast on which the baby is not sucking. You may not even feel any changes in your breasts, but you can be sure that when babies suck they receive colostrum at first and then later on milk.

Loss of Confidence

On occasion a woman nursing for the first time may experience a loss of confidence at the time when the baby has a growth spurt and a consequent increase in appetite. The breasts then seem smaller and softer and you may worry about the adequacy of your milk supply for your hungry baby. The solution is to increase the frequency of the feedings.

You may be advised by the well-meaning to force fluids to increase the milk supply. In one instance a woman I know was told to drink eight bottles of beer a day! Common sense teaches that you will need the additional fluid that you are providing to the baby, and your thirst is the best guide. Cow's milk is a suitable beverage but not a requirement.

Individual feeding times should probably be at least five minutes on each breast but again, rigid timing is not necessary or recommended. Because of the concern for sore nipples, a common occurrence in the beginning, you may be told to limit the length of the feedings. This probably makes sense if your baby is a frequent feeder but may not be advisable if your baby is sleepy most of the time and not feeding very often. Although sore nipples are common they usually do not bother women for very long.

Measures to Help with Sore Nipples

Here are a few measures that may turn out to be of value.

1. Experiment with different positions for putting the baby to the breast. If possible, ask an experienced person to observe

you and your baby during the feeding, and make what suggestions occur to her.

2. Your nipples should go deeply into the baby's mouth so you must be certain that much of your areola is also within the baby's lips. This spares the nipple itself damage from the baby's jaws.

3. Expose your nipples to the air and if possible to sunlight between feedings.

4. Washing of your nipples is unnecessary and it is unwise to use soap on them.

5. You may wish to try vitamin E oil or anhydrous lanolin (if you are not allergic to wool) on your nipples. Some patients find these measures helpful.

6. Start to nurse on the less sore side.

7. Use frequent feedings to minimize engorgement. Express some milk from the nipple to soften the areola before putting the baby to a full breast.

8. Get extra rest.

9. If your nipples become cracked or bleed, continue to breast-feed but shorten the length of the feedings and make them more frequent, so as to keep the breasts from becoming full and engorged.

Mastitis

A more serious problem is mastitis: an infection of the milk-forming glands due usually to a Staphyloccocus that has its ordinary residence on the skin. The management of the breasts, nipples, and feeding techniques listed above are all designed to minimize the chance that you will encounter this. You may be confronted with unfamiliar strains of bacteria to which you are not resistant. In that case, without other warning, you may notice that one small area of one breast is tender and the skin over it reddened. You may be extra tired and achy, and sometimes feel chills. By all means take your temperature; with these symptoms it is almost certain to be elevated. Report this promptly to your doctor or midwife. Mastitis is ideally treated by suitable antibiotics. If caught early it need not interfere with breast feeding. It may take a few days even with large doses of antibiotics for the disease to relent but you should feel better in twenty-four to thirty-six hours after starting medication. Of course the baby will get some drug, which may alter the odor of the baby's stools but otherwise will have no adverse effect.

Nipple Shields

These can be used temporarily when the nipples, unaccustomed to being wet and sucked on, become sore or cracked during the period of adjustment.

Preparation for Breast-feeding

Fortunately, as I write this it is clear that mothers in the United States are more and more choosing breast-feeding. In addition, in most hospitals women who want to nurse can get support and some education from the hospital staff. The people who have cared for you in your pregnancy should have given you some useful information during the prenatal period, and will be able, as they follow you postpartum in the hospital, to support your efforts to breast-feed. In addition, do not hesitate to ask your nurse to assist you with positioning, to watch you feed, and to make suggestions.

The mothers who have delivered by cesarean and who therefore may spend a longer time in the hospital than those who have delivered normally have both an advantage and a disadvantage. Because they have to go through the medical procedures necessary to the recovery from an abdominal operation, they may have to stay in the hospital longer than is ideal for establishing breast-feeding. On the other hand, in the hospital they have access to people who are knowledgeable about breast-feeding and who can provide the follow-up support that might not be readily available to a patient who has left the hospital one or two days after the birth. The mother who has had a cesarean has an abdominal incision and will not be quite so comfortable in holding the baby for breast-feeding as the mother who delivered normally. This is not a serious obstacle, and there are a number of simple techniques to minimize the discomfort. One is to put a pillow on the abdomen under the baby. Another is what has been referred to as the football hold, in which the baby "sits" on one hip bone, circled by the arm on the same side, with the baby's head held in the palm of the hand and its torso resting on the holder's forearm.

A very useful source of support and practical assistance with breast feeding is the La Leche League. This is an organized group of experienced women dedicated to furthering breast-feeding, whose members will give advice and assistance over the telephone, and when necessary with home visits, to mothers who need support and encouragement. Branches of the League exist in a great many communities. They are listed under the name of La Leche League in the white pages of the telephone directories of the communities where they operate. Frequently also, the hospital where you gave birth can provide support after you go home.

There are two particularly helpful and well-organized books on breast-feeding available. One is *The Breastfeeding Book*, by Máire Messenger, a British author, published by van Nostrand Reinhold in paperback. The other is *The Complete Book of Breastfeeding*, by Olds and Eiger, published by Workman.

Breast Pumps

Sometimes it becomes necessary to pump milk from the mother by mechanical means. The commonest reason is the need for mother's milk to feed those prematures born before they have developed an efficient sucking reflex. The mother pumps her own breast milk into a container, and leaves it in the newborn special-care nursery where it is fed to the baby, usually through plastic tubes passed through the nose or mouth and then down the esophagus to the stomach. The tubes may be left in place or changed with each feed. Tube feeding is safer than other methods for these tiny prematures, because it is less fatiguing than sucking on a nipple, and it protects them from breathing in oral feedings.

There are many pumps on the market now. Several are of the piston type, consisting of double plastic cylinders worked by hand. This cylinder-piston type is relatively inexpensive, and not larger or heavy. The electric pump, the prototype of which is the Egnell pump, is larger, heavier, easier to use, and more than ten times as costly. Smaller, less expensive electric pumps have come on the market under the trade name of Axicare. In most areas you can rent a pump from the local La Leche League chapter.

Breast Milk Jaundice

Breast milk has been implicated as a cause of late jaundice in a very small proportion of babies. It usually appears one to two weeks after birth and resolves with treatment and cessation of breast-feeding for up to seventy-two hours. Some newborn nurseries report an increased incidence of jaundice in breast-fed babies in the first few days of life, while others do not. "Breast milk jaundice" may result from infrequent feedings, starvation, and dehydration rather than from the breast milk itself. In hospitals where frequent-demand breast-feeding occurs, this type of jaundice is seldom a problem, although there is some concern about jaundice in the breast-fed premature.

Bottle-feeding

There are several standard prepared formulas available, all of them made from a cow's milk base. They are mostly supplemented with vitamins and iron and are available either ready-made in liquid form or as a powdered concentrate. There is probably no more need to follow a prescheduled feeding pattern with cow's milk formulas than there is in breast-feeding. I think it is important for you to individualize your baby's care, but at the same time, there are some precautions you should take. All the water that a newborn consumes should be boiled at least seven to ten minutes and then allowed to cool. In regard to the cleanliness of reused bottles, most modern dishwashers clean bottles well enough so that elaborate sterilization techniques are unnecessary, although artificial nipples may still require sterilization.

Nipples are now available that are much closer in shape to that of the human nipple during nursing than the round nipples most of us are familiar with. They have the trade name of Nuk and are also available as pacifiers.

If you are using reusable bottles for artificial feeding they should of course be emptied as soon as they are no longer in use, rinsed at once, and then run through a wash before using them again. This step is, of course, not necessary with the collapsible disposable plastic bags that are being used for bottle-feeding. Some of my patients tell me that they don't really think the plastic bag works better than the rigid bottle. The baby's individual preference is what is important, if you have to make a choice.

Rooming-In

"Rooming-in" is the name given to the practice of keeping the baby in the mother's room during the hospital stay.

It facilitates the process of bonding between the baby and its parents and at the same time materially assists in the establishment of breast-feeding. It was started in the late 1940's but had only sporadic acceptance at the beginning. By now, however, most hospitals have some provision for the practice. Babies sometimes are allowed to room-in twenty-four hours a day, but in other places round-the-clock rooming-in may conflict with local health rules designed to protect the babies from too much contact with visitors. It is my impression that there is no persuasive evidence of any more risk to the baby from visitors at the hospital than there would be at home, but old habits die hard, and hospitals understandably usually adopt a conservative course.

Returning the baby to a central nursery at night has the merit of giving the mother an opportunity for some much-needed sleep, but it may have its own risks for the babies. Specifically, the concern is for the spread of infection from one baby to another when one of them is exposed to hospital visitors, and particularly the spread of Staphylococcus infections. The usual precaution against this is careful hand washing by the mother, by the nursing staff, and by anybody else who handles the baby.

Some hospitals provide modified rooming-in, in which the baby is placed with the mother whenever she requests it and is taken back to a central nursery during visiting hours and during times when the patient is absent for hospital classes in newborn baby care.

Rooming-in of course also gives the mother an opportunity to gain experience in changing diapers and in bathing the newborn, as well as feeding. I have always looked upon bathing newborns as an extremely simple process. The real trick is to put the baby in a tub of water at body temperature, which will be reassuring to the baby, and to hold its head in such a manner that the baby's breathing is not interfered with. Since a newborn baby hardly has an opportunity to become dirty, except in the diaper area, bathing is probably more a luxury to keep the mother happy than a necessity for the baby's health.

Injuries in the Course of Childbirth

Injuries Due to Instruments

When forceps are used to deliver the baby they occasionally leave superficial bruises over the cheekbones or over an eyebrow and sometimes on an ear. These all clear up very quickly after birth and disappear after a few days. They carry no long-term implications. Occasionally a forceps blade will put pressure just in front of the baby's ear and cause swelling of the facial nerve on one side. This is the nerve that controls the muscles of the face, and a baby with this kind of injury, which is a newborn form of Bell's palsy, will be able to move the unaffected side of its face quite normally, but on the affected side the eye does not close properly and the corner of the mouth tends to sag. These changes are also transitory and have no later consequences.

When a baby is born by vacuum extraction there is a round swelling at the top of the head similar to the caput succedaneum, except for the fact that there also is a purplish discoloration due to leakage of blood into the skin of the scalp at the point where the vacuum cup was placed. The swelling itself clears up quite rapidly, at about the same speed as does a caput succedaneum. The circular area of purple, however, takes at least a week or ten days to disappear.

A baby whose shoulders are considerably broader than its head may have difficulty with the birth of the shoulders. There are obstetrical maneuvers to overcome this problem, but sometimes it has to be handled by adding the force provided by the obstetrician to that provided to the mother by her bearing down.

This force can be sufficient to fracture the clavicle, the bone that runs from the shoulder to the midline of the chest. These clavicular fractures heal completely, without later consequences, although the mother may notice a lump on the clavicle while the fracture is healing. The babies ordinarily are blissfully unaware of this fracture, since it apparently does not particularly hurt. Such clavicular fractures occur in about 2 percent of all normal births and ordinarily we are not even aware of them.

When delivery of the shoulder is difficult, there may be stretching of the bundle of nerves that runs from the spinal column in the neck down to the arm and consequently temporary loss of function of that arm. This can also occur with a breech birth if an arm becomes trapped behind the baby's head and has to be brought down by the obstetrician to facilitate delivery. The vast majority of these losses of motor function in the arm heal by themselves.

Other injuries due to instruments are described in Chapter 17.

Diseases of the Newborn

The most important problem of the newborn calling for special care is prematurity. Any of the conditions below can occur in any newborn infant, but all are more common in prematures.

Jaundice

Some babies are born with an incompletely mature liver, the organ on which the baby depends for disposing of the breakdown products of the extra blood that it has had in utero. This is the normal process by which the baby's red blood count drops in the period immediately after birth. The breakdown produces bilirubin, the pigment responsible for the yellow color of the skin in jaundice. For a normal newborn, the upper limit of bilirubin is considered to be twelve milligrams for every hundred milliliters of the baby's blood. Healthy term newborns will tolerate even much higher levels without any adverse effects. However, if the baby is ill in any way in addition to having jaundice, particularly if it is premature, it is necessary to bring down the level of bilirubin in the blood to prevent brain damage. This is most easily accomplished by exposing the skin of the baby under bright blue lights, with its eyes carefully shielded. The blue light acts on the bilirubin in the skin to change it into harmless, colorless forms.

The problem of jaundice is most severe in the babies who have blood group incompatibility with a sensitized mother and have been experiencing blood breakdown in the uterus (erythroblastosis fetalis). These babies, particularly if they are premature, may need exchange transfusion. In this process, a catheter is placed through the vein of the umbilical cord into the baby's central circulation. The baby's own blood is then removed little by little, to be replaced by equal amounts of bank blood compatible with that of the mother and free of bilirubin. In this way the bilirubin count can be brought down quite rapidly, even with severe degrees of erythroblastosis. The bank blood is broken down less rapidly than that of the baby itself. Several exchanges may be necessary before the baby is out of danger from long-term injury. Exchange transfusion is rarely necessary except for Rh incompatibility and marked degrees of prematurity.

Respiratory Distress Syndrome (RDS)

This is commonly a complication in prematures whose lungs are not sufficiently developed to remain open with only natural breathing. The air sacs tend to collapse and their lining cells to stick together, creating resistance to breathing in. These babies frequently require assistance from tubes put down into the trachea and oxygen given under positive pressure, in order to keep the lungs expanded. The tremendous strides that have been made in improving the treatment of RDS have played a major role in reducing of morbidity and mortality among small prematures. Respiratory distress syndrome in its severe forms can cause some limitation of respiratory function in later childhood. Except for tiny prematures, however, it is no longer a fatal complication.

Intracranial Hemorrhage

Another handicap of the small premature is that the blood vessels of its brain are very fragile and may bleed under the least stimulus. This is occasionally a fatal event. There is no simple relationship between the signs of such bleeding and its amount. Our ability to diagnosis intracranial hemorrhage has now been markedly improved with sonography and CAT scanning. The liability to intracranial hemorrhage is one of the reasons that normal newborns are routinely given a small dose of vitamin K, a vitamin essential to blood clotting, which is ordinarily provided by the bacteria of the intestinal tract. Those bacteria do not grow rapidly enough to have this effect until the baby is about a week old.

Convulsions

The baby who has suffered distress related to obstruction of circulation through the placenta and umbilical cord during labor has an increased liability to convulsions, which are evidence of brain injury. For that reason all babies who seem to be asphyxiated at birth must be kept under observation for convulsive disorders, and if necessary treated promptly with anticonvulsive drugs. The prognosis for such babies is not absolutely clear in the first few weeks or months, and is affected by the cause of the convulsions.

Some newborns have to be withdrawn from dependence on drugs. One such group consists of the babies born to drug-dependent women. These babies are susceptible to convulsions if drug withdrawal at birth is abrupt. It is important to know if the mother is a drug user to make proper provision for gradual withdrawal of the baby from dependency. This is ordinarily done by giving the baby one or another sedative drug and gradually tapering that off. The pediatrician must be notified if the mother is addicted to drugs. The same kind of care is given to the baby born to a mother who has been on large doses of steroids for medical conditions.

The Infants of Diabetic Mothers

A baby of excessive size, born to a mother with inadequately controlled diabetes, is likely to be susceptible to periods of hypoglycemia (lowering of the blood sugar), which can be severe enough to be fatal. Such babies are put under special observation during the first twelve to twenty-four hours of life, with repeated determinations of their blood sugar and administration of glucose when the blood sugar drops too low.

If control of the mother's diabetes has been poor, the infants tend to be born with high red-blood-cell counts; they then develop jaundice due to breakdown of the unnecessary excess blood. This results in hyperbilirubinemia, which requires treatment either with blue lights or, in more resistant cases, exchange transfusion. The large size of babies of diabetic mothers is due to deposit of fat under the skin in addition to large bone structure. When the mothers have had poor control early in pregnancy, there is a fivefold increase in congenital heart disease among the infants; abnormalities of the lower limbs, lower urinary tract, and sacrum called the caudal regression syndrome, are also observed.

Newborn Infection

As I mentioned above, the liver is not fully mature at birth. The whole immune system, in fact, is ordinarily not completely developed, since in the uterus the fetus is ordinarily not exposed to bacteria. About the only challenges that the immune system has *in utero* are those that come from virus diseases, and these only rarely come across the placenta. Organisms that cross the placenta can stimulate antibodies in the fetus, but ordinarily the immune proteins with which the fetus is endowed are those that have come passively across the placenta from the mother.

The newborn therefore is more susceptible to infection than it will ever be again in its life. Furthermore, newborns are not able to limit infections to local areas as can older children and adults and therefore generalized infections are much more likely to take place. This is one of the serious problems in the newborn, since it rapidly produces serious illness. Because of this, pediatricians are very quick to test for the evidences of sepsis, and treatment with antibiotics is frequently administered solely on a strong suspicion without waiting for proof. Most commonly in such a study, white-blood cell count and cultures of blood, spinal fluid, and, if possible, the amniotic fluid and the placenta are carried out. Although the thought of a spinal tap on a newborn tends to be frightening, these taps in newborns are fairly easily done, because the babies do not have heavily developed back muscles and the ligaments holding the vertebrae are still very flexible. With spinal fluid obtained for examination, the diagnosis of infection in the central nervous system can readily be made and can equally readily be ruled out. This will considerably influence the decision whether to initiate antibiotic therapy.

Newborn infection is associated with birth from an infected uterus, which ordinarily manifests itself by maternal fever and a marked elevation of the white count in the mother. These infections are often associated with rupture of membranes twenty-four hours or more prior to delivery. In these cases the fetus often has a high heart rate during labor and there may be signs of infection of the amniotic sac. In the newborn a suspicion of infection can be raised by either unusually high or unusually low body temperature, poor feeding, lethargy, irritability, otherwise unexplained jaundice, convulsions, vomiting, and abdominal distension. When these signs appear, ordinarily a workup for infection is undertaken and as I mentioned above, antibiotic therapy may be begun even before obtaining full laboratory proof.

The infant born to a mother with active herpes similarly needs close observation. At the time of this writing there is no established preventive therapy for herpes, but there are treatments available should signs of herpes infection make their appearance in the baby.

The baby born to the mother with the active carrier state of hepatitis B probably requires treatment with hyperimmune anti-B globulin and possibly with the recently developed hepatitis B vaccine.

Hypospadias and Cryptorchidism

Some male infants are born with the urethra opening at the base of the penis rather than out at the end where the glans is located, a condition known as hypospadias. It is more of a practical cosmetic difficulty than a threatening abnormality, although these babies are candidates for later plastic surgery.

The baby born with undescended testicles (cryptorchidism) now can be quite satisfactorily treated with a combination of hormone therapy and local plastic surgery, but it is important to make the diagnosis early so that proper planning can be done for later pediatric care.

Other Conditions

All newborns should be carefully examined for the possible presence of congenital dislocation of the hip. This failure of the head of the femur to remain in its proper socket occurs overwhelmingly in girls. It is readily diagnosed by the presence of a hip "click" felt when the legs are appropriately manipulated. With suitable positioning the hip can be encouraged to remain in its normal socket and all deformity eliminated.

Careful examination in the baby is desirable to identify the occasional newborn with some variety of trisomy, the commonest variety being Down's syndrome. This can ordinarily be recognized in the newborn state, and, although there is no treatment, appropriate counseling for the parents can be promptly initiated.

Screening for Metabolic Disorders

There are now in some communities mandatory screening blood tests for phenylketonuria, an abnormality of amino acid metabolism that causes serious mental retardation, as well as for thyroid deficiency and other inborn errors of metabolism. Suitable arrangements for this screening should be made before the baby leaves the hospital. These screenings ordinarily pick up far more positives than there are cases of disease but they do serve as an early warning system.

Parting Words to Parents

Circumcision

Urine comes out of the penis at the urethral opening, which is normally at the tip of the spongy erectile structure, the glans penis. The glans itself is covered at birth by a fold of skin, the prepuce. The skin is not firmly attached to the glans; indeed some of the shed cells from the skin itself are found under the prepuce as a sort of white cheesy material. The opening in the skin through which the urine passes is really adequate for the purpose, and infection in this area in babies is rare. As the boy becomes older and experiences erections from time to time the opening in the skin is gradually stretched and can be peeled back off the glans without material discomfort. The child in the ordinary course of events learns to keep this area clean as a part of his general hygiene.

Certain ethnic groups have practiced circumcision for at least several millennia. A good deal of anthropological evidence suggests that the practice derives from a sacrificial fertility rite and did not originate as a medical procedure. Indeed, there is no substantial historical evidence that there ever was a medical indication for circumcision. Moreover, it does not even actually simplify bodily hygiene for small boys. When the procedure is properly done, however, it has virtually no complications and no side effects and is therefore perfectly safe. With all these considerations in mind, present opinion advises against circumcision, unless there is some ethnic or religious reason to perform it.

Relationship between Parents and Infants

The decision by the Supreme Court in 1973 that abortion was a part of the right to privacy on the part of the mother, combined with the tremendous technical strides in guaranteeing the safety of abortion, has now created a situation in which we can today for the most part assume that a woman who is visibly pregnant wants the baby she is carrying, and probably so does its other parent. The relationship between the parents and the infant starts during the pregnancy, sometimes when they can hear the fetal heart for the first time through a Doppler device, sometimes when at the time of sonography they can actually see the fetus in motion, and certainly by the time that the fetus at about the sixth month becomes readily seen and felt through the mother's abdominal wall.

There is, however, still a unique status to the moment of birth and the period immediately following it. The newborn, now actually to be seen and felt and held, going through phases of crying and wiggling and then to a peaceful alertness with open eyes searching around the room, always seems like some kind of miracle. The parents are very sensitive to the baby at this point and, as we mentioned above, the baby itself sees and hears and feels and is receiving a tremendous barrage of new images and experiences. If the baby is kept close to its parents during these immediate moments, very strong and long-lasting attachments occur in a process that has been called bonding. The baby learns the smell and the sound of its mother, and in those babies who are breast-fed even the way the mother tastes. Very shortly after birth many mothers are able to identify the cry of their own baby and pick it out from the midst of other crying babies.

Bonding to the father does not proceed quite so rapidly but is ordinarily present within several days after birth, particularly if the partner has frequent access to the child. It is materially assisted by rooming-in and the father visiting in the hospital. Some of the things that have been identified as strengthening the bonding process in the early hours after birth are closeness between the baby and the parents in the first few moments following birth, skin-to-skin contact between baby and mother, stroking movements on the part of the mother, warmth and relatively dim lighting with a reduced amount of noise, early nursing, and the irreducible minimum of interruptions for such things as footprinting. The newborn baby remains alert for a half to a full hour after birth and then usually falls off into a peaceful sleep from which it wakes only when it is hungry.

These probably represent ideal circumstances, which cannot be fully achieved if the birth is by cesarean section or if the mother has been under general anesthetic for the delivery. It is also interfered with if for any reason the newborn has to be taken to a special care nursery for observation. There is no reason not to initiate the various features of bonding as soon as the mother and the baby can be brought together, however. I encourage mothers to go to the special-care nursery where their babies are. The staff there are very good about encouraging the mother to handle the baby, to stroke it and feel it, to talk to it, to attempt to establish eye contact, and all the other things that enhance bonding. If breast-feeding is practical, it can be started then and there.

Bereavement

We have become intensely aware that when a baby is stillborn or has serious congenital anomalies the parents and especially the mother are destined for a terrible letdown. Fortunately, unexpected stillbirth in normal patients has become an extremely rare event and, with genetic screening and sonography, it is most unusual for a baby to be born unexpectedly abnormal. Nevertheless, there are still occasions for the mother to go through a period of great grief. For many years, in an effort to guard the mother from this, abnormal and stillborn infants were hidden from her and, not infrequently, she was moved to a part of the hospital remote from maternity and sent home early.

We have learned that this leaves a mother with an empty feeling, compounding her disappointment at the outcome of her pregnancy. It strengthens the mother's mostly groundless suspicion that she has done something wrong, and it denies her an opportunity to get these feelings "off her chest." Mothers who have given birth to stillborn infants, even when they are deformed, if they are allowed to see the child, turn out to be able to focus on what seems to them to be beautiful about the baby and to wipe out from their memory those things that are unpleasant. Dealing with bereaved mothers as if they were normal women, allowing them to mix in the activities of a postpartum ward and to see other babies seems to facilitate their dealing with the process of grieving.

It was the unfortunate custom of some physicians in years

past to visit such a woman, pat her on the head figuratively or literally, and tell her everything was all right and that all she needed to do was go home and have another baby. Fortunately, many hospitals now have bereavement groups consisting of professionals who are attuned to the need of mothers and fathers under these painful circumstances. We have learned that it is desirable for the woman to complete the process of grieving before starting another pregnancy, so as to maximize her chance of having a happy pregnancy and delivery.

Choosing a Pediatrician

Newborn and infant care is ideally provided by pediatricians and by family doctors who are motivated to deliver this kind of service. I urge patients to try to find a physician who lives reasonably near them and who may therefore be available for house calls in the event of emergency. You might wish to interview the available physicians for your baby well before the birth so you know who they are and feel comfortable with them. It is not absolutely necessary that the doctor that you choose be on the staff of the hospital where you intend to deliver. All hospitals provide temporary pediatric consultation during the period that the mother and baby are hospitalized, and there are no difficulties in transferring care to the pediatrician selected by the parents when the baby leaves.

You might wish to look into the competence of the doctor you select by finding out whether that individual is certified by the American Board of Pediatrics or the American Academy of General Practice. It is worthwhile to go into some practical issues such as the physician's hours for well-baby care; what sort of coverage is provided for nights, weekends, and emergencies; and what fees will be involved, as well as making sure the physician's attitudes are compatible with yours on such matters as breast-feeding and the relationships between the parents and the pediatrician. If the doctor you have chosen is on the staff of the hospital where you deliver, examination of your baby at the time of its birth by someone that you now know and have already begun to trust can go a long way in being reassuring.

Taking the Baby Home

This used to be a formidable undertaking. For one thing, it was thought that an elaborate layette was called for. The babies were considered fragile and an extraordinary amount of protective clothing was considered necessary, to shield them from strangers and from large crowds of relatives. For babies who were to be bottle-fed, parents had to provide all the paraphernalia for preparing formula and sterilizing feeding equipment.

These aspects of life with baby have been greatly simplified. Disposable diapers have largely supplanted an immense trousseau of cotton diapers. But modern laundry equipment has made cloth diapers less of a chore, and diaper services are widely available. There is no question that the baby can be costumed in a frilly dress and booties and a sweater and a knit cap, but a baby can equally go home in a cotton shirt and a disposable diaper and wrapped in an appropriate soft, warm blanket. The normal healthy baby will not know the difference. And at home, you probably will find that a crib and a convenient-sized basin for bathing the baby are all the basic elements of baby furniture and furnishings you will need, at least at first.

Recommended Reading

There are many books, pamphlets, and political essays about pregnancy, exercise, and diet. I have listed below ten such books, all available in paperback, which I have enjoyed reading and from which I have learned. I do not agree with every statement, recommendation, or caution in them, but they are thoughtful and will not lead you astray. All are recently revised.

The Breastfeeding Book. Máire Messenger. Van Nostrand Reinhold, NY, 1982.
An elegantly illustrated comprehensive explanation of breast-feeding. It avoids technical language and, by systematically reviewing the problems which may arise, is consistently supportive and reassuring.

The Complete Book of Breastfeeding. Sally Olds and Marvin S. Eiger. Workman, NY, 1985.
Another fine review of preparation for and common-sense approach to breast-feeding, recently revised, with a delightful sense of humor.

Diet for a Small Planet. Frances M. Lappé. Ballantine, NY, 1982.
This volume is most helpful to women who prefer alternate diets such as vegetarian and ovo-lacto-vegetarian. Detailed guidance is provided to be certain that these diets fulfill the wide range of pregnancy needs.

Eating for Two. Isaac Cronin and Gail S. Brewer. Bantam, NY, 1983.

A thorough description of the nutritional needs of pregnancy and ways of meeting them—meals, menus, recipes, calorie counters, and further reading.

The New Pregnancy. Susan S. Lichtendorf and Phyllis L. Gillis. Bantam Books, NY, 1979.

The best presentation of pregnancy from the viewpoint of working and career women. There is an appendix listing support facilities, legal assistance, state insurance and commissioners, occupational hazards, resources, and the like.

Our Bodies, Ourselves. Revised edition. The Boston Women's Health Collective. Simon and Schuster, NY, 1985.

This volume, now thoroughly revised, originally appeared in the early 70's, written by some of the pioneers of the Women's Health Movement. Its orientation is feminist, and it contains a wealth of information in sensible and readily understood form.

The Pregnancy Exercise Book. Barbara Dale and Johanna Roeber. Pantheon Books, NY, 1982.

Among many books on this subject, this one is outstanding for its completeness and its warm illustrations.

Right from the Start. Gail S. Brewer and Janice P. Greene. Rodale Press, PA, 1981.

Readable and clear discussion of pregnancy, delivery, breast-feeding, newborn baby care, nutrition, circumcision, and many other matters.

Six Lessons for an Easier Childbirth. Elisabeth Bing. Bantam, NY, 1982.

This is the classic presentation of the Lamaze method of preparation for childbirth, written by the wonderful woman who is one of its best teachers.

When Pregnancy Fails: Families Coping with Miscarriage, Stillbirth and Infant Death. Susan O. Borg and Judith Lasker. Beacon, NY 1981.

A warm and informative discussion of every aspect of preg-

nancy failure—abortion, stillbirth, and death of an infant, subjects which often are avoided by care providers and even family.
A partial directory of support groups, counseling services, and
adoption services is included.

Index